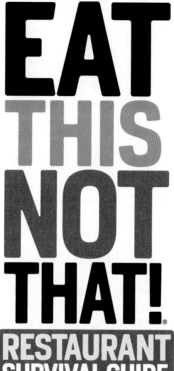

EAT THIS NOT THAT!®
RESTAURANT SURVIVAL GUIDE

The No-Diet Weight Loss Solution

BY DAVID ZINCZENKO
WITH MATT GOULDING

RODALE

Eat This, Not That! is a registered trademark of Rodale Inc.
© 2010 by Rodale Inc.

Rodale books may be purchased for business or promotional use or for special sales. For information,
please write to: Special Markets Department, Rodale Inc., 733 Third Avenue, New York, NY 10017.

Printed in the United States of America
Rodale Inc. makes every effort to use acid-free ∞, recycled paper ♻.

Book design by George Karabotsos

Cover photographs by Jeff Harris.
Food styling by Susan Sugarman. Hand model: Ashly Covington

All interior photos by Mitch Mandel and Thomas MacDonald/Rodale Images
with the exception of the following: pages 100–101, 118–119, 150–151, 152–153, 166–167, 172–173, 197,
222–223, 234–235 ©Lisa Adams; pages 72–73, 108–109, 130–131, 144–145, 146–147, 160–161,
162–163 ©Ray Kachatorian; pages 102–103 ©Orly Catz; pages 244–245, 254–255 ©Jeff Harris;
pages 252–253 ©Manny Rodriguez; pages 260–291 ©Melissa Punch

Food styling by Melissa Reiss

Library of Congress Cataloging-in-Publication Data is on file with the publisher
ISBN-10: 1–60529–540–X paperback
ISBN-13: 978–1–60529–540–4 paperback

Distributed to the trade by Macmillan
2 4 6 8 10 9 7 5 3 1   paperback

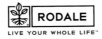

RODALE
LIVE YOUR WHOLE LIFE™

We inspire and enable people to improve their lives and the world around them

For more of our products visit **rodalestore.com** or call 800-848-4735

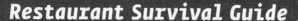

EAT THIS NOT THAT!

DEDICATION

To the millions of men and women who, like us, have manned the drive-thrus, sweated in the kitchens, and waited on and bussed the tables of America's restaurants. As the American food revolution continues, your hard work will be at its very core.

—Dave and Matt

ACKNOWLEDGMENTS

As always, it took a team of talented individuals to put this book together. Our undying thanks to all of you who have inspired this project in any way. In particular:

To the Rodale family, whose dedication to improving the lives of their readers is apparent in every book and magazine they put their name on.

To George Karabotsos and his crew of immensely talented designers, including Laura White, Mark Michaelson, Courtney Eltringham, Elizabeth Neal, and Rob Campos. You're the reason that each book looks better than the last.

To our crack team of researchers, including Clint Carter, Carolyn Kylstra, Anna Maltby, and Sophie Fitzgerald: Your relentless pursuit of the truth about our food is what makes these books vital.

To Tara Long, who spends more time in the drive-thru than anyone on the planet, all in the name of making us look good.

To the Rodale book team: Steve Perrine, Karen Rinaldi, Chris Krogermeier, Debbie McHugh, Nancy Bailey, Sara Cox, Mitch Mandel, Tom MacDonald, Troy Schnyder, Melissa Reiss, Nikki Weber, Jennifer Giandomenico, Wendy Gable, Keith Biery, Liz Krenos, Brooke Myers, Sean Sabo, and Caroline McCall. You continue to do whatever it takes to get these books done. We appreciate your heroic efforts.

Special thanks to the entire *Men's Health* staff, especially Allison Falkenberry and Brett LeVecchio, whose dedication to spreading the message helps millions of Americans lead healthier lives.

—Dave and Matt

Check out the other informative books in the *EAT THIS, NOT THAT!*® series:

Eat This, Not That! (2007)

Eat This, Not That! for Kids! (2008)

Eat This, Not That! Supermarket Survival Guide (2009)

Eat This, Not That! The Best (& Worst!) Foods in America! (2009)

Eat This, Not That! 2010 (2009)

CONTENTS

Congratulations.

You've just taken back control of your weight, your health, your wallet, and even your life.

Wait—you don't remember giving up control of those things? Nobody ever slid a sheet of paper in front of you and had you sign away the right to manage the very body you inhabit?

Well, here's the bad news: *Yes, they did.* In fact, if you're like most Americans, you probably signed that contract yesterday. And the day before. And probably the day before that. And if you're not careful, you might just sign it away tomorrow, as well.

You see, the last time a waitress handed you a menu, she might as well have been handing you a contract that says "I give total control of my body to Olive Garden/Burger King/Woody's Sports Bar/Al's Greasorama." Because once you blindly trust a food service establishment to determine what goes into your body, you've lost control. No, check that—you haven't lost it. You've given it away—voluntarily. And that's not good.

Whether you're choosing off a backlit sheet of Plexiglass on the side of a drive-thru, a ketchup-smeared laminated cardboard menu at the local diner, or an elegant paper folder laid upon your ironed tablecloth, being a patron at a restaurant is nothing less than a leap of faith. Once you put in your order, you're forking over that control to a handful of folks who have a lot less invested in your health and well-being than you do.

And gaining that control back isn't easy.

Sure, you can pour over that menu like Sherlock Holmes rummaging through a murder scene. You can pepper the waiter with questions like Bill O'Reilly grilling a left-wing politico. Heck, you can even try to peek through the swinging doors to see what's really sizzling in the kitchen. But even if you can get a good look through the greasy streaks on the door windows, you can't really know what's in your food and how many calories you're packing into your body—because often, neither the people cooking it nor the people serving it have any idea themselves. So what can you turn to for answers, and how can you take back control?

Welcome to **EAT THIS, NOT THAT! RESTAURANT SURVIVAL GUIDE.** Or, as we like to call it, the weight loss coach that fits in your pocket.

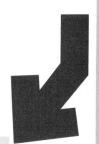

Why You Need This Book (Now, More Than Ever!)

Like we said, every order you place in a restaurant is, essentially, a leap of faith. And to be honest with you, most restaurants aren't keeping that faith. The portions and calories that American restaurants serve with each meal have skyrocketed faster than real-estate prices in a boomtown, but sadly, there's no popping this bubble. And the results are easy to see, all around us—from our out-of-control health care costs, to our national obesity crisis, to the insane development of adult-onset diabetes among our children (who were historically not at risk for the disease until our restaurants started supersizing us)!

But wait: Isn't the obesity crisis and all that comes with it caused by the lack of exercise we get, the video game/cable TV/World Wide Web world we live in, the absence of gym classes in public schools, and the fact that most new neighborhoods don't even have sidewalks where families can ride their bikes? How can we finger restaurants?

Well, it's simple: First of all, Americans actually work really hard to stay lean. Every year we spend an estimated $524 million on health and fitness books,

$18.5 billion on health club memberships, and $5.2 billion on diet foods and weight loss programs. And that's not to mention the popularity of TV shows like *The Biggest Loser* and fitness magazines like *Runner's World, Bicycling, Women's Health,* and *Men's Health.* All told, we'll burn through close to $60 billion this year alone, trying to keep the pounds off.

Yet since the 1970s, the obesity rate in this country has doubled. The average American man now eats 7 percent more calories every day than he did back when Young still got along with Crosby, Stills, and Nash. And the average American woman has fared even worse: She now takes in 22 percent more calories than in the '70s—that's enough to add a pound of flab every 11 days!

And much of the blame belongs in two places: On us, the consumers, for choosing to eat one in every four meals not at home, but on the road at a restaurant or drive-thru. And on the restaurants themselves, for choosing to make our foods fattier and more unhealthy than ever. Just look at the chart below.

So why are our restaurants so intent on ruining our health? And more important, how can we enjoy our favorite foods without suffering the consequences? The answers to those questions, and more, are right here in your hands.

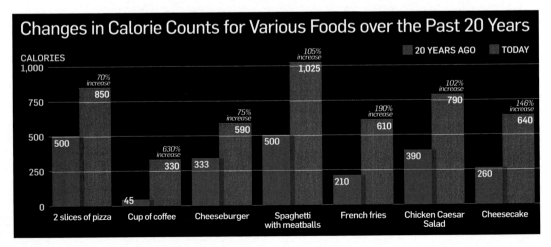

Changes in Calorie Counts for Various Foods over the Past 20 Years

Why Restaurants Make Us Fat—And How to Fight Back!

The reason food marketers seem so intent on making us fat is because the economics of the restaurant business are so completely different from any other business. For food manufacturers, it actually pays to sell us more for less—even if that "bargain" kills us.

Here's how it works: Let's say you go to your local JCPenny to buy a bathing suit. While you're there, you see a cool T-shirt that you'd also like to buy. Let's say each one costs the manufacturer about the same to make, and each one is priced similarly, at about 30 bucks. You, however, have only $50 in your pocket.

But, ooh, there's a sale! Buy one, get the other at 30 percent off! You could buy the bathing suit *and* the T-shirt. You've essentially supersized your order, and when you get home, you've got two things: a bathing suit and a T-shirt. That's a bargain!

Now, let's say you do that over and over again, until your closet is stuffed. The next time you go shopping, and you see a cool bathing suit and a cool T-shirt, you'll think twice: *I already have a lot of bathing suits and T-shirts. In fact, my closet is stuffed. I don't really need more, unless I get rid of the ones I have.*

What does this little tale have to do with our weight? It's simple: When we go into a restaurant, we use the same "shopping" thought process that we do when we hit the department store. But the results are wildly different.

For example, let's say you go to Pizza Hut because you hanker for a slice. There are a whole lot of options on their tasty-looking menu, but you're trying to decide: You could get two slices of the Meat Lover's Pan Pizza, but you're also liking the looks of the Meaty P'Zone Pizza. *Hmm.* You choose the P'Zone and eat it up. Delicious! But when you get home, what do you actually have? Not a T-shirt or a bathing suit, and not a P'Zone, either. What you have—what you've actually bought—is 1,480 calories. And that's what is now, for the most part, stuffed in your closet—the closet that is your waistline. Sounds bad, right?

But wait—what if you chose the two slices of Meat Lover's Pan Pizza? Like the T-shirt and the bathing suit, these two foods cost about the same because it costs Pizza Hut about the same to manufacture each. But when you get home, you don't have a T-shirt or a bathing suit or your two slices, either. What you have—what you're trying to stuff into your body's closet—is not 1,480 calories, but a mere 660! If you made a choice like that every day, you would lose a pound of fat off your body every 5 days. That's 15 pounds in just 2 months, simply by eating one type of Pizza Hut meat pie over another!

Surprised?

Two delicious foods, but when you pick the P'Zone, you're getting more than twice what you paid for. And while that's terrific when you're talking about bathing suits and T-shirts, and even groceries, it's not terrific when you're talking about calories. But that's what's happening every time you go to a restaurant—you're shopping for calories to stuff into your body's closet, but you have no idea how much you're actually buying. And as a result, your closet is getting bigger and bigger—and bigger.

But you can't not eat. You can't say, "This closet is too stuffed. I'll wait until I've gotten rid of some of what's in here before I buy more." So you keep going to the fast-food joints, the sit-down chain restaurants, the greasy spoons and taverns and sports bars and seafood shacks and diners and all-you-can-eat buffets because you get hungry. And each time you do, it's a complete mystery as to what you're buying and stuffing in your body's closet.

And because restaurants don't have to abide by the same rules that grocery store foods do—there are no labels that indicate fat, calories, sodium, and all the other nasty stuff that's cluttering our closets—it behooves the restaurants to give you more. Because "more" for the same price looks like a bargain when it's piled on your plate. "More" for the same price is a bargain when we're shopping for bathing suits or DVDs or sporting goods or real estate.

But we're not buying clothes or electronics or DVDs or sporting goods or real estate. And really, we're not even buying food. What we're buying when we eat at a restaurant is fat, calories, and sodium. And "more" is not a bargain—not by a long shot.

How This Book Can Help You Lose Weight Fast

If all this kind of freaks you out—and it should—then this is the book for you. Because even among all the calorie-dense, fat-padding items on the menus of America's restaurants, there are tons of delicious ways to cut hundreds, even thousands, of calories from your daily diet. And you don't have to go hungry or give up your favorite foods. (Indeed, swapping that P'Zone for the Meat Lover's Pan Pizza once a day isn't much of a sacrifice at all, is it? Especially when it means losing 90 pounds in the next 12 months!)

And every type of restaurant in America is loaded with the same kind of smart swaps. Consider:

 At Chili's, just order the Fajita Pita Chicken instead of the Chicken Crisper Bites Sandwich, and you'll save 950 calories! (That's 8.1 pounds of weight loss this month!)

 Choose McDonald's Big N' Tasty over the Burger King Triple Whopper and you'll save 790 calories! (That one swap is enough to lose more than 82 pounds of flab in the next year!)

 Head to Jamba Juice for a small Peach Perfection smoothie, but pass up The Hulk (Strawberry) at Smoothie King. You've just saved . . . oh, this is too crazy . . . 1,860 calories. (In one week—one week!—you'd lose 3¾ pounds. Do it every day for a year, you've just lost 193 pounds—or the equivalent of an entire Angelina Jolie, plus both of Brad Pitt's legs.)

Plus, think about how much easier life will get when you no longer have to scrutinize each and every menu—and then pay the price for guessing wrong! Here's what you have to look forward to:

> You'll lose weight and look better. The ordering advice in *EAT THIS, NOT THAT! RESTAURANT SURVIVAL GUIDE* is designed specifically to target belly fat—by

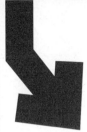

keeping your belly full of smart, healthy choices that keep your resting metabolism revving and never letting you go hungry. That means you'll be at the top of your game and burning fat all day, every day, even when you sleep!

> You'll reshape your body. Most "diets" force you to cut down on the amount of food you're eating, but that's not your goal, or ours! Instead, by keeping you full, you'll retain lean muscle while trimming away only flab—so you'll be sculpting the body you've always wanted, effortlessly!

> You'll save time and stress. What four words are more stressful to hear than "Can I help you?" (Besides, "Give me your money"?) The waitress or counter person comes to take your order, and suddenly you feel a world of pressure to make up your mind. It's easy to spout out the first thing you see—and maybe sabotage your weight loss hopes. But no longer. Now, you have the power to order quickly, smartly, and without hesitation, each and every time!

> You'll bulk up your wallet, not your waistline. There's an old saying: Look the part and you'll get the part. Well, research shows that people who are leaner and fitter are viewed as being more competent and successful than those who are overweight. Don't believe us? A Cornell University study found that people packing on an extra 64 pounds earn 9 percent less than their slimmer colleagues. And when you make smart choices at restaurants, you save money, too—because you'll quickly identify the best foods for you and be able to order them confidently, again and again.

> You'll even improve your health. The list of health problems that come as side orders with our overstuffed restaurant entrées is long and depressing: Diabetes, heart disease, high blood pressure, stroke, cancer, gout, and back pain are just the beginning. But imagine being able to sidestep them all—even if you're just pulling into the drive-thru!

The time to take back control of your weight, your health, your wallet, and your life is now.

Fortunately, the only tool you'll ever need is right in your hands!

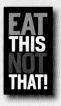

Restaurant Survival Guide

AMERICA'S TOP SWAPS

The Simplest, Smartest, Fastest Steps You Can Take to Change Your Body Forever

Wraps

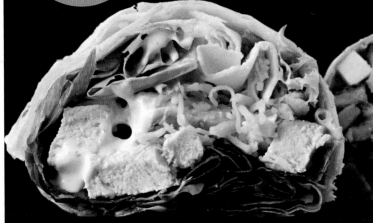

Eat This!
Eat This!
Ruby Tuesday
Grilled Chicken Wrap

436 calories
17 g fat
40 g carbohydrates

Not That!
T.G.I. Friday's
BBQ Chicken Wrap

1,540 calories

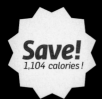

Save!
1,104 calories!

There's a reason that Friday's wrap has four times as many calories as Ruby Tuesday's: As they say, the secret's in the sauce. Or, in the case of the BBQ Chicken Wrap, the three sauces. Friday's has smothered a hunk of virtuous grilled chicken with a fat-filled trifecta consisting of their own special BBQ sauce, ranch dressing, and Jack Daniels mayo. The result: A bastardized BBQ sandwich that delivers nearly a full day's worth of calories. Ruby's rendition, on the other hand, is one of the few wraps in this country that actually lives up to the healthy hype.

Burgers

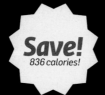

Save!
836 calories!

Not That!
**Outback Steakhouse
Outbacker Burger**

1,600 calories

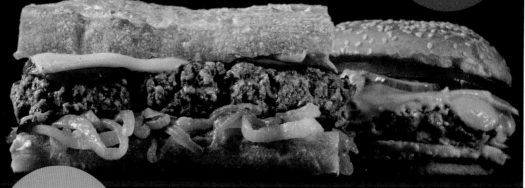

Eat This!
**Cheesecake Factory
The Factory Burger**

*737 calories
16 g saturated fat
1,018 mg sodium*

We're not sure which is more astonishing: That Outback managed to pack a simple cheeseburger with as many calories as you'll find in three of its 8-ounce prime rib steaks, or the fact that the Cheesecake Factory made an appearance on any list in this book as an "Eat This" pick. Let's start with Outback: There's nothing particularly special about this burger. It's not poached in pork fat, bathed in butter, or battered and deep fried. It's merely a patty with lettuce, tomato, pickles, onion, and cheese. Considering that it still packs more calories than three Big Macs, that prime rib is looking like a pretty good alternative. The Cheesecake Factory has its own long lineup of diet-destroying patties, but this cheese- and onion-slathered concoction surprisingly stands out as one of America's best sit-down burgers. Just don't even think of straying elsewhere on the menu.

Tacos

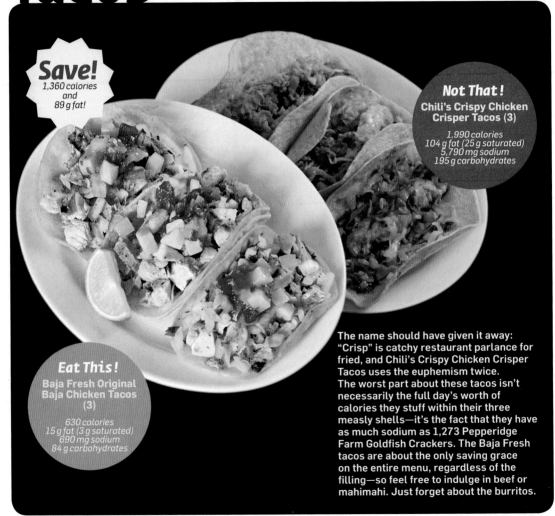

Not That!
Chili's Crispy Chicken Crisper Tacos (3)

1,990 calories
104 g fat (25 g saturated)
5,790 mg sodium
195 g carbohydrates

Eat This!
Baja Fresh Original Baja Chicken Tacos (3)

630 calories
15 g fat (3 g saturated)
690 mg sodium
84 g carbohydrates

The name should have given it away: "Crisp" is catchy restaurant parlance for fried, and Chili's Crispy Chicken Crisper Tacos uses the euphemism twice. The worst part about these tacos isn't necessarily the full day's worth of calories they stuff within their three measly shells—it's the fact that they have as much sodium as 1,273 Pepperidge Farm Goldfish Crackers. The Baja Fresh tacos are about the only saving grace on the entire menu, regardless of the filling—so feel free to indulge in beef or mahimahi. Just forget about the burritos.

Breakfast Sandwich

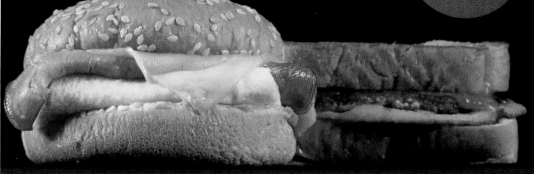

Save!
330 calories
and
30 g fat!

Not That!
**Sonic Sausage,
Egg & Cheese
Breakfast Toaster**

620 calories
42 g fat
(13 g saturated, 1 g trans)
1,380 mg sodium

Eat This!
**Burger King Ham
Omelet Sandwich**

290 calories
12 g fat (4.5 g saturated)
870 mg sodium

When it comes to lunchtime fare, Burger King has a hard time living up to its self-proclaimed royalty. But breakfast is a different story. This satisfying ham and cheese melt delivers a metabolism-rousing shot of protein without breaking the 300-calorie barrier. (Just forget about the hash browns, okay? Even a small packs 420 calories and 27 grams of fat.) Whereas BK succeeds on account of the lean ham and the well-portioned bun, Sonic fails with its reliance on a flying saucer of sausage and the thick slices of Texas Toast—which alone contain more calories (about 300) than the entire Omelet Sandwich.

Chicken Sandwich

Chick-fil-A serves up a trio of America's best chicken sandwiches, including their standard grilled version, their lightly fried rendition, and this—the best club sandwich we've ever come across. Nowhere else will you find a substantial sandwich swaddled in melted cheese and robed in bacon for fewer than 500 calories. Panera serves up plenty of respectable lunchtime fare, but full-size sandwiches are not their strong suit. Most pack more than 600 calories, and a few—including this train wreck—flirt with the catastrophic 1,000-calorie mark. Your best bet is Panera's You Pick option, where you can pair half a sandwich with a salad or a cup of soup.

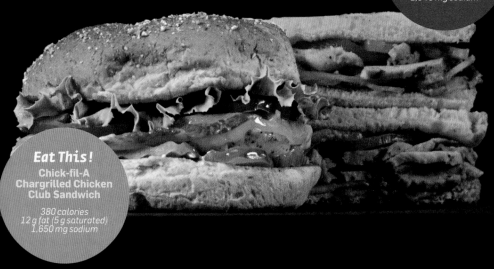

Not That!
Panera
Chipotle Chicken

980 calories
55 g fat
(15 g saturated, 1 g trans)
2,340 mg sodium

Eat This!
Chick-fil-A
Chargrilled Chicken
Club Sandwich

380 calories
12 g fat (5 g saturated)
1,650 mg sodium

Kids' Meals

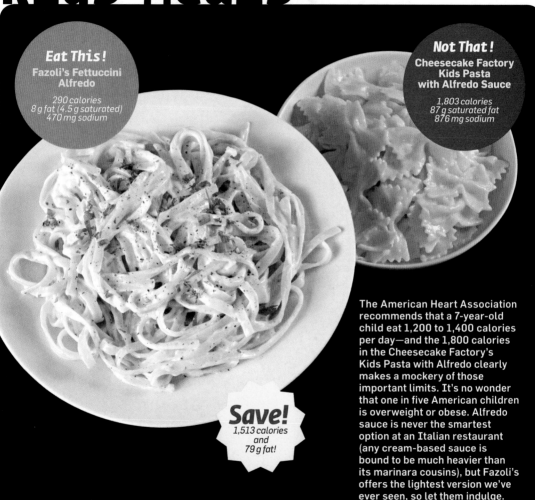

Eat This!
Fazoli's Fettuccini Alfredo

290 calories
8 g fat (4.5 g saturated)
470 mg sodium

Not That!
Cheesecake Factory Kids Pasta with Alfredo Sauce

1,803 calories
87 g saturated fat
876 mg sodium

Save!
1,513 calories
and
79 g fat!

The American Heart Association recommends that a 7-year-old child eat 1,200 to 1,400 calories per day—and the 1,800 calories in the Cheesecake Factory's Kids Pasta with Alfredo clearly makes a mockery of those important limits. It's no wonder that one in five American children is overweight or obese. Alfredo sauce is never the smartest option at an Italian restaurant (any cream-based sauce is bound to be much heavier than its marinara cousins), but Fazoli's offers the lightest version we've ever seen, so let them indulge.

Fish Sandwich

Once upon a time, the BK Big Fish was called The Whaler, until some marketing flack got harpooned and a slightly gentler moniker was applied. (We're not making this stuff up!) The fact remains, though, that even without cheese, the King's catch has 40 percent more calories and fat and more than twice as much sodium as McDonald's Filet-O.

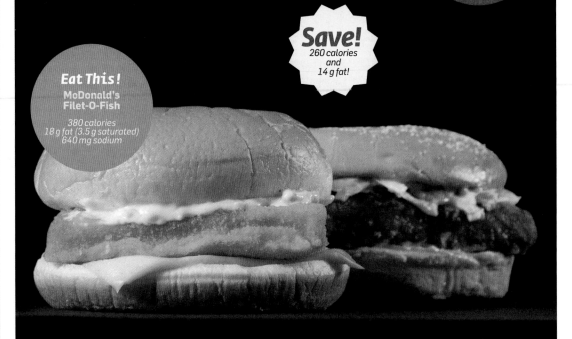

Not That!

**Burger King
BK Big Fish Sandwich**

*640 calories
32 g fat
(5 g saturated, 0.5 g trans)
1,540 mg sodium*

Save!
260 calories
and
14 g fat!

Eat This!

**McDonald's
Filet-O-Fish**

*380 calories
18 g fat (3.5 g saturated)
640 mg sodium*

Chinese

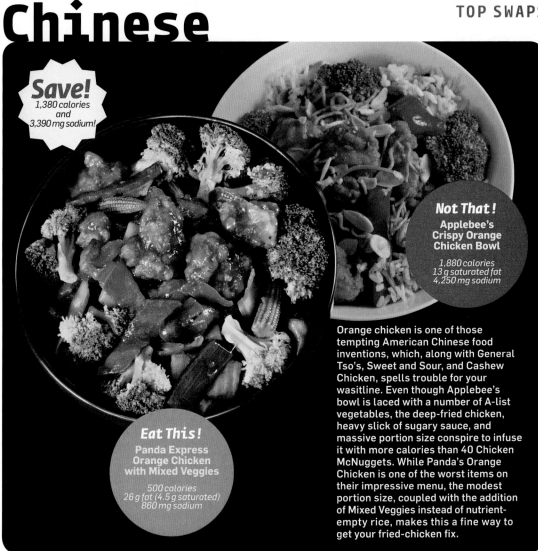

Save!
1,380 calories
and
3,390 mg sodium!

Not That!
Applebee's
Crispy Orange
Chicken Bowl

*1,880 calories
13 g saturated fat
4,250 mg sodium*

Eat This!
Panda Express
Orange Chicken
with Mixed Veggies

*500 calories
26 g fat (4.5 g saturated)
860 mg sodium*

Orange chicken is one of those tempting American Chinese food inventions, which, along with General Tso's, Sweet and Sour, and Cashew Chicken, spells trouble for your wasitline. Even though Applebee's bowl is laced with a number of A-list vegetables, the deep-fried chicken, heavy slick of sugary sauce, and massive portion size conspire to infuse it with more calories than 40 Chicken McNuggets. While Panda's Orange Chicken is one of the worst items on their impressive menu, the modest portion size, coupled with the addition of Mixed Veggies instead of nutrient-empty rice, makes this a fine way to get your fried-chicken fix.

Surf and Turf

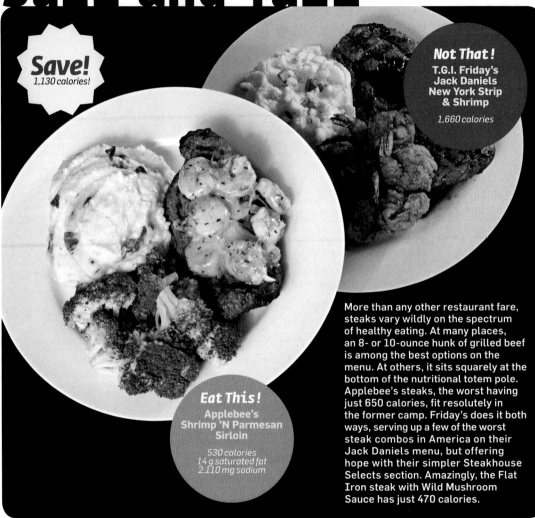

Save!
1,130 calories!

Not That!
**T.G.I. Friday's
Jack Daniels
New York Strip
& Shrimp**

1,660 calories

Eat This!
**Applebee's
Shrimp 'N Parmesan
Sirloin**

*530 calories
14 g saturated fat
2,110 mg sodium*

More than any other restaurant fare, steaks vary wildly on the spectrum of healthy eating. At many places, an 8- or 10-ounce hunk of grilled beef is among the best options on the menu. At others, it sits squarely at the bottom of the nutritional totem pole. Applebee's steaks, the worst having just 650 calories, fit resolutely in the former camp. Friday's does it both ways, serving up a few of the worst steak combos in America on their Jack Daniels menu, but offering hope with their simpler Steakhouse Selects section. Amazingly, the Flat Iron steak with Wild Mushroom Sauce has just 470 calories.

Coffee

Save!
260 calories
and
48 g sugars!

Frozen coffee drinks are the bottom feeders of the caffeine culture, gobbling up whatever precious calories they can with sugary syrups and massive dairy infusions. But Dunkin's Frozen Cappuccino with Skim Milk shows that even if you switch to the nonfat filler, you can still run up a calorie tab of more than 500 calories—that's what you should aim to take in at lunch, to give you some perspective. Starbucks Frappuccino lineup is generally the weakest part of their menu, but this Espresso option proves the exception by being lighter on the milk and the syrup than any other regular blended drink in the store.

Not That!
Dunkin' Donuts Frozen Cappuccino with Skim Milk (large)

550 calories
0 g fat
105 g sugars

Drink This!
Starbucks Espresso Frappuccino Blended Coffee (Venti)

290 calories
3.5 g fat (2.5 g saturated)
57 g sugars

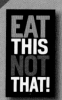

Restaurant Survival Guide

1

THE NEW RULES OF EATING OUT

In olden days of yore (which, for the purposes of this book, we'll define as anything before the Reagan administration), dinner was something you typically ate at home. And going to a restaurant was something special.

Often, it worked like this: Dad would come home tired, cranky, and hungry and wonder why dinner wasn't on the table. Mom, also cranky and hungry and exhausted from a day of putting up with you, would mutter something like "Make your own darn dinner!" Then there'd be lots of banging noises and hushed but urgent bickering in the kitchen, and Dad would emerge 10 minutes later and say, "We're going out for dinner!"

Problem solved! And since going out to dinner was such a special treat, there wasn't much call to worry about what was being served. Sure, a burger and fries might not be as nutritious as Mom's broccoli casserole, but once a week or so, that wasn't such a big deal, right? On average, Americans ate just one in seven meals outside the home in the 1970s. Indulgences are important every once in a while.

Today, however, going out to dinner isn't a special treat anymore. Today we eat one of every four meals— and get a third of our calories—at restaurants. (In fact, we take in twice as many calories from restaurants today than we did 30 years ago.) We're far more likely to chew our food while looking across at a schoolmate, a business associate, a hot date, or just a random stranger —or simply while looking over the dashboard for the on ramp—than we are to look across the family dinner table at our loved ones. And therein lies the problem: Instead of indulging ourselves every once in a while, we're indulging ourselves every single day. That's why America is getting so darn fat.

And that's why we need *EAT THIS, NOT THAT! RESTAURANT SURVIVAL GUIDE.*

How Did Food Get So Darn Fast?

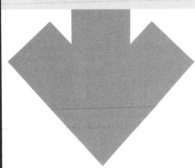

What famous person has had the biggest impact on the way you eat today?

Was it Martha Stewart, Rachael Ray, Gordon Ramsay, or any of the many cooks who dominate TV land? Was it Ray Kroc, the inventor of McDonald's and the man who made hamburgers cheaper than grapefruit? Was it Aunt Jemima maybe, or Count Chocula, or the Jolly Green Giant?

I have a different answer.

I bet the biggest influencer of the way you and I and most all Americans eat today isn't a chef, a restaurateur, or cartoon food hawker. My vote goes to Henry Ford. Here's why: Henry Ford invented the assembly-line auto factory. And, quite accidentally, he also invented assembly-line eating.

See, up until the middle of the last century, running a restaurant was a job for people who actually liked other people. You had to have a big dining space, tables and chairs, waiters and waitresses—the whole shebang. Plus, you'd have to build *relationships* with your customers. You'd see them face-to-face, see how their lives changed over the years, and you'd get to care about them and want them to be happy and healthy so they kept coming back to your establishment.

But by the 1950s, things had changed. America became known as the land of cars and, as a result, the land of drive-ins. And that meant a lot less overhead for the restaurant and a lot more customers because you no longer had to worry about clearing and resetting the tables. Customers brought their own tables—in the form of Pontiacs and Buicks and Mercurys—and when they finished eating, they just drove off, taking their tables with them. Restaurant owners knew their customers not by their faces and families, but by their grills and taillights.

Then, restaurants saw the light and took the whole concept one step further: What if, instead of parking and eating, we could get people to eat our food, in their cars, without even stopping? What if we could turn the drive-in into a drive-thru? We'd never have to get to know them and they'd never get to know us, and instead of expensive, professional waitstaffs—or even bobby soxers on roller skates— we'd just have teenagers in paper hats. And bam, the fast-food culture world was up and running, big-time.

And that's where we live today.

Now, fast-food culture has a lot to recommend it—especially if you like your coffee and McMuffin with a side of Howard Stern or NPR or Sirius Hits 1. And even more so if you like going through your day without having to talk to another human being face-to-face. But what's been lost is a culture in which our food is prepared by people who know and care about us. Nowadays, when both the help and the customers are anonymous, how much do you think the big food corporations really care about our health? Especially when there's always

another car pulling up behind ours, ready to honk if we don't get our order finished in record time?

And the weird thing is, even restaurants that aren't "fast food" seem to follow the same ethos. Whether you're in Amarillo or Athens or Augusta, a Chili's there looks just like a Chili's anywhere, and the waitress handing you a menu probably won't be working there 6 months from now. Food is so well planned out by the restaurant's giant parent company (in this case, that would be Brinker International, Inc., which also owns On the Border and Maggiano's Little Italy) that it takes no time or thought to put together the ingredients of, say, their Chicken Fajita Pita. Indeed, they don't want the people in their kitchen thinking at all—because thinking might lead to creativity. Instead, they want that food produced as identically and robotically as possible, from Maine to Georgia to Texas. The faster it's made, the faster it's served, the faster you're out the door and the next family of customers takes your seat.

The great thing about fast-food culture—speed and convenience—is also the worst thing. Speed is terrific for making it to work on time, for shutting up the kids when they're crying for dinner, and for filling that empty hole in your belly when you're just too tired to shop/cook/sit upright at a table. But when it comes to food, fast is bad for one thing—your health. And everything about fast food is fast. Consider:

We order it fast.

Instead of really thinking about what we're about to eat, we typically pick the path of least resistance—what can we order that can get the food into our bellies and us out of the line as efficiently as possible? Often, we'll just let the corporations decide for us: At hamburger chains, "combination meals" make up a whopping 31 percent of all purchases. That takes a lot of the thinking out of the process, but it adds a lot of the calories in: The average combo meal packs more than 1,200 calories, and about a third of those calories come from the predetermined sides that the restaurant corporation decided you should order.

That's bad.

It's cooked fast.

Ever notice that the different parts of a fast-food meal all sort of taste the same? The burger, the fries, the onion rings, even the shake—they all kinda taste like "fast food," rather than what they normally should taste like: broiled cow, fried potatoes, whipped ice cream. That's because fast foods are made to appeal to our taste buds in a way that inspires us to keep eating— not too meaty, not too vegetable-y, not too dairylike. Our bodies— specifically, the part of our brain called the hypothalamus— evolved to crave a variety of sweet, salty, and bitter tastes, so we would munch on one type of food, then get tired of it and look for something different. (That ensured we got a balanced diet.) But today's food marketers have created "Frankenfoods" that combine all those flavors into each food, so we don't lose interest—we just eat and eat and eat. All the fry cook has to do is dump the frozen nuggets into the boiling fat, and science does the rest.

We eat it fast, that's for sure.

Since everything sort of tastes the same, we don't stop to savor any particular flavors. Unlike a hamburger you make on the grill, a fast-food burger doesn't feature the bite of the pickle, the creamy richness of the melted cheese, the smoky tang of the grilled meat. And the speed at which we consume that food allows us to fill up on calories in an unnatural way. It takes about 20 minutes for your stomach to send the message to your brain that your hunger is satisfied and for your brain to say, "Okay, chill with the chocolate shake. We're good here." But since the average fast-food meal can be gone in 5 minutes or less, we can scarf down far more calories than we'd normally be able to. In a recent study, Japanese scientists found that people who wolfed down their food were more likely to be overweight and insulin-resistant—both early signs of future diabetes—than those who ate at a slower pace.

And worst of all, we digest it fast.

When you eat, say, an almond, your body has to earn its nutrition. Your teeth kick things off, grinding overtime to break down that little nut. Then your body has to work first to digest the protein, a process that burns calories even as it's happening, and second to digest the fiber, which slows the pace of the almond through your digestive system. All those nutrients and calories enter your body slowly, so the hormonal system that regulates energy has time to react and manage the food and to burn the energy it generates over time. But because fast-food meals are so rich in fat, carbs, and sodium and relatively low in fiber and protein, your body digests them very quickly. Suddenly, all those calories have flooded your system, and there's no way you can burn them off unless you're going mano a mano with Roger Federer right after. Instead, your body has to act fast to put them somewhere—usually, around your midsection. And that rapid process of digesting and storing calories leaves you feeling, well, guess how? Hungry and tired.

7 Habits of Highly Obese People

Why do some people simply pack on the pounds effortlessly? It's not always genetics and it's not always gluttony and you can't always blame it on lack of exercise. Indeed, getting fat is often a result of some simple—and easily correctible—bad habits, especially when it comes to dining out.

As my coauthor, Matt Goulding, and I began researching the **EAT THIS, NOT THAT!** series, we discovered plenty of egregious examples of superfattening foods in both America's supermarkets and our chain restaurants. And we learned that if you just know what to order and what to avoid, you can shave off pounds effortlessly. For example, does On the Border really need to stuff more than a day's worth of calories—2,550—into its Dos XX Fish Tacos? (Remember when fish was healthy?) And shouldn't Chili's warn parents when a selection on its kids' menu comes with 82 grams of fat, like its Pepper Pals Little Chicken Crispers does?

But it's not just the food itself. The restaurant industry has spent decades studying human behavior and figured out all sorts of subliminal ways to make us want to order and eat more. (Ever notice how all fast-food restaurants use red, yellow, and orange in their packaging and decor, but never blue, green, or purple? Think that's just a coincidence? Check out page 63 to find out.) And a lot of those psychological tricks have become ingrained in our behavior. In a study in the journal *Obesity*, researchers looked at the habits of people dining at an all-you-can-eat buffet. Those with the highest body mass index (BMI)—a measure of obesity—seemed to demonstrate a series of "fat habits."

1.
They use larger plates.

When offered two plate sizes, 98.6 percent of those with the highest BMI took the larger of the two plates to the buffet. A bigger plate tricks your eye into thinking you're not eating as much when you stuff more food onto the surface—and into your mouth. Use a smaller plate, get a smaller belly.

2.
They eat while looking at food.

Of those with high BMIs, 41.7 percent took seats that overlooked the buffet, instead of sitting in a booth or facing in a different direction. The sight of food tends to make our minds think we have more work to do, eating-wise. Keep your food stored in the fridge or stashed in the pantry, not out on the countertops.

3.
They eat with maximum efficiency.

While Chinese buffets offer chopsticks, 91.3 percent of obese patrons opt for forks. That just makes it easier to shovel in the food!

4.
They clean their plates.

Of those patrons who were heaviest, 94 percent cleaned their plates so there was nothing left. Ignore Mom's advice—let a little linger.

5.
They chew less.

Researchers actually monitored the chewing habits of the buffet-goers and discovered that the heaviest one-third among them chewed their food an average of 11.9 times before swallowing. The middle one-third chewed an average of 14 times, and the leanest one-third chewed 14.8 times.

6.
They dive in.

The leanest people in the study typically took a lap around the buffet first, to plot out what they wanted to eat. But the more overweight group charged right in; doing so means you may fill up on some less-appealing items, then have to go back to snag that one nosh you have to have but missed the first time.

7.
They skip breakfast.

A simple habit, but it raises your risk of obesity by a whopping 450 percent!

16 No-Diet Weight Loss Tips

HOW TO SHED POUNDS WITHOUT GIVING UP A SINGLE SOLITARY THING!

1 FILL UP WITH FRUIT.

Turns out, an apple a day may also keep the extra weight away. Penn State researchers discovered that people who ate a large apple 15 minutes before lunch took in 187 fewer calories during lunch than those who didn't snack beforehand. (The apples had around 128 calories. So make just that one move every Monday through Friday and you'll shed 4½ pounds in a year!) What's more, they reported feeling fuller afterward, too. Sure, the fruit is loaded with belly-filling fiber, but there's another reason apples help you feel full: They require lots of chewing, which can make you think you're eating more than you really are, says study author Julie Obbagy, PhD.

2 SLEEP AWAY FLAB.

Lack of shut-eye can cause you to overeat. University of Chicago scientists discovered that people who lost 3 hours of slumber ate about 200 more calories that day from snacks. The researchers haven't yet pinned down the mechanism but speculate that it may be simple: The longer you're awake, the longer you're exposed to food.

3 PUMP UP WITH PROTEIN.

If you hate to diet, it may be that you're just eating the wrong foods. University of Illinois researchers found that people who ate higher amounts of protein were more likely to stick to their diets for 1 year than those who ate more carbohydrates instead. The reason: "Protein is more satiating than carbohydrates are, so people weren't as hungry as those in the other group," says study author Donald L. Layman, PhD. "They also had more energy and didn't feel as tired." Turns out, the dieters who best stuck to their eating plan consumed a diet that provided 40 percent of its calories from carbohydrates and 30 percent from protein.

4 FIGHT FAT WITH FAT.

Fish isn't just good for your heart; it's good for your gut, too. That's because omega-3 fatty acids help you feel full longer, report scientists from Iceland. In the study, dieters who ate salmon felt fuller 2 hours later than those who either didn't eat seafood or had cod, a fish with little fat. The researchers found that eating foods high in omega-3s increased blood levels of leptin, a hormone that promotes satiety. Hate fish? Take a fish-oil capsule every day—one has 500 milligrams of the omega-3s DHA and EPA. It offers the same benefits as the salmon.

5 CONTROL YOUR ANXIETY.

No worries, no weight gain. Researchers from the Netherlands found that anxiety can cause you to overeat when you're not hungry. In their study, people who felt stressed after taking a difficult test consumed more sweets than people who felt relaxed after taking an easy one. "Eating sugary foods may relieve stress by releasing chemicals in the brain that increase reward feelings," says study author Femke Rutters, PhD.

6 UNPLUG YOUR TV.

Watching TV while you eat may cause you to consume more food later in the day. UK scientists found that people who watched a video during lunch ate more at a midafternoon snack than those who'd dined while away from the tube. "Watching TV during a meal can cause people to remember less about the food, so they subconsciously eat more later," says study author Suzanne Higgs, PhD.

7 MAKE FIT FRIENDS.

Keeping excess weight off can be difficult if you have heavy pals, according to a study in the journal *Obesity*. That's because you may be less likely to exercise and eat healthfully in your free time. The good news: Befriending people who are fit may help you lose weight, even if you're not consciously trying to. Why? People often emulate behaviors of close friends they look up to, says study author Ray Browning, PhD.

8 WALK AWAY FROM CHOCOLATE.

Need a simple way to avoid dessert? Go outside. Researchers in the UK found that taking a short walk can weaken chocolate cravings. In the study, regular chocolate eaters refrained from eating the treat for 3 days and then either took a 15-minute walk or stayed idle. The strollers' cravings dropped by 12 percent after a walk, but those of the couch potatoes intensified. "Like chocolate, exercise may increase the levels of feel-good chemicals in your brain, reducing a desire for sweets," says study author Adrian Taylor, PhD.

9 RESIST THE BLOB MENTALITY.

Your dining partner could be making you fat. Researchers from Eastern Illinois University have discovered that people consume 65 percent more calories when they eat with a person who opts for seconds than when they dine with a companion who doesn't. "Just being aware of it can help you avoid becoming a victim," says *Men's Health* nutrition advisor Jonny Bowden, PhD. Instead of taking seconds, opt for a cup of herbal tea after you finish your main course. It will keep your mouth busy while providing a refreshing, no-calorie end to your meal.

10 WRITE OFF THE POUNDS.

Hold yourself accountable: In a 13-week study, dieters who kept a food record for 3 weeks or longer lost 3½ pounds more than those who didn't, say researchers at the University of Arkansas. And over the long term, this strategy may be even more important for enhancing your results. "Keeping a detailed account of what you eat helps you learn how to accurately estimate portion sizes," says *Men's Health* weight loss coach, Alan Aragon, MS. To eyeball calories like an expert, log and analyze your daily meals for at least 2 weeks on a free Web site such as sparkpeople.com.

11 IGNORE YOUR SERVER.

Eastern Illinois University scientists found that people ate 85 percent more bread when their server offered them seconds. "Blame social pressure," says study advisor Karla Kennedy-Hagan, PhD. "It's harder for people to decline an offer when it comes directly from another person." Your best bet? Order soup and pass on the breadbasket altogether.

12 ORDER THE SMALL.

That "medium" soda may actually be a large. Duke University researchers have discovered that some fast-food chains are encouraging customers to buy larger soft drinks—which justifies higher prices—by increasing the number of ounces in all sizes of drinks. They know what you may not: Most people subconsciously pick the middle option without considering the actual amount, says study author Richard Staelin, PhD. Remember, 8 ounces is one serving.

13 WATCH OUT FOR WEEKENDS.

A study in the journal *Obesity* reveals that people eat an average of 236 more calories on Saturday than on any given weekday. Blame it on the break from your usual routine. "Since your day is not as structured on the weekends, neither are your eating habits," says study author Susan Racette, PhD.

14 DON'T CLEAN YOUR PLATE.

In a Cornell University study, the heaviest men said they stopped eating when they thought they had consumed the "normal" amount—for example, a heaping restaurant entrée—instead of when they started to feel full. "Focusing on the food left on your plate and not what's in your stomach influences you to keep eating," says study author Brian Wansink, PhD.

15 DRINK MORE WATER.

Thirst can masquerade as hunger, which is one reason dieters should stay hydrated. Now German researchers have found another reason: Water fuels your body's fat burners. For 90 minutes after drinking 16 ounces of chilled water, adults saw their metabolisms rise by 24 percent over their average rates. The increase is partly attributed to the energy your body generates to warm the water during digestion.

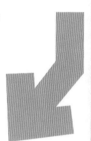

16 CUT UP YOUR FOOD.

Japanese researchers recently proved what dietitians have been saying for years: Slicing your food into strips or chunks may help you eat less. Study participants who compared equal amounts of sliced and whole vegetables rated the sliced serving as much as 27 percent larger. The end result: Believing that you are eating a larger portion of food causes you to feel more satisfied with fewer calories.

Sneaky Secrets the Restaurants Don't Want You to Know

If being an anonymous blip on a giant corporation's assembly line makes you feel like a character in some bleak sci-fi movie, we've got good news. There are plenty of ways to fight back—to enjoy all the convenience of modern restaurants and all the foods you still like to eat without paying extra money every 6 months for a new pair of pants.

You see, all major restaurant chains— from the fast-food purveyors to the sandwich shops and coffee bars to the sit-down dinner joints with their vaguely Italian/Mexican/Chinese/ whatever themes—operate with the same set of secrets, secrets they don't want their customers to know. And if you know these secrets, well, guess what? The power to eat what you want and still stay slim is in your hands.

Lucky you!

Here's how to start taking back control.

Don't get "supersized"

Sure, it *feels* like you're getting a bargain because you're getting proportionately more food for proportionately less money. But a "value meal" is only a value for two sets of people: the corporations that make the food and the corporations that make liposuction machines and heart stents. Because food is so inexpensive for manufacturers to produce on a large scale, your average fast-food emporium makes a hefty profit whenever you supersize your meal—even though you're getting an average of 73 percent more calories for only 17 percent more money. But as we pointed out in the introduction to this book, you're not actually buying more food. You're

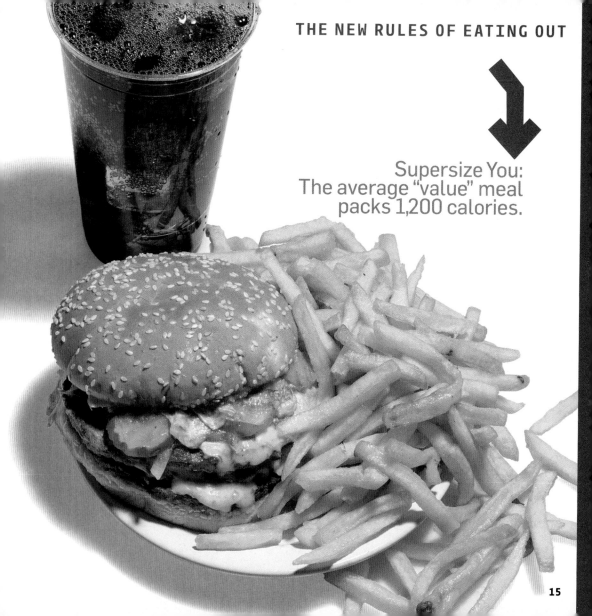

Supersize You:
The average "value" meal
packs 1,200 calories.

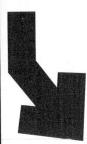

buying more calories. And that's not something you want more of. (If we were really smart, fast-food shops would be charging us more for the smaller portions!)

Remember, the waiter is a salesperson

A 2005 study published in the *Journal of Retailing and Consumer Services* found that you're more likely to order a side dish when the server verbally prompts you. ("Do you want fries with that?") Restaurants know this, and now you know it, too. When the waiter makes a suggestion, remember his job is not to make you happy. His job is to extract money from your wallet and insert fat in its place.

Don't get too excited

You eat out all the time. A 2008 study in the *International Food Research Journal* found that people are less likely to make healthy restaurant choices when they feel that they're dining out for a "special occasion." And as we said at the top of this chapter, dining out used to be special. But before you head out to your next meal, really take stock of how many times you've eaten out this week. If you're eating every meal at home and dining out truly is a once-a-week splurge, then don't worry about it so much. But if you're like most of us, eating out is probably more like a once-a-day splurge. And if that's the case, remember, there's nothing special here. Eat smart today because you'll have to do it again tomorrow.

Start small

Here's the good news: No one is going to stop you from ordering seconds. So be like any good businessperson, and start small. Here's exactly how expensive it really is whenever you go for the "bargain":

7-ELEVEN > Gulp to Double Gulp Coca-Cola Classic: 37 cents extra buys 450 more calories.

CINNABON > Minibon to Classic Cinnabon: 48 more cents buys 370 more calories.

MOVIE THEATER > Small to medium unbuttered popcorn: 71 additional cents buys you 500 more calories.

CONVENIENCE STORE > Regular to "The Big One" Snickers: 33 more cents packs on 230 more calories.

MCDONALD'S > Quarter Pounder with Cheese to Medium Quarter Pounder with

Cheese Extra Value Meal: An additional $1.41 gets you 660 more calories.

SUBWAY > 6-inch to 12-inch Tuna Sub: $1.53 more buys 420 more calories.

WENDY'S > Classic Double with Cheese to Classic Double with Cheese Old Fashioned Combo Meal: $1.57 extra buys you 600 more calories.

BASKIN ROBBINS > Chocolate Chip Ice Cream, Kids' Scoop, to Double Scoop: For another $1.62, you've added 390 calories.

The bottom line on all this? For just a hair more than 8 bucks, you've bought yourself an additional 3,620 calories. If you ate each of these once a week, and you were to switch to the smaller size each time—again, still all your favorite foods, just in a more reasonable size—you'd save about $417 a year. It's not going to buy you a new car, but it could put you on a plane to the Bahamas. But far more important than that is what it will mean to your waistline, because in saving that $417, you'll also save 188,240 calories in a year— enough to shave 54 pounds of flab off your body. (Hey, take the 400 bucks and buy some new pants!)

Know your food

Once upon a time, back when Ray Kroc was still pushing milk-shake machines, a hamburger and fries meant a wad of freshly ground chuck and a peeled, sliced, and fried potato. Now, these two iconic foods—like nearly everything we consume—has taken on a whole new meaning. Sadly, many of our favorite foods today (especially fast foods) weren't merely crafted in kitchens, they were also designed and perfected in labs. So before you mindlessly chew your way through another value meal, take these mini-mysteries (conveniently solved below) into account. Sometimes the truth is tough to swallow.

What's in a Chicken McNugget?

You'd think that a breaded lump of chicken would be pretty simple. Mostly, it would contain bread and chicken.

But the McNugget and its peers at other fast-food restaurants are much more complicated creatures than that. The "meat" in the McNugget *alone* contains seven ingredients, some of which are made up of yet more ingredients. (Nope, it's not just chicken. It's also such nonchicken-related stuff as water, wheat starch, dextrose, safflower oil, and sodium phosphates.) The "meat" also contains something called "autolyzed yeast extract." Then add another 20 ingredients that make up the breading, and you have the industrial chemical—I mean, fast-food meal—called the McNugget.

Still, McDonald's is practically all-natural compared to Wendy's Chicken Nuggets, with 30 ingredients, and Burger King Chicken Fries, with a whopping 35 ingredients.

What's in a Wendy's Frosty?

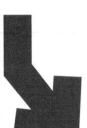

Wendy's Frosty requires 14 ingredients to create what traditional shakes achieve with only milk and ice cream. So what accounts for the double-digit ingredient list? Mostly a barrage of thickening agents that includes guar gum, cellulose gum, and carrageenan. And while that's enough to disqualify it as a milk shake in our book, it's nothing compared to the chemist's list of ingredients in the restaurant's new line of bulked-up Frankenfrosties.

Check out the Coffee Toffee Twisted Frosty, for instance. It seems harmless enough; the only additions, after all, are "coffee syrup" and "coffee toffee pieces." The problem is that those two additions collectively contain 25 extra ingredients, seven of which are sugars and three of which are oils. And get this: Rather than a classic syrup, the "coffee syrup" would more accurately be described as a blend of water, high-fructose corn syrup, and propylene glycol, a laxative chemical that's used as an emulsifier in food and a filler in electronic cigarettes. Of all 10 ingredients it takes to make the syrup, coffee doesn't show up until near the end, eight items down the list.

What's in a Filet-O-Fish?

The world's most famous fish sand wich begins as one of the ocean's ugliest creatures. Filet-O-Fish, like many of the fish patties used by fast-food chains, is made predominantly from hoki, a gnarly, crazy-eyed fish found in the cold waters off the coast of New Zealand. In the past, McDonald's has purchased up to 15 million pounds of hoki a year, each flaky fillet destined for a coat of batter, a bath of oil, a squirt of tartar, and a final resting place in a warm, squishy bun. But it seems the world's appetite for this and other fried-fish sandwiches has proven too voracious, as New Zealand has been forced to cut the allowable catch over the years in order to keep the hoki population from collapsing. Don't expect McDonald's to scale down Filet-O-Fish output anytime soon, though; other whitefish like Alaskan pollock will likely fill in the gaps left by the hoki downturn. After all, once it's battered and fried, do you really think you'll know the difference?

What's in my salami sandwich?

Salami, the mystery meat: Is it cow? Is it pig? Well, if you're talking Genoa salami, like you'd get at Subway, then it's both. Most salami is made from slaughterhouse leftovers that are gathered using "advanced meat recovery," which sounds like a rehab center for vegans but is actually a mechanical process that strips the last remaining bits of muscle off the bone so nothing is wasted. It's then processed using lactic acid, the waste product produced by bacteria in the meat. It both gives the salami its tangy flavor and cures it as well, making it an inhospitable place for other bacteria to grow. Add in a bunch of salt and spices—for a total of 15 ingredients in all—and you've got salami.

But now that you know what's in there, you might need to check yourself into an advanced meat recovery center.

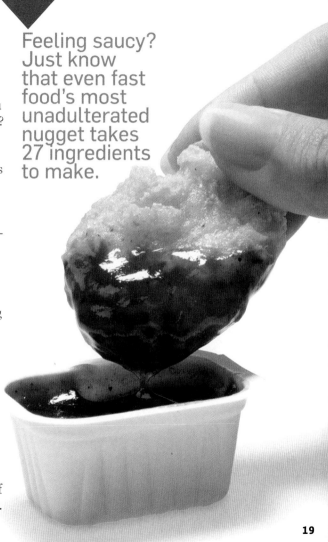

Feeling saucy? Just know that even fast food's most unadulterated nugget takes 27 ingredients to make.

THE BEST & WORST RESTAURANT FOODS IN AMERICA

Restaurant Survival Guide

2

The 20 Best Restaurant Foods in America

When it comes to finding America's standout restaurant foods, we've got some good news and some bad news. Let's start with the bad: It's considerably easier to build a list of abominable items than it is to round up a selection of truly commendable food. Some menus' vitals look more like national debt figures or Paris Hilton's monthly booze allowance than they do nutritional values that we should be putting into our bodies. It's not uncommon to find fish dishes with triple-digit fat counts, salads that gobble up an entire day's caloric allotment, and sides that stick us with an entire week's worth of cholesterol-spiking trans fat. Many restaurant chains have tried to march toward a healthier horizon, but thus far the road to nutritional salvation has been littered with some supersize setbacks. (Think McDonald's new Angus Burgers, Burger King's Burger Shots, or Pizza Hut's Stuffed Crust Pan Pizza).

The good news is that consumers actually want healthier items. When Canadian researchers asked patrons at 10 different restaurants to rate how satisfied they were with their meals, those eating low-fat foods were significantly more pleased than their fat-feeding peers. The reasons cited for their pleasant experiences ranged from "freshness" to "lack of fat and grease." What's that mean for you? Replace at least one of your usual weekly meals with any of the items on this list and you'll not only shed pounds, but you'll also walk away completely satisfied. Eating out doesn't get any better than that.

BEST BLENDED COFFEE DRINK

BEST FOODS
BEST CHINESE

Smoothie King Skinny Coffee Smoothie Mocha (20 oz)

*160 calories
2 g fat (0 g saturated)
13 g sugars
17 g protein*

When a chain that specializes in one thing—say, smoothies—takes on something outside their area of expertise—say, coffee—the results are rarely good. (Think of Domino's 1,400-calorie foray into bread-bowl pastas.) That makes this an anomaly in the world of food service. Somehow Smoothie King managed to wrangle a beverage from the hands of the coffee shops that know it best and transform it into a bona-fide nutritious treat.

The secret is in the smoothie chain's ability to keep it simple. This drink, as long as you order it "skinny," consists of nothing more than coffee, nonfat milk, and chocolate-flavored protein. The only sugar in the cup is that which occurs naturally in milk, so it comes with a shipment of calcium and amino acids in tow. That's a massive boon for your bones and muscles.

Luckily we've saved you the distress of ordering by rooting out the best Chinese entrée in America, but even if you stray from the Mushroom Chicken, there's one rule you should always follow. Regardless of restaurant, trade in the rice and noodles for either an extra entrée or—even better—a side of vegetables. You'll save hundreds of empty calories and gain a massive boost of protein and phytonutrients.

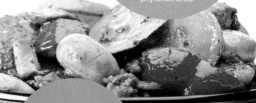

Panda Express Mushroom Chicken with Vegetables

*180 calories
10 g fat (2 g saturated)
720 mg sodium*

Here's what Chinese food has going for it: It's made without the use of cheese, butter, or cream, yet somehow it still doesn't garner much enthusiasm from nutritionists. The reason? Most notable is the one-two punch of sodium and carbohydrates. Pair the wrong entrée with the wrong carb at Panda Express, for instance, and you'll wind up with either half a day's worth of sodium or close to 400 calories in carbs. And that's assuming you limit yourself to a single-entrée plate.

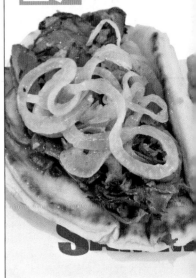

There is virtually no end to the number of side dishes a good chef can dream up, which is why it's odd that we rely so stubbornly on such a small selection. How many times have you eaten French fries alongside a hamburger? How many times was that your only decent option? Too many.

The best side dishes, of course, are unadorned vegetables, and we'll stand behind that any day of the week. But when it comes to creating something innovative and tasty that customers might actually want to eat alongside a hamburger, Wendy's has provided the perfect solution.

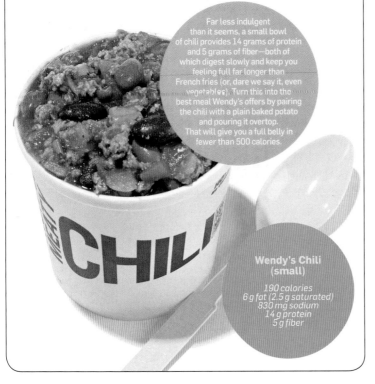

Far less indulgent than it seems, a small bowl of chili provides 14 grams of protein and 5 grams of fiber—both of which digest slowly and keep you feeling full far longer than French fries (or, dare we say it, even vegetables). Turn this into the best meal Wendy's offers by pairing the chili with a plain baked potato and pouring it overtop. That will give you a full belly in fewer than 500 calories.

Wendy's Chili (small)

190 calories
6 g fat (2.5 g saturated)
830 mg sodium
14 g protein
5 g fiber

Here's a lesson in sandwich making that you can take home to your own kitchen: The less bread you use, the more calories you have to spend on meat, cheese, and vegetables. That's the motivating force behind Quiznos Sammies: Pack as much food as possible into a small piece of flatbread. The result is a resounding success. Only one crosses 300 calories (that's the 305-calorie Italiano Sammie), and they carry up to 17 grams of protein each.

No. 16 BEST SMOOTHIE

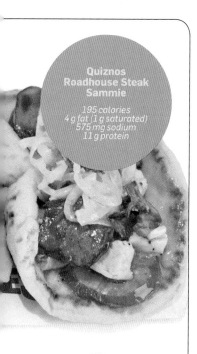

Quiznos Roadhouse Steak Sammie

195 calories
4 g fat (1 g saturated)
575 mg sodium
11 g protein

At Jamba Juice, separating the real from the pseudo-smoothies is easy; just look for the menu section dubbed "All Fruit." That's where you'll find this masterful blend of fruit and unsweetened fruit juice. You'll also find a smattering of B vitamins, 60 percent of your day's vitamin A, and 70 percent of your vitamin C in this smoothie. One caveat, though: Real fruit smoothies are essentially without protein, so order yours with a Whey Super Protein Boost and it will take the edge off your hunger.

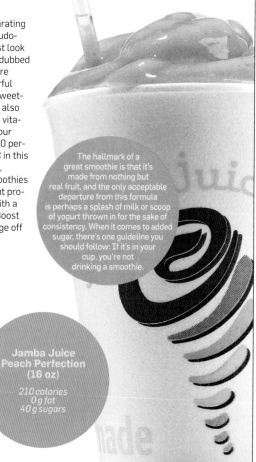

The hallmark of a great smoothie is that it's made from nothing but real fruit, and the only acceptable departure from this formula is perhaps a splash of milk or scoop of yogurt thrown in for the sake of consistency. When it comes to added sugar, there's one guideline you should follow: If it's in your cup, you're not drinking a smoothie.

Compare a Sammie with the smallest sandwiches on the menu: At a mere 5 inches, the subs average 514 calories per sandwich, more than two Roadhouses. But it's not just the diminished size that makes the Sammie the Best Sandwich; it's the flexibility. One makes for a perfect snack, two make for a commendable meal, and three for an understandable splurge.

Jamba Juice Peach Perfection (16 oz)

210 calories
0 g fat
40 g sugars

BEST TACOS

BEST DESSERT

There are at least a couple good reasons why mahimahi earns two plugs on our list. First, with only a quarter to a tenth as much fat as salmon, it's one of the leanest fish in the sea. Second, it trounces any other meat you're likely to find stuffed into a taco shell. Really, mahimahi is almost pure protein, and each one of these tacos has a whopping 12 grams, plus a good hit of healthy fat from the fresh avocado.

Baja Fresh Grilled Mahi Mahi Fish Tacos (2 tacos)

460 calories
18 g fat (3 g saturated)
600 mg sodium
24 g protein
8 g fiber

Not eating at Baja? Don't fret. There's one edict that will keep you safe at any Mexican restaurant: Stick with the tacos. They're almost always the leanest option on the menu. That's because they offer built-in portion control (especially if you opt for smaller, healthier corn tortillas); proteins that are normally grilled, rather than fried or sautéed in an abundance of oil; and a heavy reliance on healthy condiments like salsa and guacamole. Exceptions exist (we're looking at you, 2,350-calorie Dos XX Fish Tacos from On the Border!), but more often than not, tacos will be your salvation.

It's only natural: You eat, the sweet tooth flares, and you decide to order something small to calm it down. Problem is, most sit-down restaurants are trying to milk you for every buck they can, and they do that by building hulking, multilayered desserts to justify the 8-dollar price tag. As soon as you grab that dessert menu, they've got you hooked. Every major restaurant chain in the country sells desserts packing in more than 800 calories apiece, and most of them sell desserts with more than 1,200. You can bet your flat belly that these are the ones most likely to be pictured on the menu.

That's why you need a strategy, and this is what it should be: simple, small, and sweet, and Romano's sorbetto fits that to a T. It's sugar you want, not fat, and that's just what you get with sorbetto. Unlike ice cream, which carries a load of dairy fat, sorbetto uses shaved ice as a vehicle for the fruit and sugar that will satisfy your craving. It's worth the trip to Romano's just for this healthy indulgence.

No. 13 BEST FISH ENTRÉE

Even the oiliest of fish looks lean when stacked alongside your average piece of red meat, but that rule holds only when both cuts are still raw. Once a fish passes through the kitchen at a chain restaurant, all bets are off. That's where fish develop the Killer Whale Complex, a blubber-inducing bath of butter and frying oil that results in thousand-calorie plates of shrimp pasta, lobster ravioli, and fried catfish.

Want to maintain your fish's pristine nutritional profile? Here's what you do: Avoid creamy sauces and don't eat anything with breading. Oh, and ask for your fish sans butter, since most restaurants will brush them before and after cooking. Your best bet is right here: grilled mahimahi that eschews the butter treatment for cilantro-seasoned mangoes, peppers, and tomatoes instead.

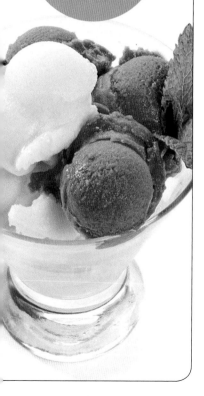

Romano's Macaroni Grill Italian Sorbetto with Biscotti

240 calories
2 g fat (0.5 g saturated)
58 g carbs

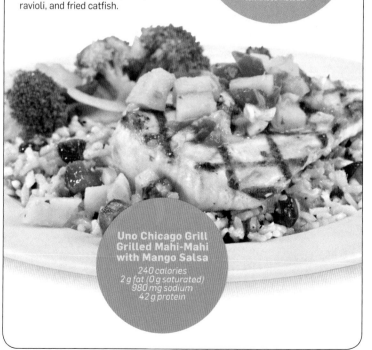

Uno Chicago Grill Grilled Mahi-Mahi with Mango Salsa

240 calories
2 g fat (0 g saturated)
980 mg sodium
42 g protein

BEST COFFEE-SHOP BREAKFAST

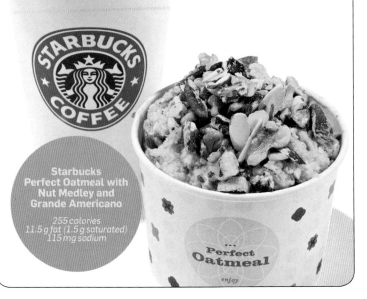

Americanos are kings of the coffee counter. Why? Because they're made from pure espresso, thinned out with a pour of hot water. The damage: 10 calories. Looking for a flavor boost? Turn to one of the many sugar-free syrups that Starbucks keeps tucked behind the counter.

Oatmeal sits right alongside eggs in the Breakfast Hall of Fame, and the reason is simple: fiber. Along with protein, fiber is your best weapon for fighting hunger, and it's also the nutrient people have the hardest time working into their diet. A USDA study found that few people meet their daily quota, and the overweight subjects consumed, on average, less than half their recommended amount, which is about 30 grams a day. Not only does a low fiber intake increase your risk of heart disease and cancer, but studies show it also increases your risk of vitamin inadequacy.

Starbucks Perfect Oatmeal with Nut Medley and Grande Americano

255 calories
11.5 g fat (1.5 g saturated)
115 mg sodium

BEST KIDS' MEAL

So why Applebee's Corn Dog? Sure you can do better by pushing the Grilled Chicken Sandwich and Steamed Broccoli, but ultimately kids today, just like kids 20 years ago, want foods that they can jab into the air like a mock saber and smear across their plates like swamp sludge. The goal is to combine low calories with high stimulation. That being said, if you can get your kid to go the broccoli route, go for it!

Childhood obesity rates have more than doubled in the past 20 years, which is especially scary when you consider that studies show heavy children are more likely to grow into overweight adults. According to the USDA, a moderately active child between the ages of 4 and 8 should consume between

No. 10 BEST FAST-FOOD BREAKFAST

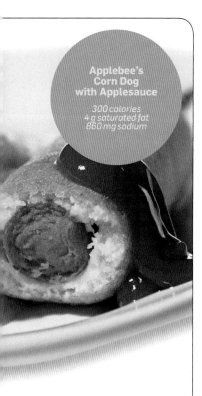

Applebee's Corn Dog with Applesauce

300 calories
4 g saturated fat
860 mg sodium

What happens when there's no McDonald's within striking distance? Well, here's your crib sheet, a list of our favorite breakfast sandwiches: Burger King's Ham Omelet Sandwich with 290 calories and 13 grams of protein, Jack in the Box's Breakfast Jack with 300 calories and 16 grams of protein, and Starbucks Egg White Turkey Bacon and Cheddar Breakfast Sandwich with 340 calories and 22 grams of protein. Write these sandwiches down and stick them in your glove box, or just keep Cheat Sheets at the end of this chapter ever close at hand.

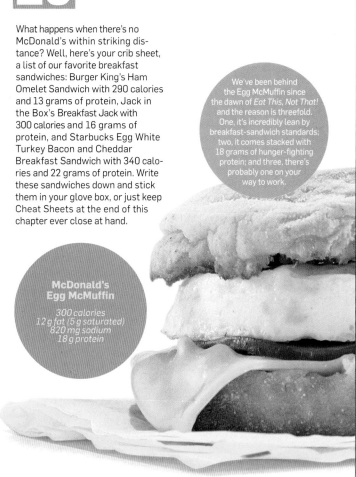

We've been behind the Egg McMuffin since the dawn of *Eat This, Not That!* and the reason is threefold. One, it's incredibly lean by breakfast-sandwich standards; two, it comes stacked with 18 grams of hunger-fighting protein; and three, there's probably one on your way to work.

McDonald's Egg McMuffin

300 calories
12 g fat (5 g saturated)
820 mg sodium
18 g protein

1,400 and 1,600 calories per day. That means one bad meal—say an 800-calorie basket of chicken fingers and fries—can gobble up more than half your child's calories for the day. It's no coincidence, then, that meals like that are today equally as common as the weight problems they precipitate.

BEST PIZZA

BEST DRIVE-THRU MEXICAN

Here's what every child should be taught in health class: how to order a pizza. Seriously, the one-time humble pie has undergone a majorly fattening overhaul from its Italian roots, and now every American is gobbling up some 23 pounds a year. That means the difference between this pie and, say, a Deep Dish Pepperoni might make the difference between Han Solo and Jabba the Hutt.

Rules for ordering a good pie: First and foremost, build it on a thin crust. At Papa John's, for instance, ordering your crust Thin over Pan will save you 170 calories per slice. Second, skip all the traditional meats—pepperoni, sausage, beef, and bacon. Instead aim for the lean protein of chicken and ham. And last, round out your meal with at least one fruit or vegetable. That's why this Hawaiian-style pie is our favorite.

Domino's Thin Crust Ham and Pineapple Pizza (2 slices)
310 calories
14 g fat (5 g saturated)
680 mg sodium

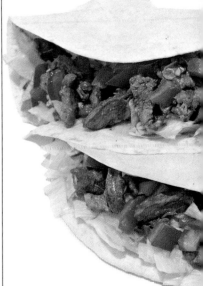

Taco Bell's Fresco Menu represents the sort of drive-thru innovation we welcome with open windows. The four tacos and four burritos on the menu abandon cheese and oil-based sauces in favor of TB's fat-free, flavor-packed Fiesta Salsa. So you're not just losing fat; you're also gaining a host of disease-fighting antioxidants.

BEST APPETIZER

Want to ruin your chances of survival at a sit-down restaurant? Flip to the appetizer menu and pick one at random. Chances are, you'll end up with a plate of deep-fried something-or-other buried under a mound of cheese, bacon, and/or oily sauce. Appetizers like that are the norm, and at restaurants like Outback, they can mean starting your meal with anywhere from 1,000 to 2,000 calories.

Luckily, there's another angle to the appetizer conundrum. The calories in this ahi starter come almost entirely from protein and healthy fat. Multiple studies have highlighted the advanced appetite-squashing ability of these two vital nutrients, and nowhere is that more important than at a place like Outback, where 3,000-calorie ribs and 2,000-calorie desserts lurk, waiting to ensnare famished diners.

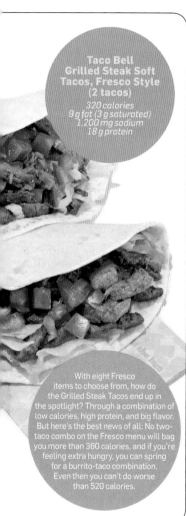

Taco Bell Grilled Steak Soft Tacos, Fresco Style (2 tacos)
320 calories
9 g fat (3 g saturated)
1,200 mg sodium
18 g protein

With eight Fresco items to choose from, how do the Grilled Steak Tacos end up in the spotlight? Through a combination of low calories, high protein, and big flavor. But here's the best news of all: No two-taco combo on the Fresco menu will bag you more than 360 calories, and if you're feeling extra hungry, you can spring for a burrito-taco combination. Even then you can't do worse than 520 calories.

Outback Steakhouse Seared Ahi Tuna
325 calories
21 g fat (2.5 g saturated)
1,351 mg sodium

BEST DRIVE-THRU MEAL

BEST PASTA

Chick-fil-A Chargrilled Chicken Sandwich with medium Fruit Cup and Unsweetened Iced Tea
360 calories
3 g fat (0.5 g saturated)
1,320 mg sodium

When it comes to ordering pasta out, the simpler the better. While flourishes like sun-dried tomatoes, grilled chicken, and pesto may seem like safe add-ons, they're telltale signs of overwrought, oversize bowls of noodles likely to cost you the better part of your day's caloric allowance. This classic red sauce pasta from Olive Garden couldn't be more straightforward—and there's something perfectly satisfying about that.

Join The
Chicken Wave Fo
A Ch
in Fre

Surprise, surprise, you *can* get a healthy meal in the drive-thru lane. Here you have a full meal for 360 calories, and between the chicken and fruit, it provides 27 grams of protein, 40 percent of your day's vitamin A, and more than 2 days of your vitamin C. Choose this over a Big Mac with medium fries twice a week, and in a year's time, you'll have cut almost 17 pounds of flab off your belly.

Numerous studies show that people who regularly eat fast food carry around more extra body fat and are at a higher risk for diabetes than their home-eating peers. The problem is meals eaten out are generally light on fruits and vegetables and heavy on cheeseburgers, fries, and sodas. Spend your calories at places like Chick-fil-A, where fresh fruits and vegetables are as common as fried potatoes, and you'll tip the balance in your favor.

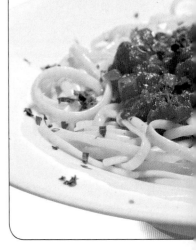

No. 4 BEST KIDS' FAST FOOD

More than steak, chicken, and even burgers, finding a bowl of healthy pasta at a restaurant is a truly challenging feat. Who would guess that there'd be 1,200 calories in a Mac Grill dish called Pollo Limone Rustica? Or that the California Pizza Kitchen's Asparagus & Spinach Spaghettini would be carrying 1,116 greasy calories? Blame the fact that American establishments tend to dish out more than twice as much pasta per bowl as you'd find in a typical Italian trattoria.

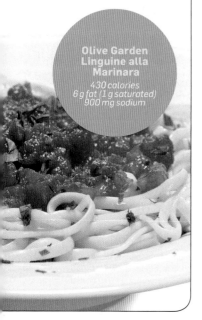

Olive Garden Linguine alla Marinara
*430 calories
6 g fat (1 g saturated)
900 mg sodium*

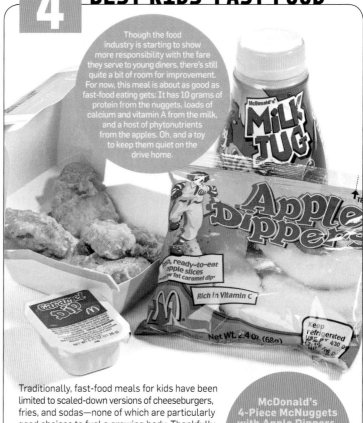

Though the food industry is starting to show more responsibility with the fare they serve to young diners, there's still quite a bit of room for improvement. For now, this meal is about as good as fast-food eating gets: It has 10 grams of protein from the nuggets, loads of calcium and vitamin A from the milk, and a host of phytonutrients from the apples. Oh, and a toy to keep them quiet on the drive home.

Traditionally, fast-food meals for kids have been limited to scaled-down versions of cheeseburgers, fries, and sodas—none of which are particularly good choices to fuel a growing body. Thankfully, shifts in consumer expectations have forced the quick-serve titans to sprinkle in a few healthy options, which is why it's no longer uncommon to see menus featuring milk, mandarin oranges, and apples cut to resemble French fries (you gotta hook 'em somehow).

McDonald's 4-Piece McNuggets with Apple Dippers, Caramel Dip, and 1% Milk
*390 calories
15 g fat (4 g saturated)
570 mg sodium*

33

BEST FAST-FOOD BURGER

Surprisingly, the burgers at fast-food restaurants are in considerably better shape than their cousins over at the sit-down diner, but that doesn't mean they're immune from belt-busting calorie hikes. Far from it: Jack in the Box offers a burger with 1,010 calories. Burger King has one with 1,250. And Hardee's serves up a terrifying 1,420-calorie burger tower. Want to have your burger and eat it, too? Keep it to a quarter-pound of meat, choose between cheese and mayonnaise, and load on the produce.

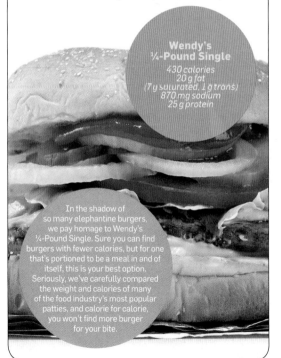

**Wendy's
¼-Pound Single**
*430 calories
20 g fat
(7 g saturated, 1 g trans)
870 mg sodium
25 g protein*

In the shadow of so many elephantine burgers, we pay homage to Wendy's ¼-Pound Single. Sure you can find burgers with fewer calories, but for one that's portioned to be a meal in and of itself, this is your best option. Seriously, we've carefully compared the weight and calories of many of the food industry's most popular patties, and calorie for calorie, you won't find more burger for your bite.

BEST SALAD

This salad harkens back to the days when salads were reliably lean fare. For starters, Chipotle's ingredients are better than those at any other Mexican restaurant in the country: The meat is hormone-free, the beans are often organic, and everything is prepared fresh daily. There is one key, though, to unlocking this salad as the best in the country. You must ask to have the usual vinaigrette replaced with salsa.

**Chipotle
Grilled Steak Salad
with Black Beans,
Guac, and
Green Salsa**
*485 calories
20.5 g fat (4 g saturated)
995 mg sodium
41 g protein*

Wondering what happened to the salad-as-health-food concept? Just as the bowls of greens grew bigger, their accoutrements grew ever more deleterious: shredded cheese, fried chicken, bacon bits, half a dozen different iterations of ranch dressing. Rare today is the entrée-size salad with fewer than 800 calories—and that's especially true if it happens to be a Mexican salad. More often than not, these battered greens are stuffed inside of a deep-fried tortilla shell, completely demolishing any remnants of a healthy reputation.

No. 1
BEST SIT-DOWN BURGER

The sit-down hamburger is, to put it mildly, the best example of America's misguided bigger-is-better mentality. What once consisted of a modest fistful of ground chuck placed neatly on a bun with ketchup and mustard has today transmogrified into a colossal pileup of cheese, bacon, mayonnaise, guacamole, and whatever else the heavy-handed chef decides to toss on. That's bad news for your waistline, especially considering that industry estimates put the country's per-capita burger consumption at around 150 per year.

To be fair, Red Robin is as guilty as any other chain of jumping on the burgeoning burger bandwagon. Their beef-and-bun mash-ups can stretch well beyond 1,000 calories and feature superfluous add-ons such as onion straws, tortilla strips, and fried jalapeño rings. That makes the Natural Burger—featuring only lettuce, tomato, onions, and beef on a sesame seed bun— the menu's only attempt to return to the obsolescent burgers of yore.

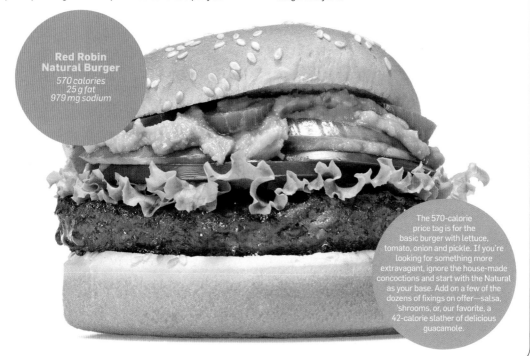

Red Robin Natural Burger
570 calories
25 g fat
979 mg sodium

The 570-calorie price tag is for the basic burger with lettuce, tomato, onion and pickle. If you're looking for something more extravagant, ignore the house-made concoctions and start with the Natural as your base. Add on a few of the dozens of fixings on offer—salsa, 'shrooms, or, our favorite, a 42-calorie slather of delicious guacamole.

The 20 Worst Restaurant Foods in America

Indulge. Go ahead. You're here, aren't you? That makes this a special occasion, and on special occasions, it's okay to let go a little. At least that's the message that seems to be bellowing from every glossy menu board and red-striped tablecloth at your local restaurant chain. The problem with this advice is that Americans today eat out more than four times per week, and when it comes to gauging the nutrition of these meals, we are demonstrably ill equipped for the task. For instance, in 2007, researchers asked patrons in both McDonald's and Subway to guess how many calories were in the meals they'd just finished eating. Those eating at McDonald's guessed an average of 744. Those at Subway guessed 585. Turns out both were low, but here's the rub: Eaters at both restaurants were sitting in front of 1,000 calories of food. Those at Subway thought their plates were healthier just because they were at Subway!

The point is that it's easier to bite off more than you think you're chewing. Some of the meals on this list can skyrocket your day's caloric intake 1,500 calories beyond what you should be eating. Do that just once a week and you're facing 22 extra pounds of flab in a year's time. Think about that the next time someone tells you to relax a little and have some chili cheese fries.

No. 20 ◆ WORST SIDE

It doesn't take a nutritionist to identify the hazards of a grease-soaked, cheese-slathered sack of deep-fried potatoes, but by appearance alone, nobody could guess what's really at stake when you order this side from Jack's. The American Heart Association recommends that people cap their trans fat intake at 1 percent of total calories. For people on a 2,000-calorie diet, that's about 2 grams per day. See the problem? This sack crushes that number with six times your daily intake—not to mention nearly half your day's calories.

Jack in the Box Bacon Cheddar Wedges

*760 calories
53 g fat
(17 g saturated, 13 g trans)
963 mg sodium*

The danger with trans fat is that it raises LDL cholesterol and increases your risk for heart disease and stroke. So why do some chains insist on keeping it around? Because it's cheap and versatile. The good news is that most of the big players have switched over to better frying oil, but there are still a few chains that refuse to budge—namely Jack in the Box, White Castle, and Church's Chicken. In fact, the only side at Jack's that's free of trans fat is the salad.

Eat This Instead!

Grilled Chicken Strips (4) with Fire Roasted Salsa

*185 calories
2 g fat (0.5 g saturated)
805 mg sodium*

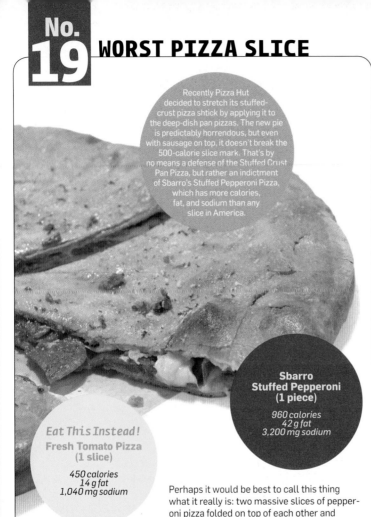

Recently Pizza Hut decided to stretch its stuffed-crust pizza shtick by applying it to the deep-dish pan pizzas. The new pie is predictably horrendous, but even with sausage on top, it doesn't break the 500-calorie slice mark. That's by no means a defense of the Stuffed Crust Pan Pizza, but rather an indictment of Sbarro's Stuffed Pepperoni Pizza, which has more calories, fat, and sodium than any slice in America.

Eat This Instead!
Regular Fries
½ serving

310 calories
15 g fat (3 g saturated)
45 mg sodium

**Sbarro
Stuffed Pepperoni
(1 piece)**

960 calories
42 g fat
3,200 mg sodium

Eat This Instead!
**Fresh Tomato Pizza
(1 slice)**

450 calories
14 g fat
1,040 mg sodium

Perhaps it would be best to call this thing what it really is: two massive slices of pepperoni pizza folded on top of each other and painted with oil. Now, unless you're preparing to play Santa at the local mall this Christmas, you should plan on finding a better lunch.

Besides the fact that Five Guys very publicly played host to President Obama and his burger-hungry entourage, it has one claim to fame that is unmatched by almost any other burger chain in the country: It's built an entire menu without a single gram of trans fat. We applaud them for that, but it seems as though the chain is a little too proud of its trans-fat-free oil. Hence the wheelbarrow of fries.

No. 17 WORST FOOD INVENTION

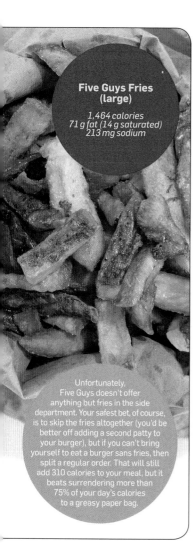

Five Guys Fries (large)

1,464 calories
71 g fat (14 g saturated)
213 mg sodium

Unfortunately, Five Guys doesn't offer anything but fries in the side department. Your safest bet, of course, is to skip the fries altogether (you'd be better off adding a second patty to your burger), but if you can't bring yourself to eat a burger sans fries, then split a regular order. That will still add 310 calories to your meal, but it beats surrendering more than 75% of your day's calories to a greasy paper bag.

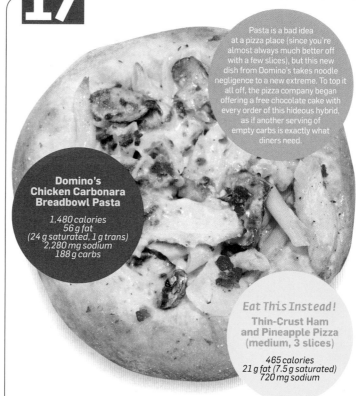

Pasta is a bad idea at a pizza place (since you're almost always much better off with a few slices), but this new dish from Domino's takes noodle negligence to a new extreme. To top it all off, the pizza company began offering a free chocolate cake with every order of this hideous hybrid, as if another serving of empty carbs is exactly what diners need.

Domino's Chicken Carbonara Breadbowl Pasta

1,480 calories
56 g fat
(24 g saturated, 1 g trans)
2,280 mg sodium
188 g carbs

Eat This Instead!

Thin-Crust Ham and Pineapple Pizza (medium, 3 slices)

465 calories
21 g fat (7.5 g saturated)
720 mg sodium

Here's the breakdown: The noodles here contribute 200 calories, the sauce and toppings another 440. And finally, the bread bowl itself contributes a staggering 840 calories and 138 grams of carbohydrates. It's like eating 12 slices of Pepperidge Farm White Sandwich Bread alongside your pasta dish, and all of those calories are the kind that spike your blood sugar and force your body to store away more fat. We used to harp on Panera's Sourdough Soup Bowl, but it looks tame next to the Domino's disaster.

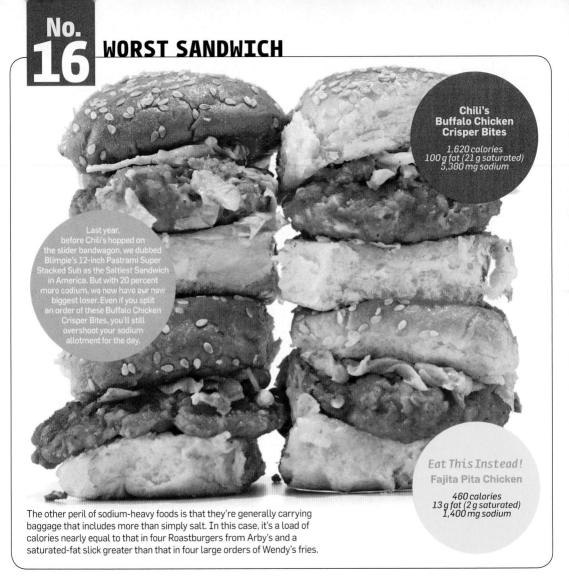

Chili's Buffalo Chicken Crisper Bites

1,620 calories
100 g fat (21 g saturated)
5,300 mg sodium

Last year, before Chili's hopped on the slider bandwagon, we dubbed Blimpie's 12-inch Pastrami Super Stacked Sub as the Saltiest Sandwich in America. But with 20 percent more sodium, we now have our new biggest loser. Even if you split an order of these Buffalo Chicken Crisper Bites, you'll still overshoot your sodium allotment for the day.

Eat This Instead!

Fajita Pita Chicken

460 calories
13 g fat (2 g saturated)
1,400 mg sodium

The other peril of sodium-heavy foods is that they're generally carrying baggage that includes more than simply salt. In this case, it's a load of calories nearly equal to that in four Roastburgers from Arby's and a saturated-fat slick greater than that in four large orders of Wendy's fries.

No. 15 WORST WRAP

This wrap seems to have been engineered with the goal of packing in extra calories. It employs a one-two punch of the two fattiest sauces known to man: ranch dressing and mayonnaise. And if that's not enough, it's served with even more ranch on the side to satisfy all your dipping fancies. You'd be better off housing three Big Macs than tussling with this felonious fowl.

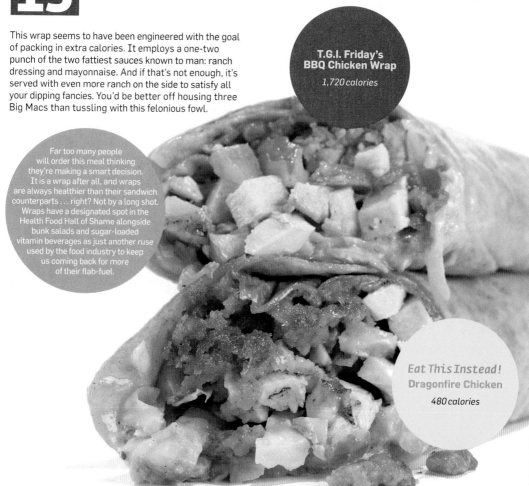

T.G.I. Friday's BBQ Chicken Wrap

1,720 calories

Far too many people will order this meal thinking they're making a smart decision. It is a wrap after all, and wraps are always healthier than their sandwich counterparts ... right? Not by a long shot. Wraps have a designated spot in the Health Food Hall of Shame alongside bunk salads and sugar-loaded vitamin beverages as just another ruse used by the food industry to keep us coming back for more of their flab-fuel.

Eat This Instead!
Dragonfire Chicken

480 calories

WORST KIDS' MEAL

Unfortunately the Cheesecake Factory's kids' menu follows the same trend as the rest of the menu: Oversize and flooded with calories. That's why the average kids' entrée packs 839 calories. In fact, the leanest kids' meal on the menu happens to be the one with "butter" in the name. If you want some actual nutrition, though, push for the Pasta with Marinara. It's nearly as low in calories and offers a bounty of antioxidants.

It's bad enough to stick this much fat into an adult-size meal, but for a child? That ought to be deemed criminally negligent. This cream- and cheese-infused pasta bowl is bloated with more saturated fat than a full-grown adult should eat in 4 days, and more calories than you'd find in 40 Chicken McNuggets.

**Cheesecake Factory
Kids' Pasta
with Alfredo Sauce**

*1,803 calories
86 g saturated fat
876 mg sodium
70 g carbohydrates*

Eat This Instead!

**Kids' Pasta
with Marinara Sauce**

*517 calories
1 g saturated fat
569 mg sodium
78 g carbohydrates*

No. 13 WORST BURGER

Applebee's Quesadilla Burger

1,820 calories
46 g saturated fat
4,410 mg sodium

The state of burgers in America is a sad affair indeed. Our predisposition toward towering hunks of beef has overtaken nutritional prudence, and now burgers with more than 1,000 calories are available on the menu at every major sit-down hamburger joint in the country. How can you defend yourself? Avoid hybrid-type burgers like this one, skip the bacon and cheese, or just resign yourself to a lean steak instead.

Eat This Instead!
House Sirloin (9 oz)

350 calories
5 g saturated fat
970 mg sodium

Nobody orders a burger thinking it's healthy eating, and as an occasional treat, that's not a problem. But if you knew for a fact that said burger had 2 days' worth of sodium and more than 2 days' worth of saturated fat stuffed between those two soggy pieces of bread, would you even consider it? Probably not. Blame it on the massive patty, the Mexi-ranch sauce, and, oh, the cheese- and bacon-crusted quesadilla "bun" that holds this hybrid hellraiser together.

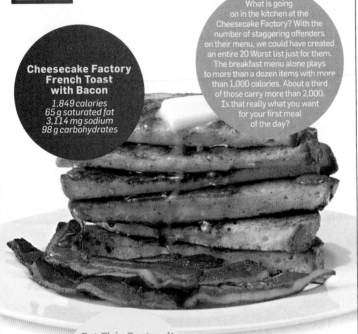

Cheesecake Factory French Toast with Bacon

1,849 calories
65 g saturated fat
3,114 mg sodium
98 g carbohydrates

What is going on in the kitchen at the Cheesecake Factory? With the number of staggering offenders on their menu, we could have created an entire 20 Worst list just for them. The breakfast menu alone plays to more than a dozen items with more than 1,000 calories. About a third of those carry more than 2,000. Is that really what you want for your first meal of the day?

Eat This Instead!

Factory Create-an-Omelette with Spinach, Tomatoes, and Mushrooms

529 calories
10 g saturated fat
780 mg sodium
8 g carbohydrates

So here's the best way to defang a bloated menu like this one: Go for something you can control. Cheesecake's Create-an-Omelette allows you to fashion a breakfast with eggs and your choice of fillings. Stick with the veggies and you'll come out still standing.

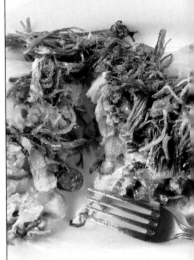

It's rare that we ever come across an omelet with fewer than 600 calories. That's because an abundance of oil and a battery of cheese and meat have become the norm at sit-down restaurants. Want an omelet you can feel good about? Tell your server you want yours prepared with two eggs, no oil, and with half the amount of cheese they normally use. You'll save up to 400 calories with that simple strategy.

No. 10 WORST DRINK

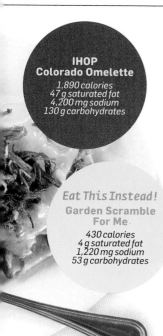

IHOP
Colorado Omelette

1,890 calories
47 g saturated fat
4,200 mg sodium
130 g carbohydrates

Eat This Instead!
Garden Scramble For Me

430 calories
4 g saturated fat
1,220 mg sodium
53 g carbohydrates

Life is filled with hard truths. Your football team isn't infallible. Extended warranties are scams. The bathroom will need to be cleaned even if you don't make a mess. And here's one more: There's no such thing as a healthy milk shake. With their Sinless line, Cold Stone has made a valiant effort at a lighter shake, but even those pack a minimum of 490 calories into the smallest cups.

Cold Stone
PB&C Shake
(Gotta Have It size)

2,010 calories
131 g fat (68 g saturated,
2.5 g trans)
880 mg sodium
153 g sugars

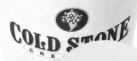

Eat This Instead!
Sinless Strawberry Bananza Smoothie
(Love It size)

220 calories
1.5 g fat (0 g saturated)
34 g sugars

Colorado is the leanest state in America, so it seems unlikely that its citizens are eating many of these omelets. Nevertheless, IHOP claims the Centennial State as the source of inspiration for this egregious egg envelope. The state's Attorney General might consider pursuing libel charges against the restaurant—after all, their namesake dish packs more calories than six Egg McMuffins.

There were dozens of contenders in line for this dishonorable distinction, but Cold Stone's PB&C is the only drink in America to stretch across the 2,000-calorie mark. The combination of peanut butter—good in small amounts, horrendous when liquefied in bathtub-size quantities—and chocolate ice cream outpaces even the worst cookie- and candy-strewn shakes that clutter Cold Stone's embarrassing shake menu. Suck this thing down and you've just blasted away a day's worth of calories, more than 3 days' worth of saturated fat, and almost as much sugar as an entire 15-ounce box of Chewy Chips Ahoy! Cookies.

45

WORST DESSERT

Here's the rule: Never order more than one dessert for the whole table, and as long as you're at Outback, limit your selection to the cheesecake. Also be warned that if you decide to add any raspberry or chocolate sauce on top, you're risking an extra 300 to 550 calories. The point is to treat your taste buds, not punish your gut.

We'll concede that desserts are intended to be decadent, but there's a dramatic difference between indulgence and recklessness. Add one of these ice-cream–covered chocolate cinder blocks onto the end of one meal per week and you're looking at more than 2 extra pounds of body fat each month. Think that extra flab is just inconvenient? Actually, according to numerous studies, it increases your risk of developing a host of conditions from diabetes and high blood pressure to esophageal cancer. Some of those risks are magnified when you factor in the 4½ days' worth of saturated fat gluing this thing together like toxic cement.

Outback Steakhouse Chocolate Thunder from Down Under

2,020 calories
88 g saturated fat
161 g carbohydrates

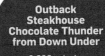

Eat This Instead!
Cheesecake

737 calories
15 g saturated fat
105 g carbohydrates

No. 8

WORST CHINESE FOOD MEAL

To be fair, P.F. Chang's does suggest splitting entrées and making use of their Lazy Susan to share with the table. Problem is, Americans have a hard time shaking the ratio of one entrée to one diner, making their menu a perilous dinner proposition. Figure one entrée per two people instead, and make use of their openness to tweaks and substitutions. "Wok velvetted," for example, is a technique they offer with many of their entrées that replaces the sea of wok oil with broth, dramatically lowering the dish's caloric price tag. Ask which entrées take well to the technique and order accordingly.

P.F. Chang's Crispy Honey Shrimp

2,110 calories
70 g fat (10 g saturated)
1,815 mg sodium
290 g carbs

Chang's menu sounds innocent enough: "Lightly battered and tossed in a flavorful sauce." But with it being one of the most calorie-laden meals in the entire country, it seems fair to call this description a mild understatement. More accurate might be something like, "cooked with a day's worth of fat and served with more carbohydrates than you'd find in an entire box of Triscuit crackers!" Okay, so maybe they won't follow our lead on that one, but it would be nice to see a little more transparency.

Eat This Instead!
Orange Peel Shrimp

546 calories
21 g fat (3 g saturated)
2,382 mg sodium

WORST SEAFOOD DISH

This trend of frying all seafood is particularly concerning at Culver's, since it's not balanced by a single grilled fillet. If you want a piece of fish at Culver's, you have to take it fried. What's worse, though, is that when you order a dinner, Culver's buries your plate under a mess of sides that are equally as harmful as the fish. By the time they're done loading on the fries, dinner roll, coleslaw, tarter sauce, and butter, you're facing a full day's worth of calories, sodium, and saturated fat crammed into one meal.

**Culver's
North Atlantic Cod
Filet Meal (3 pieces)**

*2,121 calories
135 g fat (21 g saturated,
2 g trans)
2,568 mg sodium*

Fish is one of the world's healthiest protein sources, right? If only eating out were so simple. While it's true that seafood has the potential to be the best option on the menu, it too often ends up being one of the worst. See, people don't always love fish's natural flavor, so to make it more palatable to finicky customers, some restaurants routinely deep-fry anything that spent time in salty waters.

Eat This Instead!
**Tuna Salad on Grilled
Sourdough**

*484 calories
26 g fat (7 g saturated,
0 g trans)
1,008 mg sodium*

No. 6

WORST SALAD

California Pizza Kitchen Thai Crunch Salad with Fresh Avocado

2,238 calories

Eat This Instead!
Chinese Chicken Salad (half portion)

503 calories

Shredded carrots, edamame, cabbage, fresh avocado: The menu reads like an Intro to Nutrition class at the local junior college. If that's the case, CPK is flunking out of school, since this seemingly harmless salad will saddle you with more calories than 3 pounds' worth of sirloin from Applebee's. Blame the two different dressings, the shower of fried wonton strips, and the sewer cap–size plate.

How is it that restaurants are able to make dangerously oversize salads and sell them to the kind of customers who wouldn't even dream of eating a cheeseburger? Simple: They use public perception against the public. People assume salads are healthy—or at least that they're healthier than cheeseburgers and pizza. Turns out that with today's heavy-handed techniques, that assumption is wrong as often as it's right.

WORST TACOS

On the Border Dos XX Fish Tacos with Creamy Red Chile Sauce

2,350 calories
152 g fat (31 g saturated)
4,060 mg sodium

Mexican food doesn't have to be served with such dire consequences. What you want to do is build a plate that centers on vegetables or lean meats. Skip out on anything that's fried and try to sub out your flour tortillas and rice for corn tortillas and beans. And whatever sauce they try to stick you with, just know that nothing beats regular salsa—neither in terms of flavor nor nutrition.

Eat This Instead!

Pico Shrimp Tacos with Black Beans and Grilled Veggies

490 calories
5 g fat (1 g saturated)
1,650 mg sodium

How many Taco Bell Crunchy Tacos could you eat for this many calories? Ten. Plus one Steak Baja Gordita Supreme. Basically, it's a perversion of Mexican cuisine that adds up to more food than you'd ever dream of wolfing down in one sitting, and On the Border achieves it through a heavy load of greasy beer-battered fish and a fat-riddled cream sauce to boot.

WORST STEAK DINNER

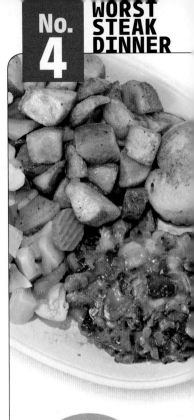

Unfortunately, IHOP's menu is riddled with overwrought calorie traps like this, so if you want to play it safe, turn your attention toward the "IHOP For Me" menu. There you'll find a host of meals with fewer than 600 calories, not one of which has more than 11 grams of saturated fat.

No. 3 WORST APPETIZER

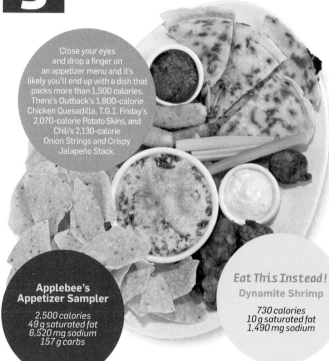

IHOP
Top Sirloin Steak

2,380 calories
42 g saturated fat
5,220 mg sodium

Eat This Instead!

Balsamic Glazed
Chicken For Me

510 calories
20 g fat (3 g saturated)
1,770 mg sodium

Close your eyes and drop a finger on an appetizer menu and it's likely you'll end up with a dish that packs more than 1,500 calories. There's Outback's 1,800-calorie Chicken Quesadilla, T.G.I. Friday's 2,070-calorie Potato Skins, and Chili's 2,130-calorie Onion Strings and Crispy Jalapeño Stack.

Applebee's
Appetizer Sampler

2,500 calories
49 g saturated fat
6,520 mg sodium
157 g carbs

Eat This Instead!

Dynamite Shrimp

730 calories
10 g saturated fat
1,490 mg sodium

In the world of beef, sirloin is one of the good guys. Unless it's not, which is the case at IHOP. But don't blame the beef. Here, as is so often the case with commercially prepared steaks, the meat suffers by association. IHOP adds an inexplicable blanket of provolone cheese and a heaping scoop of fried potatoes and buttered toast to the party. The result of these add-ons is six Milky Ways' worth of saturated fat and five full Pringles cans' worth of sodium.

Nothing spells nutritional doom more decidedly than a "sampler" platter. The idea is that by eating only a little bit of a bad thing, you won't suffer severe caloric consequences. That's true in theory, but not when you're eating a little bit of several bad things—in this case mozzarella sticks, spinach and artichoke dip with chips, cheese quesadilla, and Buffalo wings. Truth is, the traditional sampler is actually little more than a roundup of all the worst appetizers, and ordering it will almost certainly saddle you with more calories than any one of those appetizers would have on its own.

Eat This Instead!

Pizzette Margherita

609 calories
13 g saturated fat
1,005 mg sodium
45 g carbohydrates

Cheesecake Factory Bistro Shrimp Pasta

2,819 calories
77 g saturated fat
1,008 mg sodium
184 g carbohydrates

Problem is, this is just the tip of the Cheesecake Factory iceberg. The rest is hidden beneath wholesome-sounding names, waiting for an opportunity to sink your chances of a flat stomach. As it turns out, when you order a regular dinner entrée at Cheesecake Factory, you're more likely to get one in excess of 2,000 calories than you are to get one with fewer than 1,000.

How would you feel if someone asked you to eat three full orders of Fettuccine Alfredo and three bread sticks from Fazoli's? Or how about three Big Macs and three medium orders of fries from McDonald's? Or 14 Original Doughnuts from Krispy Kreme? Like the rest of the sane world, you'd balk at the idea. It's ludicrous, for sure, but the truth is that any of these options would actually save you calories over this horrendous glut of oil and cream from the Cheesecake Factory.

No. 1 WORST FOOD IN AMERICA

We hope the guys at Guinness World Records are paying attention: Outback now holds the dubious distinction of serving the first nationally available entrée in America to pack more than 3,000 calories. Congratulations.

Outback Steakhouse Baby Back Ribs (full rack)

3,021 calories
242 g fat
(90 g saturated fat)
4,648 mg sodium

Eat This Instead!

Teriyaki Marinated Sirloin (9 oz)

418 calories
12 g fat (4 g saturated)
1,832 mg sodium

Sad to say it, but there's no such thing as a lean rack of ribs. Still, it is possible to get your face-painting fix without burning through more saturated fat than 11 Mexican Pizzas from Taco Bell. The first step is to stop looking at ribs through Fred Flintstone's eyes. Limit yourself to a half rack and then set your sights on a couple of healthy sides. Step two? Order ribs prepared with dry rubs or have the sauce served on the side. That way you can avoid the dessert's worth of sugar that's poured over the top of these troubled bones.

The Eat This, Not That! No-Diet Cheat Sheets

SATISFY YOUR HUNGER SMARTLY
WITH THESE AT-A-GLANCE CRAVING SELECTORS

BREAKFAST SANDWICHES

		CALORIES	FAT (G)	SATURATED (G)	TRANS (G)	SODIUM (MG)
1.	Dunkin' Donuts Turkey Sausage Flatbread	280	6	2.5	0	820
2.	McDonald's Egg McMuffin	300	12	5	0	820
3.	Jack in the Box Bacon Breakfast Jack	300	14	5	0	730
4.	Burger King Ham, Egg & Cheese Croissan'wich	340	17	7	0	1,200
5.	Starbucks Bacon, Gouda Cheese, Egg Fritatta on Artisan Roll	380	20	8	0	1,050
6.	Hardee's Frisco Breakfast Sandwich	420	20	7	0	1,340
7.	Chick-fil-A Chicken Biscuit	450	20	8	0	1,310
8.	Carl's Jr. Sourdough Breakfast Sandwich	450	21	8	0	1,470
9.	Panera Bacon, Egg, and Cheese Breakfast Sandwich	510	24	10	0.5	1,060
10.	Sonic Bacon, Egg and Cheese Breakfast Toaster	530	32.5	10	0.5	1,440
11.	Hardee's Monster Biscuit	710	51	17	0	2,250
12.	Au Bon Pain Sausage, Egg, and Cheddar on Asiago Bagel	810	47	23	0.5	1,540

(Some restaurants do not disclose complete nutritional data.)

PASTA

	CALORIES	FAT (G)	SATURATED (G)	TRANS (G)	SODIUM (MG)
1. Romano's Macaroni Grill Capellini Pomodoro	390	14	2	0	980
2. Olive Garden Linguine alla Marinara	430	6	1	0	900
3. Domino's Italian Sausage Marinara	670	32	15	0.5	1,760
4. Olive Garden Chicken Marsala	770	37	5	0	1,800
5. Romano's Macaroni Grill Spaghetti & Meatballs with Bolognese Sauce	880	118	14	0	2,400
6. Fazoli's Chicken Broccoli Penne Bake	920	42	24	1	2,310
7. T.G.I. Friday's Bruschetta Chicken Pasta	990				
8. Red Lobster Chef's Signature Lobster and Shrimp Pasta (full portion)	1,020	50	22	0	2,180
9. Applebee's Three-Cheese Chicken Penne	1,300		33		2,960
10. Outback Walhalla Pasta with Grilled Chicken	1,393		43		3,600
11. California Pizza Kitchen Garlic Cream Fettuccine with Chicken & Shrimp	1,728				
12. Cheesecake Factory Bistro Chicken Pasta	2,819		77		1,008

FAST-FOOD BURGERS (MINIMUM ¼-LB PATTY)

	CALORIES	FAT (G)	SATURATED (G)	TRANS (G)	SODIUM (MG)
1. McDonald's Quarter-Pounder	410	19	7	1	730
2. Wendy's ¼-Pound Single	430	20	7	1	870
3. Carl's Jr. Big Hamburger	460	17	8	0.5	1,090
4. McDonald's Big N' Tasty	460	24	8	1.5	720
5. McDonald's Big Mac	540	29	10	1.5	1,040
6. Dairy Queen ¼-lb Classic GrillBurger with Cheese	560	28	12	0.5	1,090
7. Sonic Sonic Burger with ketchup	560	26	9	1	820
8. Jack in the Box Jumbo Jack	580	33	11	1	920
9. Burger King Whopper	670	40	11	1.5	1,020
10. Five Guys Hamburger	700	43	19.5	0	430
11. A&W Papa Burger	720	42	15	4	1,390
12. Hardee's Six Dollar ThickBurger	1,060	73	28	0	1,950

RESTAURANT BURGERS

		CALORIES	FAT (G)	SATURATED (G)	TRANS (G)	SODIUM (MG)
1.	Red Robin Natural Burger	570	25			979
2.	Cheesecake Factory The Factory Burger	737		16		1,018
3.	Applebee's Hamburger	770		15		1,170
4.	Chili's Oldtimer	820	44	2	0	1,310
5.	Chili's Mushroom Swiss	1,070	67	18	0	1,670
6.	Uno Chicago Grill Uno Burger	1,080	72	28	4	1,620
7.	Ruby Tuesday Ruby's Classic Burger	1,090	75			
8.	Outback Bacon Cheese Burger	1,113		28		2,127
9.	Denny's Western Burger	1,300	82	30	3	2,700
10.	Cheesecake Factory The Classic Burger	1,375	28			1,592
11.	T.G.I. Friday's Jack Daniels Burger	1,540				
12.	Applebee's Quesadilla Burger	1,820	46			4,410

FISH

		CALORIES	FAT (G)	SATURATED (G)	TRANS (G)	SODIUM (MG)
1.	Uno Chicago Grill Grilled Mahi Mahi with Mango Salsa	240	2	0	0	980
2.	Red Lobster Broiled Sole	245	3.5	0.5	0	320
3.	Applebee's Cajun Lime Tilapia	310	6	1.5	0	2,160
4.	Ruby Tuesday Asian Glazed Salmon	433	27			
5.	Olive Garden Herb-Grilled Salmon	510	6	6	0	760
6.	Outback Fresh Tilapia with Pure Lump Crab Meat	510	14	5	0	58
7.	Chili's Southwest Cedar Plank Tilapia	600	31	4.5	0	1,750
8.	P.F. Chang's Mahi Mahi	650	32	8	0	1,498
9.	Applebee's Garlic Herb Salmon	740	11			2,630
10.	Romano's Macaroni Grill Grilled Halibut	770	34	11	0	1,100
11.	T.G.I. Friday's Honey Pecan Salmon	810				
12.	Cheesecake Factory Wasabi Crusted Ahi Tuna	1,750	58			1,302

CHICKEN SANDWICHES

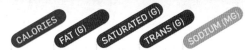

		CALORIES	FAT (G)	SATURATED (G)	TRANS (G)	SODIUM (MG)
1.	Chick-fil-A Chargrilled Chicken Sandwich	260	3	0.5	0	1,300
2.	Hardee's BBQ Chicken Sandwich	320	6	1	0	1,200
3.	Wendy's Crispy Chicken Sandwich	360	18	3.5	0	710
4.	Arby's Roasted Chicken Fillet Sandwich	380	16	3	0	920
5.	KFC Tender Roast Sandwich	400	15	3	0	810
6.	Jack in the Box Chicken Sandwich	400	21	4.5	2.5	740
7.	McDonald's Premium Grilled Chicken Classic Sandwich	420	10	2	0	1,190
8.	Sonic Crispy Chicken Sandwich	560	32	5	0	780
9.	Dunkin' Donuts Chicken Bruschetta Sandwich	580	26	7	0	1,200
10.	Dairy Queen Grilled Flame Thrower Chicken Sandwich	590	36	9	0	1,480
11.	Burger King Original Chicken Sandwich	630	39	7	0.5	1,390
12.	Carl's Jr. Bacon Swiss Crispy Chicken	750	40	9	0	1,990

STEAKS

		CALORIES	FAT (G)	SATURATED (G)	TRANS (G)	SODIUM (MG)
1.	Denny's Top Sirloin Steak	220	6	2	0	600
2.	Applebee's 9 oz. House Sirloin	350		5		970
3.	Chili's Classic Sirloin	370	27	7	0	1,270
4.	Ruby Tuesday Bayou Sirloin	387		16		
5.	P.F. Chang's Asian Marinated New York Strip	558	30	12	0	864
6.	Romano's Macaroni Grill Bistecca Filet	590	17	7	0	650
7.	Outback New York Strip	713		17		694
8.	Denny's T-Bone Steak	740	56	25	0	740
9.	Olive Garden Steak Toscano	880	43	14	0	1,700
10.	IHOP T-Bone Steak	970	24			1,160
11.	T.G.I. Friday's Championship BBQ New York Strip	1,570				
12.	Cheesecake Factory Carne Asada Skirt Steak	1,703		24		3,695

ENTRÉE SALADS (WITH DRESSING)

		CALORIES	FAT (G)	SATURATED (G)	TRANS (G)	SODIUM (MG)
1.	Chipotle's Barbacoa Salad with Black Beans and Tomato Salsa (no vinaigrette)	320	8	2.5	0	1,235
2.	Panera Full Asian Sesame Chicken Salad	410	19	3.5	0	900
3.	Romano's Macaroni Grill Scallops and Spinach Salad	420	19	4	0	1,510
4.	Bob Evans Wildfire Grilled Chicken Salad	440	19	6	0	963
5.	Boston Market Market Chopped Salad	480	40	8	1	1,640
6.	Chili's Garlic & Lime Grilled Shrimp Salad	630	40	11	0	1,850
7.	Outback Queensland Salad with Thousand Island	1,376		31		4,239
8.	Applebee's Oriental Chicken Salad	1,430		16		1,920
9.	Cheesecake Factory Caesar Salad with Chicken	1,510		16		1,453
10.	IHOP Chicken, Spinach, and Apple Salad	1,600		30		2,850
11.	T.G.I. Friday's Santa Fe Chicken Salad	1,000				
12.	California Pizza Kitchen Thai Crunch Salad with Avocado	2,338				

FRIES

		CALORIES	FAT (G)	SATURATED (G)	TRANS (G)	SODIUM (MG)
1.	Sonic Regular Fries	220	9	1.5	0	100
2.	KFC Potato Wedges	260	13	2.5	0	740
3.	Dairy Queen Regular Fries	310	13	2	0	640
4.	McDonald's Medium French Fries	380	19	2.5	0	270
5.	In-N-Out French Fries	400	18	5	0	245
6.	Wendy's Medium Fries	420	20	4	0	380
7.	Chick-fil-A Waffle Potato Fries	420	24	5	0	120
8.	Carl's Jr. Medium Natural-Cut Fries	460	22	4.5	0	1,180
9.	Jack in the Box Medium Natural-Cut Fries	460	24	6	7	850
10.	Burger King Medium Fries	480	23	5	0	820
11.	Arby's Medium Curly Fries	500	29	5	0.5	1,160
12.	Five Guys Regular Fries	620	30	6	0	90

SUNDAES

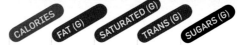

	CALORIES	FAT (G)	SATURATED (G)	TRANS (G)	SUGARS (G)
1. **A&W Hot Fudge Sundae**	350	11	6	0	15
2. **Uno Chicago Grill Mini Hot Chocolate Brownie Sundae**	370	16	8	0	38
3. **McDonald's Hot Fudge Sundae with Peanuts**	375	13.5	7.5	0	48
4. **Dairy Queen Medium Chocolate Sundae**	400	10	6	0	59
5. **Bob Evans Strawberry Sundae**	419	20	14	0	44
6. **Baskin-Robbins Banana Royale Sundae**	620	28	19	0	73
7. **IHOP Hot Fudge Brownie Sundae**	630		18		
8. **Red Robin Hot Fudge Sundae**	803	38			
9. **Baskin-Robbins Oreo Outrageous Sundae**	1,130	55	27	0	120
10. **Outback Sydney's Sinful Sundae**	1,361		62		
11. **Uno Chicago Grill Uno Deep Dish Sundae**	1,400	68	36	0	136
12. **Applebee's Chocolate Chip Cookie Sundae**	1,620		43		

KIDS' ENTRÉES

	CALORIES	FAT (G)	SATURATED (G)	TRANS (G)	SODIUM (MG)
1. **Red Lobster Popcorn Shrimp**	140	7	1	0	620
2. **McDonald's 4-piece Chicken McNuggets**	190	12	2	0	400
3. **Red Robin Rad Robin Burger**	276	12			370
4. **Fazoli's Kids' Spaghetti with meatballs**	300	7	2.5	0	570
5. **Chili's Pepper Pals Little Mouth Burger**	440	23	8	0	420
6. **Romano's Macaroni Grill Kids' Spaghetti with Meatballs and Meat Sauce**	610	29	10	0	1,550
7. **Baja Fresh Kids' Chicken Taquitos**	630	33	7	1	990
8. **Outback Kids' Kookaburra Chicken Fingers**	676		12		1,942
9. **Applebee's Kids' Two Mini Cheeseburgers**	740	15			2,120
10. **On the Border Kids' Cheese Quesadilla**	850	66	26	0	1,250
11. **Ruby Tuesday Kids' Mini Burgers**	917	46			
12. **Cheesecake Factory Kids' Pasta with Alfredo Sauce**	1,803	87			876

EAT THIS NOT THAT!

3

AT YOUR FAVORITE RESTAURANTS

Criss Angel.
David Blaine.
David Copperfield.
Ronald McDonald.

What do all these clowns have in common?

They all want to trick your mind, confuse you, convince you that you are seeing things that aren't there—or not seeing things that are.

The first three use the power of suggestion and illusion to make you believe they can walk through walls, endure impossible feats of endurance, and escape from near-certain death traps. They want to fool your eyes and trick your mind.

Ronald McDonald, on the other hand, uses the same powers of suggestion and illusion, but he doesn't want to trick your mind. He wants to trick your tummy. And his friends Wendy, Burger King, and the Colonel— plus their fancier compatriots at Chili's, Outback, and other sit-down restaurants—have the same tricks.

For example, ask yourself this: Why do all the menus, logos, French fry and burger packages, and even Ronald's costume consist of only three colors: red, yellow, and orange (with a little white thrown in)? If you were starting a new fast-food restaurant and calling it, say, Wendy's, wouldn't you want to stay away from Mickey D's logo? Come up with something origi-nal maybe? A nice purple cow or a blue dinosaur or a green leprechaun as your mascot, instead of a girl with red hair who looked so much like... Ronald McDonald?

In fact, no. Because food purveyors know that "warm" colors such as red, yellow, and orange stimulate appetite, while "cool" colors such as purple, blue, and green tend to subdue it. (That's why buying yourself a set of blue plates is a great way to pull a Copperfield on yourself—you trick yourself into eating less.) Pretty sneaky, right? So the next time you go to your favorite restaurant and order too much, eat too much, and leave thinking *Why did I do that?*, don't put so much blame on yourself. It wasn't your fault.

You were tricked. And since the average American consumes 4.2 commercially prepared meals a week, you're getting tricked over and over again.

Well, there's good news. The simple swaps in this chapter will keep you happy, not hungry; full, not fat; satisfied, not supersized. Here's your guide to eating all your favorite restaurant foods—and losing all the weight you want!

A&W

Did You Know?

● Even though A&W announced in 2007 that they'd decided to remove trans fat from their hash browns and fries, the big changes were made primarily in their Canadian locations. Sadly, the US menu has one of the worst trans-fat problems in the entire food industry.

● In February 2009, A&W announced that it would launch a new prototype restaurant that combines drive-thru, drive-in, and dine-inside styles.

DIP DECODER
(per 1-oz dipping cup)

BBQ
40 calories,
0 g fat

HONEY MUSTARD
100 calories,
6 g fat (1.5 g saturated)

RANCH
160 calories,
17 g fat (2.5 g saturated)

Eat This
Coney (Chili) Dog

340 calories
20 g fat
(9 g saturated,
1.5 g trans)
900 mg sodium

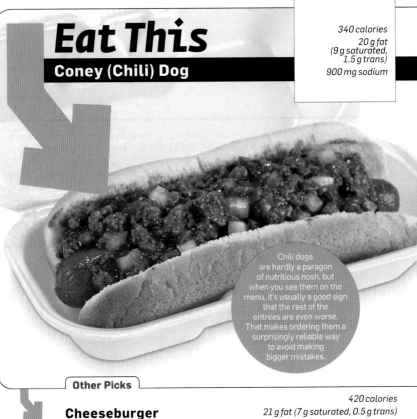

Chili dogs are hardly a paragon of nutritious nosh, but when you see them on the menu, it's usually a good sign that the rest of the entrées are even worse. That makes ordering them a surprisingly reliable way to avoid making bigger mistakes.

Other Picks

Cheeseburger

420 calories
21 g fat (7 g saturated, 0.5 g trans)
1,040 mg sodium

Corn Dog Nuggets
(regular, 8)

280 calories
13 g fat (3 g saturated, 0.5 g trans)
830 mg sodium

A&W Root Beer Float
(small, 16 oz)

330 calories
5 g fat (3 g saturated)
57 g sugars

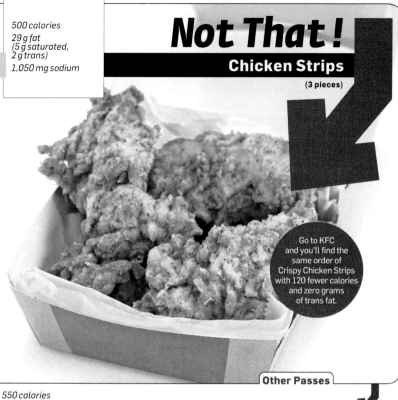

500 calories
29 g fat
(5 g saturated,
2 g trans)
1,050 mg sodium

Not That!
Chicken Strips
(3 pieces)

Go to KFC and you'll find the same order of Crispy Chicken Strips with 120 fewer calories and zero grams of trans fat.

Other Passes

550 calories
25 g fat (4.5 g saturated, 1.5 g trans)
1,130 mg sodium

Crispy Chicken Sandwich

350 calories
16 g fat (3.5 g saturated, 4.5 g trans)
710 mg sodium

Breaded Onion Rings
(regular)

720 calories
31 g fat (19 g saturated, 1 g trans)
57 g sugars

Vanilla Milkshake
(small, 16 oz)

65

Applebee's

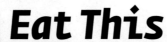

Did You Know?

● Applebee's is one of the last chain restaurants that refuses to offer comprehensive nutritional data for their food. Luckily, new California legislation has forced them and their ilk—including IHOP, Friday's, the Cheesecake Factory—to list calories, saturated fat, and sodium on their in-store menus.

MENU MAGIC

Exciting-sounding entrées like the Chicken Fajita Rollup and the Chili Cheese Nachos weigh in at 1,450 and 1,680 calories, respectively. Want big flavor without all the calories? Stick with the 9-ounce Sirloin and Seasonal Veggies. Top it with either Grilled Onions, Sautéed Garlic and Mushrooms or Shrimp 'N Parmesan. You'll down a dose of flavor in the 400- to 600-calorie range.

Eat This
Steak & Grilled Shrimp

390 calories*
6 g saturated fat
1,890 mg sodium

* Applebee's refuses to provide full nutritional information for all of its menu items.

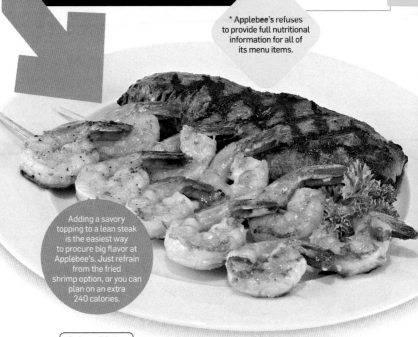

Adding a savory topping to a lean steak is the easiest way to procure big flavor at Applebee's. Just refrain from the fried shrimp option, or you can plan on an extra 240 calories.

Other Picks

Bruschetta Chicken Sandwich

530 calories
3.5 g saturated fat
1,500 mg sodium

Garlic Herb Chicken

370 calories
1 g saturated
1,930 mg sodium

1,040 calories*
11 g saturated fat
2,380 mg sodium

Not That!

Grilled Shrimp and Spinach Salad

Half of the salads on Applebee's menu break the 1,000-calorie barrier, making them just as dubious as any other menu item. If a field of greens is calling your name, limit yourself to a half order, or choose the Weight Watchers Grilled Chili-Lime Chicken Salad—it's the only salad with fewer than 700 calories.

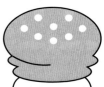

SALT LICK

SIZZLING STEAK FAJITAS

5,900 mg sodium
1,300 calories
27 g saturated fat

Thanks to California's new menu nutrition legislation, we now know that Applebee's has been loading their dishes with days' worth of sodium. No wonder they didn't want to give up the goods! This fajita dish is the restaurant's worst offender, but other dishes are nearly as bad.

GUILTY PLEASURE

Bacon Cheese Chicken Grill

710 calories
11 g saturated fat
1,920 mg sodium

This is about as indulgent as you can get at Applebee's without incurring serious caloric repercussions. Just order something other than fries as your side. Otherwise, you're right back in the red zone.

Other Passes

1,550 calories
10 g saturated fat
2,530 mg sodium

Oriental Chicken Rollup

1,210 calories
16 g saturated fat
4,490 mg sodium

Fiesta Lime Chicken

67

Applebee's (Continued)

Did You Know?

● A class-action lawsuit was filed against Applebee's and Weight Watchers in 2009, claiming fraud and conspiracy to keep nutrition content hidden. A Scripps Howard News Service investigation revealed that the actual calorie and fat counts of Applebee's Weight Watchers menu items were up to three times higher than advertised.

MENU MISNOMER

Spinach & Artichoke Dip

1,530 calories
27.5 g saturated fat
2,320 mg sodium

Don't be surprised to see three-fourths of your day's calories in an appetizer named after two vegetables. As used in dip, spinach and artichoke's only purpose is to provide texture and a sense of virtue to what's otherwise a massive puddle of fat from cheese and cream. Never trust a dip if you can't read the ingredients list.

Eat This

Margherita Chicken

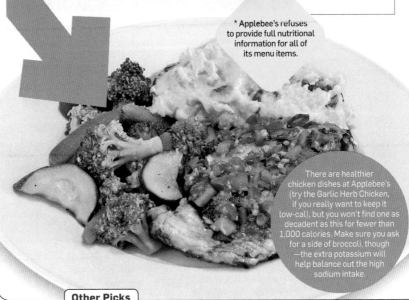

700 calories*
8 g saturated fat
2,420 mg sodium

* Applebee's refuses to provide full nutritional information for all of its menu items.

There are healthier chicken dishes at Applebee's (try the Garlic Herb Chicken, if you really want to keep it low-cal), but you won't find one as decadent as this for fewer than 1,000 calories. Make sure you ask for a side of broccoli, though —the extra potassium will help balance out the high sodium intake.

Other Picks

Dynamite Shrimp

730 calories
10 g saturated fat
1,490 mg sodium

Hot Fudge Sundae Shooter

320 calories
10 g saturated fat
39 g carbohydrates

Mango Martini

190 calories

1,880 calories*
13 g saturated fat
4,250 mg sodium

Not That!
Crispy Orange Chicken Bowl

No matter how many vegetables you throw in with it, fried chicken coated in viscous sauce of any kind will never be an even moderately decent meal. Order a drink, and you've just hit your entire day's calorie allotment in one sitting.

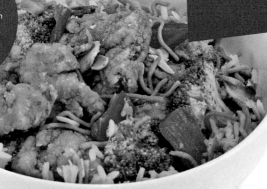

WEAPON OF MASS DESTRUCTION
Crispy Orange Chicken Bowl

1,880 calories
13 g saturated fat
4,250 mg sodium

Going by the menu description, you'd think this meal was a paragon of nutrition: "Rice topped with almonds, sautéed vegetables, and a spicy-sweet glaze." Too bad the Applebee's menu can't be trusted. Sure, the word "crispy" alludes to a load of fat, but that doesn't explain how this entrée packs in nearly an entire day's worth of calories.

STEALTH HEALTH FOOD
Grilled Shrimp

220 calories
3 g saturated fat
1,220 mg sodium

If you ask them to, Applebee's will add grilled shrimp to any entrée. That's good news for children, because shrimp is loaded with vitamin D, and New York researchers recently determined that 70 percent of kids aren't meeting their requirements.

Other Passes

1,420 calories
23 g saturated fat
4,990 mg sodium

Classic Boneless Buffalo Wings

1,620 calories
43 g saturated fat
212 g carbohydrates

Chocolate Chip Cookie Sundae

340 calories

Pomegranate Margarita

69

Arby's

Did You Know?

● Arby's roast beef is slow-cooked in the store for 4 hours. Like most supermarket roast beefs, though, Arby's injects theirs with water, salt, and preservatives to keep it fresh longer. The upside: Arby's roast beef is still impressively lean. Just be sure to skip the large Beef 'n Cheddar and the Market Fresh Roast Beef.

Eat This
Bacon Cheddar Roastburger

440 calories
18 g fat
(8 g saturated, 1 g trans)
1,427 mg sodium

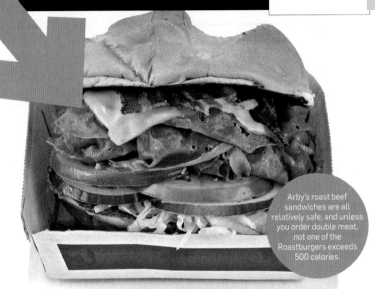

Arby's roast beef sandwiches are all relatively safe, and unless you order double meat, not one of the Roastburgers exceeds 500 calories.

Other Picks

Ham & Swiss Melt

268 calories
8 g fat (3 g saturated)
1,042 mg sodium

Super Roast Beef

399 calories
19 g fat (6 g saturated, 1 g trans)
1,061 mg sodium

Grilled Chopped Chicken Salad
with Balsamic Vinaigrette

380 calories
24 g fat (8 g saturated)
1,120 mg sodium

779 calories
45 g fat
(11 g saturated,
0.5 g trans)
1,571 mg sodium

Not That!

Ultimate BLT
Market Fresh Sandwich

This isn't even the worst of the Market Fresh Sandwiches; the Pecan Chicken Salad weighs in at a hefty 870 calories. The lesson? Trust the ingredients, not the name. "Market Fresh" is little more than a marketing ploy to persuade consumers to indulge without guilt.

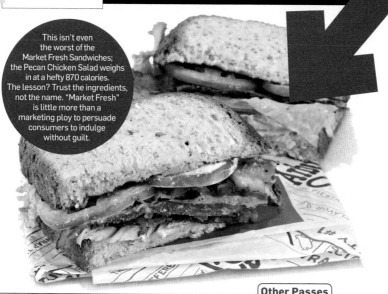

Other Passes

691 calories
31 g fat (8 g saturated, 0.5 g trans)
1,952 mg sodium

Roast Ham & Swiss
Market Fresh Sandwich

610 calories
30 g fat (9 g saturated, 1 g trans)
1,549 mg sodium

Philly Beef Toasted Sub

560 calories
43 g fat (15 g saturated)
2,030 mg sodium

Chopped Italian Salad
with Balsamic Vinaigrette

GUILTY PLEASURE

Bacon & Bleu Roastburger

466 calories
26 g fat
(9 g saturated, 1 g trans)
1,375 mg sodium

Just like a regular hamburger, Arby's Roastburgers are piled with lettuce, tomato, and onion. The difference is that Arby's replaces the beef patty with roast beef, which clears off enough excessive fat to make room for the indulgence of pepper bacon and blue cheese. If this were a real burger, you could expect it to weigh in with at least 700 calories.

Arby's (Continued)

Did You Know?

● In 2006, Arby's became the first fast-food establishment to announce that it would eliminate trans fat from its French fries. Looks like they've since gone back on their word, since their Curly Fries once again pack the dangerous fat.

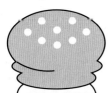

SALT LICK

SAUSAGE GRAVY BISCUIT

4,700 mg sodium
1,040 calories
60 g fat (22 g saturated, 2 g trans)

Nothing like waking up to 2 full days' worth of sodium. Sausage and gravy both carry dizzying sodium loads; nix them both from the morning routine and opt for anything on a croissant.

Eat This

Bacon, Egg, and Cheese Croissant

378 calories
25 g fat (12 g saturated)
850 mg sodium

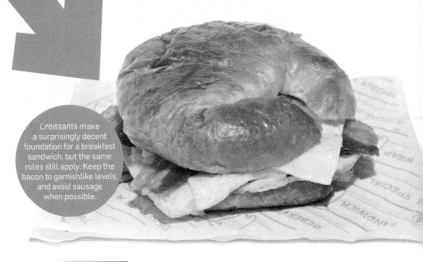

Croissants make a surprisingly decent foundation for a breakfast sandwich, but the same rules still apply: Keep the bacon to garnishlike levels, and avoid sausage when possible.

Other Picks

Popcorn Chicken
(regular, 5) with Buffalo Sauce

374 calories
17 g fat (2 g saturated)
1,712 mg sodium

Jalapeno Bites
(regular, 5)

305 calories
21 g fat (9 g saturated, 1 g trans)
526 mg sodium

Cherry Turnover
without icing

231 calories
12 g fat (6 g saturated)
8 g sugars

575 calories
31 g fat
(10 g saturated,
1 g trans)
2,005 mg sodium

Not That!

Ham, Egg, & Cheese Wrap

Ever since wraps became erroneously associated with healthy eating, restaurants have been slowly beefing up the amount of cheese and sauce they stuff inside. The reasoning is simple: The perception of health might make you test it out, but the surreptitious loads of fat and salt will keep you coming back for more.

230

The number of calories in the Buttermilk Ranch Dressing. That's just 20 fewer calories than in the entire Turkey Club Salad it's meant to dress.

HIDDEN DANGER

Mozzarella Sticks
(large, 6)

Nobody expects fried cheese to be a health food, but more than 100 calories per stick? If you order this as a companion to your sandwich, chances are you just more than doubled the caloric impact of your meal—not to mention exceeded your recommended daily intake of saturated fat. If you must eat fried foods, stick to small orders.

Other Passes

498 calories
20 g fat (7 g saturated)
1,540 mg sodium

Roast Chicken Club

496 calories
29 g fat (5 g saturated, 0.5 g trans)
1,160 mg sodium

Curly Fries
(medium)

570 calories
18 g fat (11 g saturated, 0.5 g trans)
85 g sugars

Vanilla Shake

637 calories
42 g fat
(19 g saturated,
1.5 g trans)
2,047 mg sodium

73

Atlanta Bread Compa

Did You Know?

● Atlanta Bread Company offers 15 different types of sandwich bread—from sourdough to pumpernickel to Asiago Cheese Strip. The healthiest option is the Asiago Loaf at 80 calories and 14 grams of carbohydrates per slice; the worst is Panini Bread, at 430 calories and 78 grams of carbs per serving (half a loaf).

CREAM CHEESE DECODER
(2 oz)

RASPBERRY
100 calories,
8 g fat (5 g saturated)

CHIVE
170 calories,
15 g fat (10 g saturated)

VEGETABLE
180 calories,
15 g fat (10 g saturated)

HONEY RAISIN WALNUT
190 calories,
14 g fat (9 g saturated)

PLAIN
190 calories,
19 g fat (13 g saturated)

Eat This

Chicken Waldorf Sandwich

450 calories
29 g fat
(4.5 g saturated)
510 mg sodium

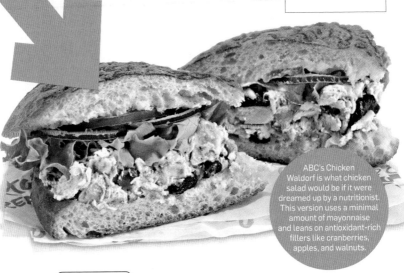

ABC's Chicken Waldorf is what chicken salad would be if it were dreamed up by a nutritionist. This version uses a minimal amount of mayonnaise and leans on antioxidant-rich fillers like cranberries, apples, and walnuts.

Other Picks

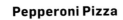

Pepperoni Pizza

400 calories
10 g fat (5 g saturated)
790 mg sodium

Morning Classic
with Bacon

420 calories
21 g fat (7 g saturated)
1,190 mg sodium

Blueberry Muffin

320 calories
15 g fat (2.5 g saturated)
26 g sugars

ny

780 calories
41 g fat
(11 g saturated)
1,660 mg sodium

Not That!

Bistro Chicken Press Sandwich

This sandwich is lined with pesto, which ordinarily we approve of for its load of healthy fats. Unfortunately, here that pesto is muddled with an aggressive application of mayo, bloating this into the fattiest chicken sandwich on the menu.

Other Passes

840 calories
33 g fat (7 g saturated)
1,700 mg sodium

Chicken Pesto Calzone

750 calories
43 g fat (15 g saturated)
1,890 mg sodium

Sausage, Egg & Cheese Sandwich

610 calories
36 g fat (5 g saturated)
38 g sugars

Banana Nut Muffin

Au Bon Pain

Did You Know?

● There's no excuse for eating poorly at Au Bon Pain. Back in 2003, while many establishments were busy hiding their nutritional information, Au Bon Pain launched their Nutrition Kiosks program. Each restaurant has at least one touch-screen kiosk that instantly provides nutritional information for every item on the Au Bon Pain menu.

Eat This

Thai Peanut Chicken Wrap

530 calories
15 g fat
(2 g saturated)
1,340 mg sodium

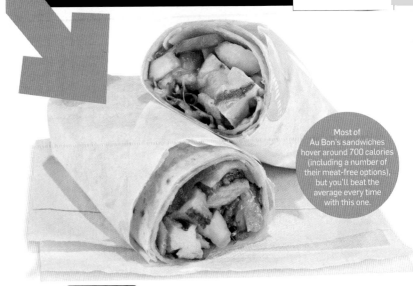

Most of Au Bon's sandwiches hover around 700 calories (including a number of their meat-free options), but you'll beat the average every time with this one.

Other Picks

Chicken Gumbo Soup
(medium, 12 oz)

180 calories
8 g fat (1 g saturated)
880 mg sodium

Thai Peanut Chicken Salad
with Thai Peanut Dressing

400 calories
16 g fat (1 g saturated)
1,020 mg sodium

Raspberry Mousse

150 calories
6 g fat (4 g saturated)
13 g sugars

780 calories
40 g fat
(16 g saturated)
2,270 mg sodium

Not That!

Prosciutto
Mozzarella Sandwich

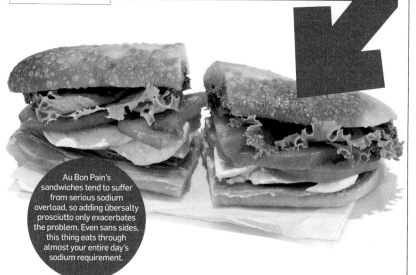

Au Bon Pain's sandwiches tend to suffer from serious sodium overload, so adding übersalty prosciutto only exacerbates the problem. Even sans sides, this thing eats through almost your entire day's sodium requirement.

Other Passes

350 calories
20 g fat (10 g saturated)
990 mg sodium

Baked Stuffed Potato Soup
(medium, 12 oz)

580 calories
41 g fat (12 g saturated)
1,220 mg sodium

Smoked Turkey Cobb Salad
with Pomegranate Vinaigrette

250 calories
3 g fat (2 g saturated)
43 g sugars

Low Fat Blueberry Yogurt
with Blueberries (small, 8.5 oz)

Auntie Anne's

Did You Know?

● Auntie Anne is a real person. She launched the business as an Amish housewife and later sold it for $293 million. Today, the company makes more than 500,000 pretzels every 2 days. That's enough dough to feed the entire population of Auntie Anne's hometown in Lancaster County, PA.

STEALTH HEALTH FOOD
Marinara Sauce

20 calories
0.5 g fat
330 mg sodium

The basic ingredient in marinara is cooked tomato, and studies have shown that people who eat tomato-rich diets have lower cholesterol and a lower risk for heart disease. This is partly due to the antioxidant lycopene, which is responsible for the tomato's color. The cooked tomatoes in marinara provide more lycopene than raw tomatoes do, so make this your dip of choice.

Eat This

Raisin Pretzel
with Cream Cheese

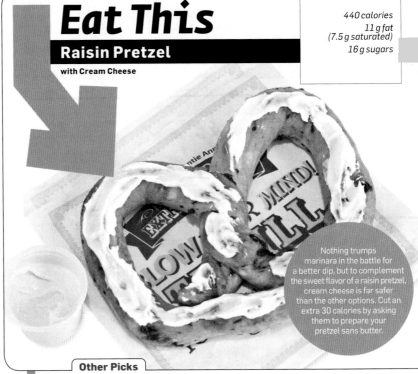

440 calories
11 g fat
(7.5 g saturated)
16 g sugars

Nothing trumps marinara in the battle for a better dip, but to complement the sweet flavor of a raisin pretzel, cream cheese is far safer than the other options. Cut an extra 30 calories by asking them to prepare your pretzel sans butter.

Other Picks

Pretzel Dog

360 calories
20 g fat (9 g saturated, 0.5 g trans)
740 mg sodium

Original Pretzel
with heated Marinara Sauce (2 oz)

360 calories
5.5 g fat (3 g saturated)
1,320 mg sodium

Piña Colada Dutch Ice
(14 oz)

210 calories
0 g fat
48 g sugars

600 calories
12 g fat
(7 g saturated)
61 g sugars

Not That !

Cinnamon Sugar Pretzel

with Sweet Dip

The combination of the sweetest pretzel with the sweetest dip (there are 32 grams of sugar in that little cup!) makes this the most nefarious option for your blood sugar.

WEAPON OF MASS DESTRUCTION
Pepperoni Pizza with Cheese Topping

650 calories
27 g fat (12 g saturated)
1,120 mg sodium

A massive load of saturated fat makes this the worst food item on Auntie Anne's menu. You could cut the fat by half—and save calories—by eating two full Garlic Pretzels with Marinara Sauce, instead.

DIP DECODER
(per serving)

SWEET MUSTARD
60 calories,
2 g fat (1 g saturated),
9 g sugars

CREAM CHEESE
80 calories,
6 g fat (4.5 g saturated)

MELTED CHEESE
80 calories,
6 g fat (1 g saturated)

CHEESE SAUCE
100 calories,
8 g fat (3 g saturated)

HOT SALSA CHEESE
110 calories,
8 g fat (3.5 g saturated)

CARAMEL
130 calories,
3 g fat (1.5 g saturated),
19 g sugars

Other Passes

480 calories
16 g fat (8 g saturated)
860 mg sodium

Pepperoni Pretzel

510 calories
18 g fat (7 g saturated)
1,440 mg sodium

Sesame Pretzel
with Hot Salsa Cheese (1.4 oz)

360 calories
17 g fat (11 g saturated, 1 g trans)
38 g sugars

Mocha Dutch Latte
(14 oz)

Baja Fresh

Did You Know?

● Baja Fresh doesn't keep a microwave, freezer, or can opener in any of its 300-plus locations. This Cali-Mex chain prides itself on preparing everything—from a half-dozen salsas to the marinated hormone-free meats—fresh on-site. But what's great for your palate isn't always great for your gut: Baja earned a D+ on our 2009 Restaurant Report Card.

38

The amount of saturated fat, in grams, in the average quesadilla at Baja Fresh. A healthy person should max out at 20 grams for the day.

Eat This

Chicken Torta
without Chips

620 calories
23 g fat
(6 g saturated)
1,330 mg sodium

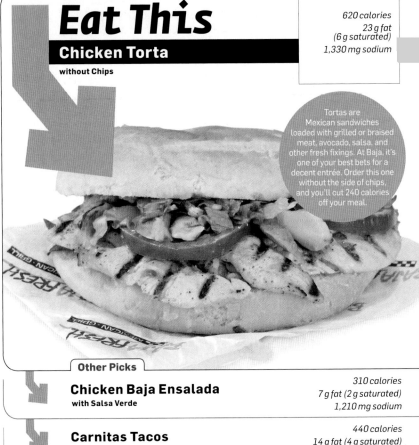

Tortas are Mexican sandwiches loaded with grilled or braised meat, avocado, salsa, and other fresh fixings. At Baja, it's one of your best bets for a decent entrée. Order this one without the side of chips, and you'll cut 240 calories off your meal.

Other Picks

Chicken Baja Ensalada
with Salsa Verde

310 calories
7 g fat (2 g saturated)
1,210 mg sodium

Carnitas Tacos
(2)

440 calories
14 g fat (4 g saturated)
560 mg sodium

Shrimp Soft Tacos
(2)

460 calories
20 g fat (9 g saturated)
1,280 mg sodium

1,330 calories
80 g fat
(37 g saturated,
2.5 trans)
2,590 mg sodium

Not That!
Chicken Quesadilla

Quesadillas are second only to nachos in terms of belt-breaking potential. There's not one on the menu—not even the veggie quesadilla—with fewer than 1,200 calories.

Other Passes

980 calories
52 g fat (20 g saturated)
1,770 mg sodium

Cabo Style Salad Burrito

830 calories
20 g fat (6 g saturated)
2,420 mg sodium

Carnitas Burrito Mexicano

1,120 calories
32 g fat (10 g saturated)
3,410 mg sodium

Shrimp Fajitas
with Flour Tortillas

MENU MAGIC

At places like Baja and Chipotle, where food is prepared fresh before your eyes, take advantage and come up with your own creations. Start with a serving of lean protein—mahimahi and chicken are best—and flank it with the Veggie Mix and a barrage of salsas. You'll net about 80 grams of protein for fewer than 500 calories.

BAD BREED

NACHOS

There's not a single good Nacho option on the entire Baja Fresh menu. The "best" of the bunch comes with your daily limit of both calories and sodium, and twice your daily limit of artery-clogging trans fat.

MENU DECODER

● **ENCHILADO STYLE:** A burrito variation that adds 630 calories and 40 grams of fat by adding a signature salsa and extra cheese on top and nachos on the side.

Baskin-Robbins

Did You Know?

- Baskin-Robbins finally removed its entire premium line of shakes from national menus this year. We happily said good-bye to the former Worst Drink in America, the 2,600-calorie Chocolate Oreo Shake.

- The scoop shop was twice sued for shortchanging customers who bought hand-packed ice cream in pint-size containers, first in 1985 and then once again in 2007.

MENU MAGIC

Choose a treat from the Grab-N-Go cooler. The stand-alone freezer is loaded with ready-to-eat goodies, and in general, they're far less dangerous than the regular shop items. Look for the 260-calorie Brownie a la Mode or, even better, the 50-calorie Fruit Blast Bars.

Eat This

Oreo Cookies 'n Cream Ice Cream

(2 scoops) in a Cake Cone

365 calories
18 g fat
(10 g saturated)
34 g sugars

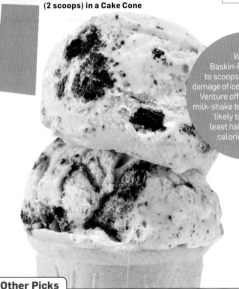

When at Baskin-Robbins, stick to scoops to mitigate the damage of ice cream indulgence. Venture off into sundae and milk-shake territory, and you're likely to sacrifice at least half of your daily calories in return.

Other Picks

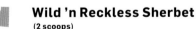

Wild 'n Reckless Sherbet
(2 scoops)

160 calories
2 g fat (1.5 g saturated)
33 g sugars

Cappuccino Blast
made with soft serve ice cream (16 oz)

280 calories
9 g fat (6 g saturated)
21 g sugars

Peach Passion Fruit Blast (small, 16 oz)

270 calories
0 g fat
65 g sugars

1,130 calories
55 g fat
(27 g saturated,
1 g trans)
120 g sugars

Not That!
Oreo Outrageous Sundae

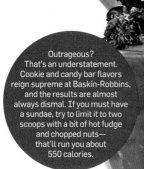

Outrageous? That's an understatement. Cookie and candy bar flavors reign supreme at Baskin-Robbins, and the results are almost always dismal. If you must have a sundae, try to limit it to two scoops with a bit of hot fudge and chopped nuts—that'll run you about 550 calories.

Other Passes

280 calories
14 g fat (9 g saturated)
28 g sugars

Strawberry Shortcake Ice Cream
(2 scoops)

670 calories
33 g fat (21 g saturated, 1 g trans)
73 g sugars

Vanilla Shake
(small, 16 oz)

420 calories
1 g fat
92 g sugars

Peach Passion Banana Fruit Blast Smoothie **(small, 16 oz)**

HIDDEN DANGER

Large Mango Fruit Blast Smoothie

A bathtub-size cup is only part of the problem here. The more concerning issue is the torrent of sucrose that's used to spike the "mango base" in this smoothie. You'd have to eat 3 pounds of actual mangoes to get that much sugar naturally. And what's more, Baskin's smoothies are dyed with artificial colors that have been linked to hyperactivity in children. Not so smooth now, huh?

870 calories
3 g fat
202 g sugars

CONE DECODER

CAKE CONE
25 calories, 0 g fat,
0 g sugars

SUGAR CONE
45 calories, 0.5 g fat,
3 g sugars

WAFFLE CONE
160 calories, 4 g fat,
13 g sugars

Ben & Jerry's

Did You Know?

● Despite being sold to Unilever for $326 million in 2000, Ben & Jerry's still lives up to its tie-dyed hippie aesthetic and dedicated environmentalism. Their dairy comes from cows that haven't been injected with rBGH, a genetically engineered growth hormone, and they rely mostly on a Vermont-based family-farmers co-op for their supplies of cream and milk.

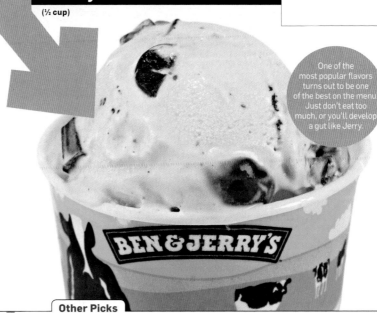

Eat This

Cherry Garcia Ice Cream
(½ cup)

200 calories
11 g fat
(8 g saturated)
20 g sugars

One of the most popular flavors turns out to be one of the best on the menu. Just don't eat too much, or you'll develop a gut like Jerry.

BEN & JERRY'S

Other Picks

Chocolate Therapy
(½ cup)

210 calories
12 g fat (7 g saturated)
19 g sugars

Berry Berry Extraordinary Sorbet
(½ cup)

100 calories
0 g fat
23 g sugars

Coffee Ice Cream
(½ cup)

190 calories
11 g fat (8 g saturated)
16 g sugars

340 calories
24 g fat
(12 g saturated)
24 g sugars

Not That!

Peanut Butter Cup Ice Cream

(½ cup)

There's only one peanut butter ice cream in the country with more calories than this one, and that's Häagen-Dazs Chocolate Peanut Butter. But as far as saturated fat goes, this one is the national loser.

BEN & JERRY'S

Other Passes

250 calories
17 g fat (9 g saturated)
21 g sugars

New York Super Fudge Chunk Ice Cream (½ cup)

140 calories
1.5 g fat (1 g saturated)
20 g sugars

Black Raspberry Swirl Frozen Yogurt (½ cup)

230 calories
14 g fat (10 g saturated)
21 g sugars

Coffee Coffee Buzz Buzz Buzz Ice Cream (½ cup)

FOOD COURT

THE CRIME
Two scoops of Chubby Hubby ice cream
(660 calories)

THE PUNISHMENT
Five 45-minute yoga sessions

SUGAR DECODER

● **INVERT SUGAR:**
Table sugar that's been split into components glucose and fructose. Tastes sweeter than regular sugar and is used to retard crystallization in ice cream.

● **BROWN SUGAR:**
White sucrose that retains a measure of surface molasses, giving it a darker color and deeper flavor.

● **LIQUID SUGAR:**
Granulated white sugar dissolved into water. By far the most common sweetener in B&J's ice creams, usually appearing as the second or third ingredient.

Blimpie

Did You Know?

● Blimpie is a better place for breakfast than it is for lunch or dinner. They offer an impressive line of A.M. entrées, with most falling under 500 calories. Avoid the biscuits and paninis and concentrate instead on the Bluffins and burritos, and all will be well with your morning.

CONDIMENT CATASTROPHE

Oil Blend
(0.5 oz)

130 calories
14 g fat (2 g saturated)
0 mg sodium

There's nothing more dangerous than an apathetic sandwich maker with a bottle of oil in his hand, and many of Blimpie's subs get this treatment whether you ask for it or not. With 130 calories in each ½ ounce, you can imagine how fast that adds up when poured on with careless indifference. Save yourself the needless fat by asking them to skip the oil treatment.

Eat This

Roast Beef & Provolone

(6" wheat)

385 calories
12 g fat
(5 g saturated)
990 mg sodium

Roast beef doesn't have the same lean reputation as turkey and chicken, but in truth, most cuts are nearly as reliable as either of those poultry choices. Feel free to make it the anchor of any sandwich you order.

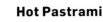

Other Picks

Hot Pastrami
(6" regular)

435 calories
16 g fat (7 g saturated)
1,354 mg sodium

Guacamole, onion, lettuce, and tomato on Jalapeño Cheddar Bread
with spicy brown mustard (6")

287 calories
8 g fat (3 g saturated)
636 mg sodium

Ham, Egg & Cheese Bluffin

280 calories
11 g fat (6 g saturated)
1,049 mg sodium

684 calories
36 g fat
(12 g saturated)
1,928 mg sodium

Not That!

Roast Beef & Cheddar Wrap

(regular)

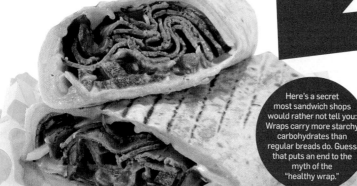

Here's a secret most sandwich shops would rather not tell you: Wraps carry more starchy carbohydrates than regular breads do. Guess that puts an end to the myth of the "healthy wrap."

WEAPON OF MASS DESTRUCTION
12" Super Stacked BLT

1,265 calories
82 g fat (18 g saturated)
2,870 mg sodium

We've always been fans of the BLT—it's an oft-overlooked sandwich with a reasonable nutritional profile. Not the case here. There's more fat in this super-stacker than in 13 Spicy Chicken Soft Tacos from Taco Bell. Surprisingly enough, the only sandwich with more saturated fat is the 12" Veggie Supreme, with 33 grams.

GUILTY PLEASURE

Pasta Fagioli with Sausage Soup

150 calories
5 g fat (2 g saturated)
910 mg sodium

It's usually best to avoid meals that center on sausage—the most dubious meat in a restaurant's arsenal. See, most chefs haven't learned to use rich ingredients in moderation. Let this sausage soup be an example to them: It delivers moderate numbers in every nutritional category.

Other Passes

607 calories
32 g fat (14 g saturated)
2,072 mg sodium

Meatball
(6" regular)

593 calories
30 g fat (10 g saturated)
1,766 mg sodium

Special Vegetarian
(6" regular)

773 calories
24 g fat (9 g saturated)
2,368 mg sodium

Breakfast Panini (6")

Bob Evans

MENU MAGIC

Build a better breakfast from à la carte items. Choose any two from this list.

SMOKED HAM
99 calories

STRAWBERRY BANANA PARFAIT
151 calories

ONE PIECE OF FRENCH TOAST
164 calories

BOWL OF OATMEAL
167 calories

TWO SCRAMBLED EGGS
168 calories

Eat This

Western Omelet
with egg lites

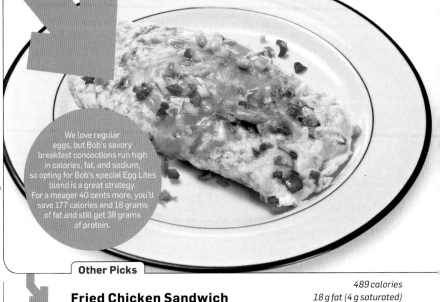

310 calories
14 g fat
(8 g saturated)
1,453 mg sodium

We love regular eggs, but Bob's savory breakfast concoctions run high in calories, fat, and sodium, so opting for Bob's special Egg Lites blend is a great strategy. For a meager 40 cents more, you'll save 177 calories and 18 grams of fat and still get 38 grams of protein.

Other Picks

Fried Chicken Sandwich

489 calories
18 g fat (4 g saturated)
1,109 mg sodium

Salmon Fillet in garlic butter
with baked potato and broccoli florets

564 calories
18 g fat (3 g saturated)
730 mg sodium

Open-Faced Roast Beef

476 calories
24 g fat (8 g saturated)
1,041 mg sodium

677 calories
33g fat
(13 g saturated)
1,716 mg sodium

Not That!

Border Scramble Burrito

with egg whites

Someone call the border police: This soggy mess of a burrito is a repeated nutritional felon. Even with egg whites as the main filler, it still manages to pack in more calories than two Egg McMuffins and as much saturated fat as 13 strips of bacon.

Other Passes

583 calories
31 g fat (11 g saturated, 1 g trans)
1,420 mg sodium

Grilled Chicken Club Sandwich

975 calories
54 g fat (20 g saturated, 2 g trans)
1,715 mg sodium

Garden Vegetable & Salmon Alfredo

1,008 calories
43 g fat (11 g saturated)
3,686 mg sodium

Steak Tip Stir-Fry

MEET YOUR MATCH

Knife and Fork Meatloaf Sandwich
(3,182 mg sodium)
=
18 small tubs of Pringles

Bojangles'

Did You Know?

● Bojangles', with more than 400 locations throughout 11 states (predominantly in the South), has one of the country's most loyal fast-food followings. In fact, the *Wall Street Journal* named it one of the top 25 franchises in America across all industries.

● Bojangles' takes their biscuits very seriously. They bake half a million of them a day and hold an annual Master Baker Biscuit Maker Challenge. The winner—judged on consistency, color, size, and texture— wins $1,000.

Eat This

Cajun Spiced Chicken Breast
with Cajun Pintos

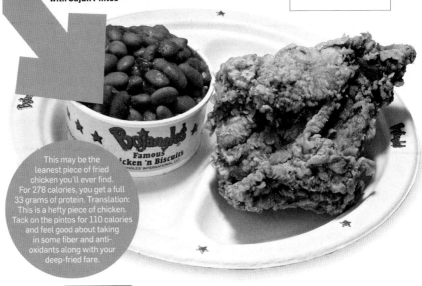

388 calories
17 g fat (0 g saturated)
1,045 mg sodium

This may be the leanest piece of fried chicken you'll ever find. For 278 calories, you get a full 33 grams of protein. Translation: This is a hefty piece of chicken. Tack on the pintos for 110 calories and feel good about taking in some fiber and anti-oxidants along with your deep-fried fare.

Other Picks

Sausage Biscuit Sandwich

350 calories
23 g fat (7 g saturated)
810 mg sodium

Chicken Breast and Leg
with Marinated Cole Slaw

536 calories
36 g fat
1,549 mg sodium

Buffalo Bites

180 calories
5 g fat (2 g saturated)
720 mg sodium

654 calories
42 g fat (5 g saturated)
945 mg sodium

Not That!

Cajun Spiced Chicken Thigh

with Seasoned Fries

Along with the wings, chicken thighs tend to be the fattiest part on the bird, meaning less protein and more calories per piece. Here, you'll end up with 200 extra calories and less than half the protein than if you go with the more satisfying breast-beans combo.

Other Passes

649 calories
49 g fat (13 g saturated)
1,126 mg sodium

Steak Biscuit Sandwich

985 calories
74 g fat
2,123 mg sodium

3 Pc. Dinner
(1 leg and 2 thighs with biscuit)

337 calories
16 g fat (6 g saturated)
629 mg sodium

Chicken Supremes

Boston Market

Did You Know?

● In an attempt to add regional diversity to its New England-centric menu, Boston Market channeled down-home Southern cooking and recently introduced the suspicious sounding Crispy Crunchy Chicken to its lineup. What's surprising is that this fried fowl dish actually has about 300 fewer calories than their Boston Chicken Carvers, which are seemingly harmless rotisserie chicken sandwiches.

MENU MISNOMER

Cinnamon Apples

210 calories
3 g fat
42 g sugars

Cinnamon and super-sweetened candied apples would be a more appropriate name. Between sugar and brown sugar, this side dish has the same sweet kick as six Cinnamon Twist Doughnuts from Krispy Kreme. This is no side; this is dessert.

Eat This

Dark Chicken Individual Meal

(3 pieces) with Fresh Vegetable Stuffing

580 calories
30 g fat
(7 g saturated)
1,850 mg sodium

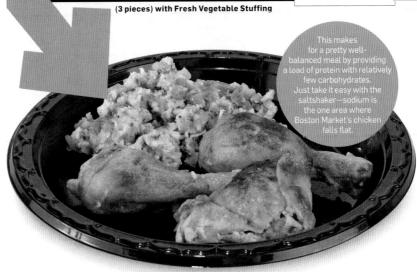

This makes for a pretty well-balanced meal by providing a load of protein with relatively few carbohydrates. Just take it easy with the saltshaker—sodium is the one area where Boston Market's chicken falls flat.

Other Picks

Rotisserie Chicken Open-Faced Sandwich

320 calories
8 g fat (2.5 g saturated)
1,630 mg sodium

Roasted Turkey
with baked beans

450 calories
4.5 g fat (1 g saturated)
1,635 mg sodium

Beef Brisket Family Meal
(¼ brisket)

280 calories
20 g fat (1.5 g saturated)
260 mg sodium

800 calories
41 g fat
(7 g saturated,
5 g trans)
1,900 mg sodium

Not That!

Classic Chicken Salad Sandwich

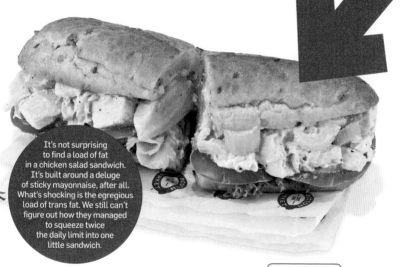

It's not surprising to find a load of fat in a chicken salad sandwich. It's built around a deluge of sticky mayonnaise, after all. What's shocking is the egregious load of trans fat. We still can't figure out how they managed to squeeze twice the daily limit into one little sandwich.

WEAPON OF MASS DESTRUCTION
Pastry Top Chicken Pot Pie

800 calories
48 g fat
(18 g saturated, 7 g trans)
1,090 mg sodium

We've been harping on potpies for years, and this is why. The flakiness in the crust comes from vegetable shortening, and it saddles this entrée with three times the acceptable daily limit for trans fat. Until the food industry learns that their tops can be made with butter and nonhydrogenated oil, stay away from potpies.

MENU MAGIC

Be skeptical of restaurant handouts. The cornbread's complimentary at Boston Market, but that doesn't mean it won't cost your waistline. Tell your server to keep it off your plate and you'll save 180 calories and 1.5 grams of trans fat—which is enough to make the difference between a good one and a bad one.

Other Passes

1,020 calories
82 g fat (15 g saturated, 2 g trans)
3,970 mg sodium

Market Chopped Salad
with Rotisserie Chicken

820 calories
42 g fat (11 g saturated)
2,040 mg sodium

¼ White Meat BBQ Chicken
with potato salad

480 calories
36 g fat (16 g saturated, 1.5 g trans)
1,030 mg sodium

Meatloaf Family Meal
(⅛ meat loaf)

Burger King

Did You Know?

● In May 2007, the Center for Science in the Public Interest sued Burger King for moving too slowly to remove trans fat from its menus. BK responded with a promise to phase out all trans fat by the end of 2008. However, as of July 2009, BK still averaged 2 grams of trans fat per Whopper sandwich.

MENU MAGIC

The simplest way to save calories at any burger joint is to replace the mayo with ketchup, BBQ sauce, or mustard. Nowhere is that move more important than at BK, where mayo comes with 180 calories. In fact, you'd be better off skipping the mayo and making it a BLT-topped burger, instead; it'll save you 120 calories. One swap like this a day will save you nearly a pound of body fat each month.

Eat This

Chicken Tenders

(8 pieces) with Barbecue Sauce

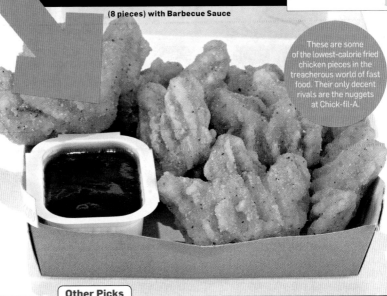

400 calories
21 g fat
(4 g saturated)
920 mg sodium

These are some of the lowest-calorie fried chicken pieces in the treacherous world of fast food. Their only decent rivals are the nuggets at Chick-fil-A.

Other Picks

Double Hamburger

420 calories
22 g fat (9 g saturated, 1 g trans)
590 mg sodium

BK Burger Shots
(2)

220 calories
10 g fat (4 g saturated, 0.5 g trans)
420 mg sodium

Tendergrill Chicken Sandwich
without mayo

380 calories
9 g fat (2 g saturated)
1,130 mg sodium

800 calories
46 g fat
(8 g saturated,
0.5 g trans)
1,640 mg sodium

Not That!

Tendercrisp Chicken Sandwich

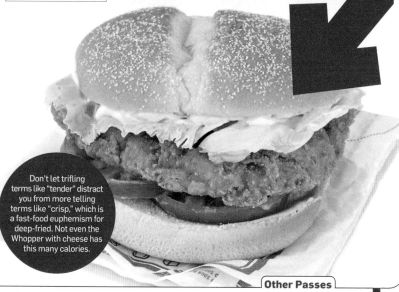

Don't let trifling terms like "tender" distract you from more telling terms like "crisp," which is a fast-food euphemism for deep-fried. Not even the Whopper with cheese has this many calories.

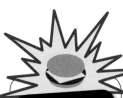

BURGER BOMB

Angry Whopper

880 calories
55 g fat
(48 g saturated, 2 g trans)
1,680 mg sodium

Why so angry, King? This spicy new take on their classic burger only adds fuel to the fire. With bacon, pepper Jack cheese, and oily dressing rounding out the new flavor profile, it seems like it would be more apt to call it Chubby, instead. This burger does, after all, have 210 more calories than an original Whopper.

Other Passes

670 calories
40 g fat (11 g saturated, 1.5 g trans)
1,020 mg sodium

Whopper

340 calories
16 g fat (7 g saturated, 0.5 g trans)
770 mg sodium

Cheeseburger

480 calories
30 g fat (6 g saturated)
1,390 mg sodium

Tendergrill Chicken Salad
with honey mustard dressing

FOOD COURT

THE CRIME
Triple Whopper with Cheese
(1,250 calories)

THE PUNISHMENT
Pedal vigorously on a stationary bike for 1 hour and 40 minutes

Burger King (Continued)

Did You Know?

● Burger King's new BK Fresh Apple Fries are fresh-cut, skinless red apples sliced to resemble real fries. They provide a full serving of fruit and are meant to increase fruit intake in children. Other kid-friendly tactics at Burger King include limiting sodium in kids' menu items to less than 600 milligrams apiece.

● Burger King sells 6.6 million burgers every day worldwide.

BAD BREED

FRIES

No major fast-food burger joint has worse fries than Burger King. Not McDonald's, not Wendy's, and not Hardee's. Burger King's fries are so bad, in fact, that you could actually save calories by eating an entire Double Hamburger instead of a medium order of the salt-soaked side dish. Better still, skip both and count yourself 450 calories smaller.

Eat This

Ham Omelet Sandwich

290 calories
12 g fat
(4.5 g saturated)
870 mg sodium

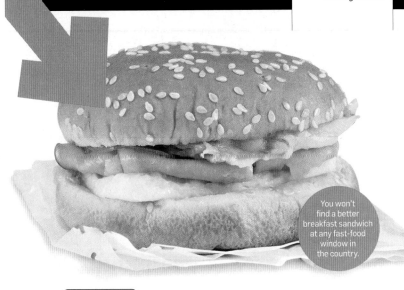

You won't find a better breakfast sandwich at any fast-food window in the country.

Other Picks

French Toast Sticks
(3 pieces) with syrup

310 calories
11 g fat (2 g saturated)
22 g sugars

Cheesy Tots Potatoes
(6 pieces)

220 calories
12 g fat (4 g saturated)
630 mg sodium

Icee Coca Cola
(small, 16 oz)

110 calories
0 g fat
31 g sugars

420 calories
31 g fat
(10 g saturated,
0.5 g trans)
910 mg sodium

Not That!

Sausage and Cheese BK Breakfast Shots

(2 sandwiches)

Sausage is the clear loser in the battle of the breakfast meats. The sooner you learn to skip it, the sooner you can start dropping pounds.

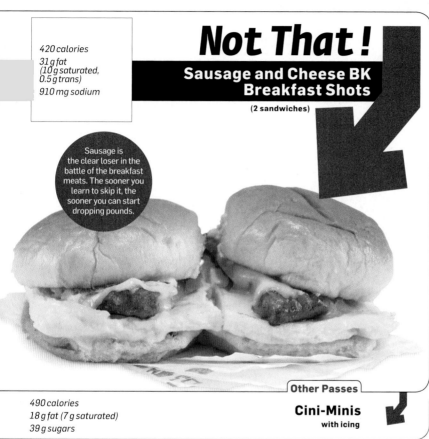

Other Passes

490 calories 18 g fat (7 g saturated) 39 g sugars	**Cini-Minis** with icing
340 calories 17 g fat (3.5 g saturated) 590 mg sodium	**French Fries** (small)
700 calories 26 g fat (16 g saturated, 0.5 g trans) 105 g sugars	**Oreo BK Chocolate Sundae Shake** (small, 16 oz)

CONDIMENT CATASTROPHE

Crispy Onions

110 calories
7 g fat
60 mg sodium

These abused onions are breaded, fried, and then stuffed into sandwiches like Angry Whoppers and Steakhouse Burgers, pushing both into the caloric danger zone. Keep them off anything you order. Doing so won't turn a burger into a tofu sandwich, but a little damage control certainly doesn't hurt.

DANGEROUS DESSERTS

Medium Strawberry Oreo BK Sundae Shake

980 calories
34 g fat
(21 g saturated, 1 g trans)
153 g sugars

See those registered trademark symbols riding next to the words "Oreo" and "BK" on the cup? It's probably not a good sign when you need two of them just to print the name of a beverage. This medium shake has about half your day's calories, more than a day's worth of saturated fat, and more sugar than you'd find in 2 pints of Ben & Jerry's decadent Chocolate Therapy ice cream.

California Pizza Kit

Did You Know?

● Founded in 1986, California Pizza Kitchen took its culinary cue from Wolfgang Puck's famous Spago restaurant, located just up the road from the original Beverly Hills CPK location. Puck made a name for himself in the '80s with a portfolio of inventive pizzas and pastas, and CPK has been known for the same ever since. A word to the wise: Indulge in the pizza, but pass on the pasta.

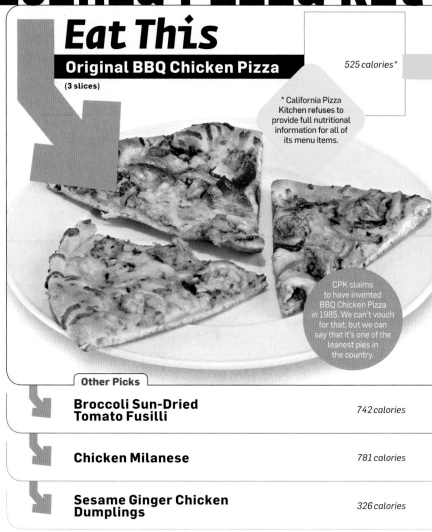

Eat This

Original BBQ Chicken Pizza

(3 slices)

525 calories*

* California Pizza Kitchen refuses to provide full nutritional information for all of its menu items.

CPK claims to have invented BBQ Chicken Pizza in 1985. We can't vouch for that, but we can say that it's one of the leanest pies in the country.

Other Picks

Broccoli Sun-Dried Tomato Fusilli	*742 calories*
Chicken Milanese	*781 calories*
Sesame Ginger Chicken Dumplings	*326 calories*

chen

1,269 calories*

Not That!
BBQ Chicken Chopped Salad

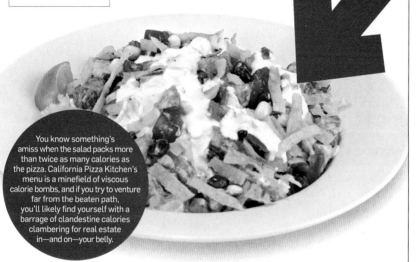

You know something's amiss when the salad packs more than twice as many calories as the pizza. California Pizza Kitchen's menu is a minefield of viscous calorie bombs, and if you try to venture far from the beaten path, you'll likely find yourself with a barrage of clandestine calories clambering for real estate in—and on—your belly.

WEAPON OF MASS DESTRUCTION
Thai Crunch Salad

2,115 calories

Blame for this caloric monster rests with an army of fried wonton strips buried in the body of the salad and a topping of rice sticks coated in TWO dressings. If your salad crunches beyond the snap of crispy lettuce, you can no longer consider it healthy.

HIDDEN DANGER

Ginger Salmon

Salmon and ginger, on their own, are paragons of nutritious eating. So how does CPK manage to mutilate them so severely? Step one is the employment of a high-calorie Sweet Ginger Sauce, and step two is piling the plate high with a profusion of oily Mandarin noodles.

1,345 calories

Other Passes

1,223 calories — **Tomato Basil Spaghettini**

1,535 calories — **Chicken Piccata**

1,180 calories — **Avocado Club Egg Rolls**

Captain D's

Did You Know?

● A 2008 Captain D's commercial targeted competitor Red Lobster's prices. An actor stood outside a Red Lobster, asking patrons how much they spent on their meal. The point: Eat the same food at Captain D's for $30 less. As a result, the Captain was served with a cease and desist order from the Lobster's legal squad.

STEALTH HEALTH FOOD
Coleslaw

170 calories
12 g fat (2 g saturated)
310 mg sodium

Thanks to mayonnaise mistreatment, coleslaw isn't generally the safest bet. But when you find a good one, you'd be wise to take it. The cabbage that constitutes the slaw contains a chemical called sulforaphane, which has been shown to bind with other agents to form cancer-inhibiting compounds inside your body. Not a bad bonus for a side dish.

Eat This

Shrimp Skewers Dinner

with Side Salad and Roasted Red Potatoes

630 calories
17 g fat
(6 g saturated, 1 g trans)
1,770 mg sodium

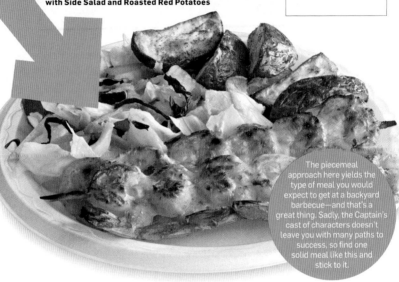

The piecemeal approach here yields the type of meal you would expect to get at a backyard barbecue—and that's a great thing. Sadly, the Captain's cast of characters doesn't leave you with many paths to success, so find one solid meal like this and stick to it.

Other Picks

Fish Snack Smacker
(no tartar sauce) with macaroni and cheese

470 calories
20 g fat (8 g saturated, 1 g trans)
1,305 mg sodium

Baked Potato
with sour cream

290 calories
6 g fat (4 g saturated)
25 mg sodium

Chocolate Cake

300 calories
11 g fat (2 g saturated, 1 g trans)
35 g sugars

1,160 calories
51 g fat
(22 g saturated,
5 g trans)
1,630 mg sodium

Not That!
Bite Size Shrimp Dinner
with Hush Puppies and Cole Slaw

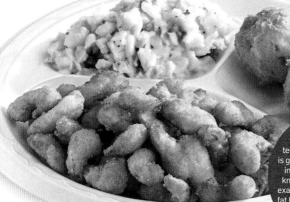

Unfortunately, the name alone doesn't tell you whether this entrée is grilled or fried, so be sure to inquire if you don't already know. This meal is a perfect example of a belly full of trans fat hiding under a wholesome-sounding dish: a Captain's specialty.

LITTLE TRICK

Bypass the Captain's typical carb-loaded fare: Combine a couple items from the Add-a-Piece menu with a veggie side. Your top picks: a Chicken Tender and a Stuffed Crab Shell, with broccoli on the side. That's only 310 calories and 16 grams of fat.

Other Passes

710 calories
36 g fat (11 g saturated, 1 g trans)
1,540 mg sodium

Chicken Ranch Sandwich

400 calories
26 g fat (11 g saturated, 2 g trans)
650 mg sodium

Hush Puppies
(4)

470 calories
26 g fat (4 g saturated, 4 g trans)
25 g sugars

Pecan Pie

Carl's Jr.

Did You Know?

● Carl's parent company, CKE, has led the charge in celebrating gluttony. After Jay Leno lambasted them for using "meat as a condiment," they took his words and used them in burger promotions.

● Carl's Jr. tried to market a cheeseburger topped with a hot dog as a 4th of July special, but ultimately pulled it from the menu.

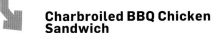

MENU MAGIC

"Veg It."
At Carl's Jr., you put a vegetarian spin on a Six Dollar Burger by ordering it sans meat. The option works best for the big-flavor Guacamole and Portobello varieties, both of which offer plenty more than just a hamburger between the buns. The best part about going meatless? You drop about 300 calories.

Eat This

Single Teriyaki Burger

610 calories
29 g fat
(11 g saturated,
0.5 g trans)
1,020 mg sodium

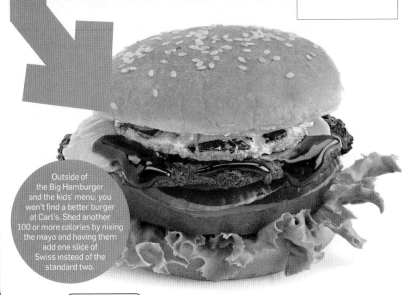

Outside of the Big Hamburger and the kids' menu, you won't find a better burger at Carl's. Shed another 100 or more calories by nixing the mayo and having them add one slice of Swiss instead of the standard two.

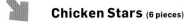

Other Picks

Charbroiled BBQ Chicken Sandwich

380 calories
7 g fat (1.5 g saturated)
1,010 mg sodium

Chicken Stars (6 pieces)

320 calories
24 g fat (6 g saturated)
460 mg sodium

Sourdough Breakfast Sandwich

450 calories
21 g fat (8 g saturated)
1,470 mg sodium

890 calories
54 g fat
(20 g saturated,
2 g trans)
2,040 mg sodium

Not That!

Six Dollar Burger

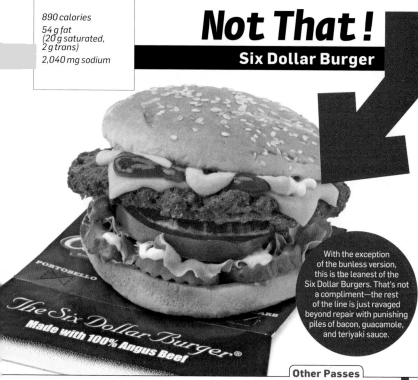

PORTOBELLO

The Six Dollar Burger
Made with 100% Angus Beef

With the exception of the bunless version, this is the leanest of the Six Dollar Burgers. That's not a compliment—the rest of the line is just ravaged beyond repair with punishing piles of bacon, guacamole, and teriyaki sauce.

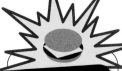

BURGER BOMB

Double Guacamole Bacon Burger

1,090 calories
74 g fat (27 g saturated)
1,770 mg sodium

In a menu ravaged by heavy burger artillery, this is currently Carl's most explosive weapon. Guac can be a great substitution for mayo on a burger, but Carl's slathers the green stuff on top of another fatty spread, then flanks it with bacon strips and multiple slices of pepper Jack. You'd be better off eating 20 strips of bacon. Seriously.

Other Passes

710 calories
37 g fat (6 g saturated)
1,280 mg sodium

Carl's Catch Fish Sandwich

530 calories
28 g fat (4.5 g saturated)
590 mg sodium

Onion Rings

780 calories
49 g fat (16 g saturated)
1,480 mg sodium

Loaded Breakfast Burrito

320 ◆

The calories saved by switching from an Original Six Dollar Burger to a Low Carb Six Dollar Burger.

Carrabba's

Did You Know?

● Carrabba's has joined a handful of other restaurants in providing a range of gluten-free menu items—a measure more establishments should adopt immediately. Unfortunately, Carrabba's has also joined a handful of other restaurants that don't provide nutritional information for their products online.

ATTACK OF THE APPETIZER

Antipasti Platter

1,520–1,960 calories

This platter's biggest caloric contributor is the only plate that isn't fried. The Grilled Bruschette changes daily, but it can pack a staggering 1,570 calories when you order it on its own.

Eat This

Manicotti

640 calories*

* Carrabba's refuses to provide full nutritional information for all of its menu items.

In a blind taste test, you'd be hard-pressed to tell the difference between these two popular plates. So why fork over the extra 710 calories? You could eat this cheesy dish, make yourself an ice cream sundae at home, and still go to bed having saved 400 calories. Make a swap like this twice a week and shed nearly 12 pounds in a year.

Other Picks

Margherita Pizza (½ pizza)   440 calories

Chicken Gratella   400 calories

Lobster Ravioli   740 calories

1,360 calories*

Not That!

Lasagne

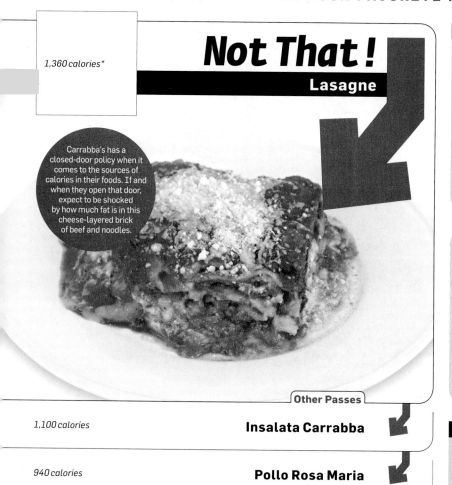

Carrabba's has a closed-door policy when it comes to the sources of calories in their foods. If and when they open that door, expect to be shocked by how much fat is in this cheese-layered brick of beef and noodles.

Other Passes

1,100 calories — **Insalata Carrabba**

940 calories — **Pollo Rosa Maria**

1,770 calories — **Pasta Weesie**

GUILTY PLEASURE

Rustica Pizza
(⅓ pizza)

575 calories

Pizza parlors take note: This is how you work sausage and two cheeses onto a pie without tipping it past 600 calories per serving. Eggplant and bell peppers help take up space to offset more cheese and sausage. The bonus is twofold: fewer calories and a more interesting culinary experience.

570

The caloric cost of tacking on meatballs to spaghetti. That's like topping your pasta with an entire Big Mac. Ay Carrabba!

FOOD COURT

THE CRIME
Rigatoni Martino with side Caesar Salad
(2,050 calories)

THE PUNISHMENT
3,285 sit-ups

Cheesecake Factory

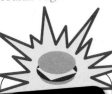

BURGER BOMB

Ranch House Burger

1,941 calories
48 g saturated fat
2,877 mg sodium

Please welcome our newest inductee to the list of Worst Burgers in America. It has nearly a full day's worth of calories, more than a day's worth of sodium, and 2½ days' worth of saturated fat.

Eat This

The Factory Burger

*Cheesecake Factory refuses to provide full nutritional information for all of its menu items.

737 calories*
15 g saturated fat
1,018 mg sodium

Surprisingly, this is one of the best burgers offered at any sit-down restaurant in America, and so long as you swap out the fries for something healthier, it's also one of the safest entrées you'll find on Cheesecake Factory's misguided menu.

Other Picks

Seared Tuna Tataki Salad

442 calories
3 g saturated fat
1,386 mg sodium

Chicken Pot Stickers
(½ order)

192 calories
1 g saturated fat
1,174 mg sodium

Energy Breakfast

714 calories
4 g saturated fat
1,304 mg sodium

1,752 calories*
28 g saturated fat
2,309 mg sodium

Not That!

Grilled Chicken and Avocado Club

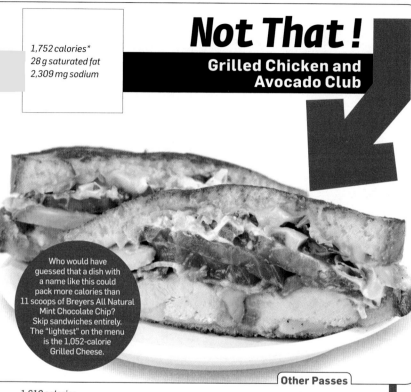

Who would have guessed that a dish with a name like this could pack more calories than 11 scoops of Breyers All Natural Mint Chocolate Chip? Skip sandwiches entirely. The "lightest" on the menu is the 1,052-calorie Grilled Cheese.

Other Passes

1,610 calories
49 g saturated fat
1,075 mg sodium

Wasabi Crusted Ahi Tuna

565 calories
10.5 g saturated fat
490 mg sodium

Fire-Roasted Fresh Artichoke
(½ order)

1,876 calories
40 g saturated fat
4,777 mg sodium

Sunrise Fiesta Burrito

Chevys Fresh Mex

Did You Know?

● Chevys takes the "Fresh" part of their name seriously: They make their salsas from scratch each day; their soft tortillas are made consistently throughout the day on a tortilla press called El Machino; and when you order guacamole, they come and smash avocados at your table. Unfortunately, "fresh" and "healthy" have little correlation here. No full dinner entrée contains less than 900 calories.

Eat This

Sea Bass Tacos

without Tamalito or Rice

729 calories
25 g fat
(7 g saturated)
2,501 mg sodium

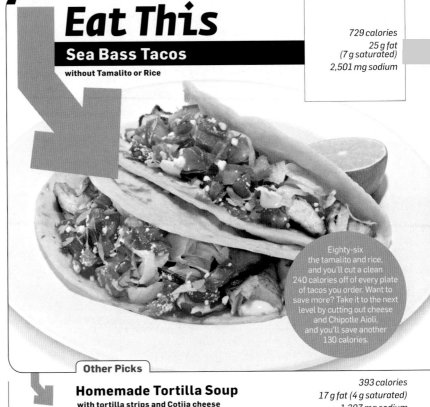

Eighty-six the tamalito and rice, and you'll cut a clean 240 calories off of every plate of tacos you order. Want to save more? Take it to the next level by cutting out cheese and Chipotle Aioli, and you'll save another 130 calories.

Other Picks

Homemade Tortilla Soup
with tortilla strips and Cotija cheese

393 calories
17 g fat (4 g saturated)
1,397 mg sodium

Santa Fe Chopped Salad
without bacon

518 calories
27 g fat (12 g saturated)
1,203 mg sodium

Black Beans
with cheese and pico de gallo

190 calories
2 g fat (1 g saturated)
930 mg sodium

1,452 calories
70 g fat
(30 g saturated)
4,693 mg sodium

Not That!

Juicy Shrimp Fajitas

with Tortillas

Fajita fixings are routinely tossed in a frying pan with loads of oil, so rarely will you find a restaurant that serves any worth eating. Take Chevys, for example. Ordering fajitas here means piling onto your plate as much saturated fat as six Snickers bars and nearly as much sodium as five full cans of Pringles.

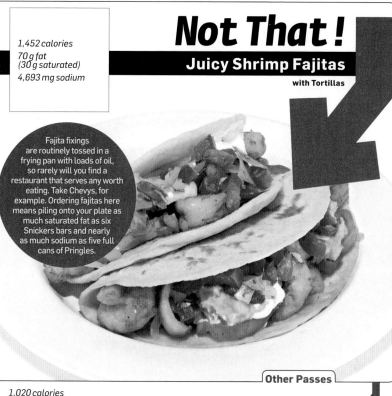

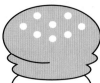

SALT LICK

GRANDE CHIMI BEEF

4,590 mg sodium
1,730 calories
90 g fat (44 g saturated)

This big brackish chimichanga packs in twice your daily limit of sodium, almost an entire day's worth of calories, and as much saturated fat as 44 bacon strips.

HIDDEN DANGER

El Machino Tortilla

We applaud Chevys for making their tortillas fresh daily, but that doesn't mean you can eat them with impunity. Cut down on the number of tortillas you use by stuffing each one to its maximum capacity—if there's no mess, you're not doing it right.

140 calories
4 g fat
(2 g saturated)
300 mg sodium

Other Passes

1,020 calories
34 g fat (9 g saturated)
2,710 mg sodium

Grilled Chicken Tacos

1,551 calories
94 g fat (37 g saturated)
2,480 mg sodium

Tostada Salad
with chicken

278 calories
14 g fat (5 g saturated)
775 mg sodium

Refried Beans
with pico de gallo without cheese

Chick-fil-A

Did You Know?

● This mega-chain closes on Sundays. Why? S. Truett Cathy, Chick-fil-A's founder, believes in a business model that respects spirituality and allows employees a day of rest with their families. "Corporate America needs faith in something more than the bottom line," he once said.

● Chick-fil-A makes biscuits and coleslaw from scratch daily. They also fresh-squeeze the lemonade and fillet and bread the chicken by hand.

MEET YOUR MATCH

Strawberry Milkshake
(100 g sugars)
=
5 Hostess Twinkies

Eat This

Chick-fil-A Chargrilled Chicken Club Sandwich

380 calories
11 g fat (5 g saturated)
1,560 mg sodium

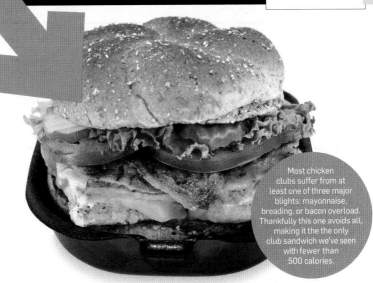

Most chicken clubs suffer from at least one of three major blights: mayonnaise, breading, or bacon overload. Thankfully this one avoids all, making it the the only club sandwich we've seen with fewer than 500 calories.

Other Picks

Chargrilled Chicken Sandwich

270 calories
3 g fat (1 g saturated)
1,270 mg sodium

Chick-n-Minis (4)

350 calories
14 g fat (3.5 g saturated)
790 mg sodium

Nuggets
(8) with honey mustard sauce

305 calories
13 g fat (2.5 g saturated)
990 mg sodium

480 calories
16 g fat (7 g saturated)
1,810 mg sodium

Not That!

Chicken Caesar Cool Wrap

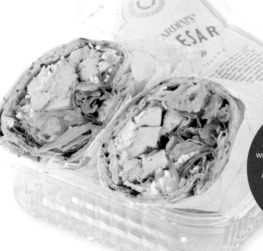

Chick-fil-A joins two of the most overrated "health" foods—wraps and Caesar salad—into one handheld package. At some establishments, it would still be a "this," but at Chick-fil-A, it's one of the worst items on the menu.

SAUCE SELECTOR
(1 oz)

BUFFALO
10 calories, 0 g fat,
420 mg sodium

BARBECUE
45 calories,
0 g fat,
9 g sugars

HONEY MUSTARD
45 calories, 0 g fat,
10 g sugars

POLYNESIAN
110 calories,
6 g fat,
13 g sugars

CHICK-FIL-A
140 calories, 13 g fat,
6 g sugars

Other Passes

500 calories
20 g fat (3.5 g saturated)
1,220 mg sodium

Chicken Salad Sandwich

500 calories
20 g fat (7 g saturated)
1,260 mg sodium

Chicken, Egg & Cheese on a Sunflower Multigrain Bagel

510 calories
22 g fat (6 g saturated)
1,370 mg sodium

Chick-n-Strips Salad
with fat-free honey mustard dressing

Chili's

Did You Know?

● Before Norman Brinker bought the chain in 1983, more than 80 percent of Chili's business was in burgers. Today, only 10 of the more than 175 items on the menu are burgers. (And they average 1,148 calories each.)

MENU MAGIC

In July 2009, Chili's introduced a $20 fixed-price meal for two that includes an appetizer, dessert, and two entrées. Order at random and you'll each average 2,311 calories per meal. Your best bet: order the three least caloric options—the Bottomless Tostada Chips and Salsa (470 calories), a half rack of original ribs (490 calories), and three Key Lime Sweet Shots (240 calories each). You'll consume 1,085 calories each, which won't totally destroy your diets.

Eat This

Southwestern Cedar Plank Tilapia

600 calories
27 g fat
(4 g saturated)
1,820 mg sodium

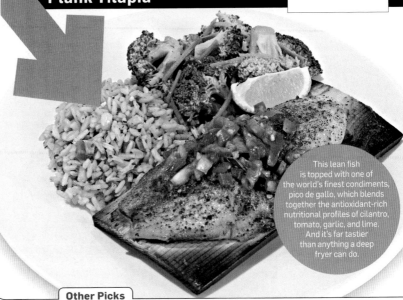

This lean fish is topped with one of the world's finest condiments, pico de gallo, which blends together the antioxidant-rich nutritional profiles of cilantro, tomato, garlic, and lime. And it's far tastier than anything a deep fryer can do.

Other Picks

Guiltless Carne Asada Steak

370 calories
10 g fat (8 g saturated)
1,440 mg sodium

Original Ribs
(½ rack)

490 calories
34 g fat (12 g saturated)
2,050 mg sodium

Fajita Pita Beef Sandwich

490 calories
21 g fat (4 g saturated)
1,540 mg sodium

1,080 calories
71 g fat
(16 g saturated)
2,650 mg sodium

Not That!
Southwestern Cobb Salad

The lettuce in this salad only serves to lend a lean look to a disastrous dish. The greens certainly aren't responsible for the glut of fat and sodium—that would be the work of fried chicken, bacon, and avocado-flavored ranch dressing.

Other Passes

610 calories
11 g fat (2 g saturated)
1,790 mg sodium

Guiltless Black Bean Burger

700 calories
34 g fat (12 g saturated)
2,540 mg sodium

Honey-Chipotle Ribs
(½ rack)

850 calories
35 g fat (7.5 g saturated)
3,520 mg sodium

Classic Steak Fajitas
with 3 tortillas

4,125

Milligrams of sodium in the average fajita plate with three flour tortillas. That's nearly 2 days' worth.

GUILTY PLEASURE

Half Rack Original Ribs

490 calories
34 g fat (12 g saturated)
2,050 mg sodium

You're probably safe with the occasional rib rack, but limit yourself to a half and stick to the original recipe. Every new flavor from there on out just piles on eye-popping amounts of sugar, fat, and salt.

FOOD COURT

THE CRIME
Create Your Own Combo Meal with Grilled Salmon and Sirloin
(1,170 calories)

THE PUNISHMENT
4 hours and 45 minutes vacuuming

113

Chili's (Continued)

Eat This
Oldtimer Big Mouth Burger

820 calories
44 g fat
(12 g saturated)
1,310 mg sodium

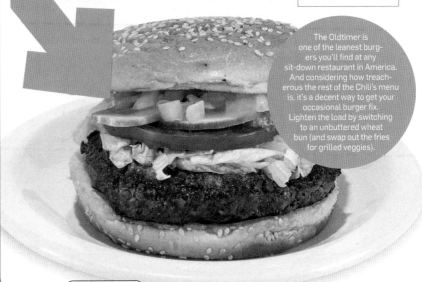

The Oldtimer is one of the leanest burgers you'll find at any sit-down restaurant in America. And considering how treacherous the rest of the Chili's menu is, it's a decent way to get your occasional burger fix. Lighten the load by switching to an unbuttered wheat bun (and swap out the fries for grilled veggies).

Other Picks

Chili's Classic Sirloin topped with Spicy Garlic Shrimp
(3), with garlic toast and seasonal veggies

670 calories
46.5 g fat (12 g saturated)
2,130 mg sodium

Broccoli Cheese Soup
(bowl)

250 calories
16 g fat (7 g saturated)
1,310 mg sodium

Sweet Shot Key Lime Pie

240 calories
12 g fat (8 g saturated)
30 g carbohydrates

1,580 calories
97 g fat
(28 g saturated)
2,930 mg sodium

Not That!

Big Mouth Burger Bites

(4)

Sliders and "small" bites are the most troubling trend in the restaurant industry today. That's because they give the illusion of portion control, but the reality is that bites and sliders almost always contain more calories than the original full-size dishes that inspired their creation.

Other Passes

1,320 calories
76 g fat (38 g saturated)
3,560 mg sodium

Grilled Shrimp Alfredo
with garlic toast

510 calories
35 g fat (21 g saturated)
1,790 mg sodium

Baked Potato Soup
(bowl)

700 calories
42 g fat (26 g saturated)
67 g carbohydrates

Cheesecake

CHICKEN CRISPERS

It takes more than a clever name to undo the harmful effects of thick breading on deep-fried chicken. That's why not one regular Chicken Crispers entrée has fewer than 1,490 calories, and the worst of them—the Crispy Chicken Crisper Tacos—has 1,990 calories. Equally bad is the fact that they average 106.5 grams of fat and 4,050 milligrams of sodium apiece.

SMART SIDES

Marinated Portobella Mushroom

90 calories
8 g fat
(1 g saturated)
75 mg sodium

Mushrooms are an underappreciated stealth-health food. Besides being a low-calorie source of big meaty flavor, they're also the only items in the produce department that can compete with seafood in terms of selenium content. Why should you care? Because selenium is a powerful antioxidant that improves health on several fronts: It may fight prostate cancer, boost the quality of cardiovascular systems, fight bacterial infections, and maybe even help prevent dandruff, among other things.

Did You Know?

● In 2009, Chipotle will serve more than 60 million pounds of naturally raised meat. 100 percent of their pork and chicken and 60 percent of their beef come from animals that were raised in humane conditions, never fed antibiotics or hormones, and fed a pure vegetarian diet.

● Chipotle tested a new menu with smaller-size, lower-priced items in April 2009. We're hoping it goes national.

THE SALSA SELECTOR

GREEN TOMATILLO
15 calories, 0 g fat, 230 mg sodium

TOMATO
20 calories, 0 g fat, 470 mg sodium

RED TOMATILLO
40 calories, 1 g fat, 510 mg sodium

CORN
80 calories, 1.5 g fat, 410 mg sodium

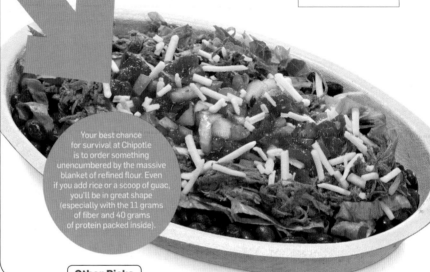

Eat This

Barbacoa Burrito Bowl

with black beans, cheese, lettuce, and tomato salsa

410 calories
17 g fat
(8 g saturated)
1,410 mg sodium

Your best chance for survival at Chipotle is to order something unencumbered by the massive blanket of refined flour. Even if you add rice or a scoop of guac, you'll be in great shape (especially with the 11 grams of fiber and 40 grams of protein packed inside).

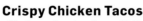

Other Picks

Crispy Chicken Tacos
with cheese, tomato salsa, and lettuce

495 calories
21 g fat (8.5 g saturated)
1,050 mg sodium

Steak Salad
with black beans, cheese, and green tomatillo salsa

435 calories
16 g fat (7 g saturated)
985 mg sodium

Guacamole
with 3 crispy taco shells

330 calories
19 g fat (3.5 g saturated)
220 mg sodium

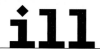

720 calories
41.5 g fat
(11 g saturated)
2,010 mg sodium

Not That!

Chicken Salad

with black beans, red salsa, cheese, and chipotle-honey vinaigrette

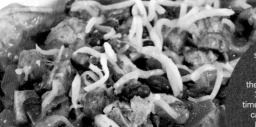

If you're seeking solace in salads at Chipotle, be sure to pass on the one and only vinaigrette on the menu. With 260 calories and 25 grams of fat, it has three times more calories than the most caloric salsa at Chipotle. Your best bet is to turn the tangy green salsa (just 15 calories per serving) into your dressing and spend the 245 calories you save elsewhere.

Other Passes

810 calories
30.5 g fat (12.5 g saturated)
1,480 mg sodium

Chicken Fajita Burrito
with sour cream and corn salsa

830 calories
35.5 g fat (10.5 g saturated)
1,950 mg sodium

Vegetarian Burrito with black beans, cheese, guacamole, and red tomatillo salsa

610 calories
28 g fat (3.5 g saturated)
930 mg sodium

Chips
with red salsa

FOOD COURT

THE CRIME
Carnitas Burrito with Black Beans, Cheese, Sour Cream, and Corn Salsa
(1,030 calories)

THE PUNISHMENT
5 hours of house cleaning

Church's Chicken

Did You Know?

● Church's still uses partially hydrogenated oils in their fryers, which means nearly everything on the menu comes washed in more trans fat than you should consume in a day. Beware: The fries are among the worst menu offenders.

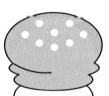

SALT LICK

PREMIUM HOMESTYLE FILLET

with brown gravy (3 oz)

6,691 mg sodium
630 calories
21 g fat
(7 g saturated, 4 g trans)

This dish has more sodium than 80 cups of Newman's Own Butter Boom Popcorn. Blame lies largely with the gravy.

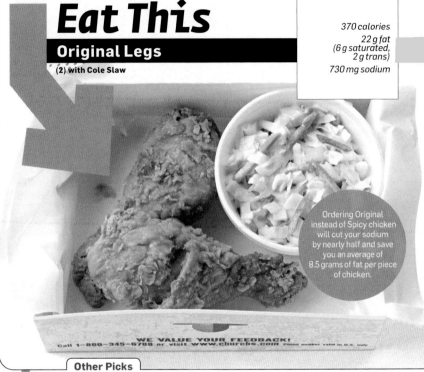

Eat This

Original Legs
(2) with Cole Slaw

370 calories
22 g fat
(6 g saturated, 2 g trans)
730 mg sodium

Ordering Original instead of Spicy chicken will cut your sodium by nearly half and save you an average of 8.5 grams of fat per piece of chicken.

WE VALUE YOUR FEEDBACK!
Call 1-866-345-6788 or visit www.churchs.com

Other Picks

Spicy Chicken Sandwich

456 calories
21 g fat (4 g saturated)
1,292 mg sodium

Nuggets
(5) with purple pepper sauce

207 calories
7 g fat (2 g saturated)
785 mg sodium

Caramel Churro

140 calories
7 g fat (2 g saturated)
4 g sugars

Not That!

Spicy Thigh

with Fried Okra

830 calories
57 g fat
(16 g saturated,
6 g trans)
1,625 mg sodium

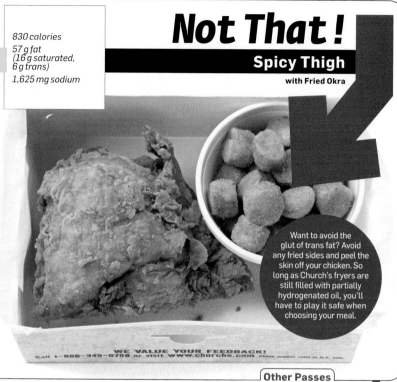

Want to avoid the glut of trans fat? Avoid any fried sides and peel the skin off your chicken. So long as Church's fryers are still filled with partially hydrogenated oil, you'll have to play it safe when choosing your meal.

WE VALUE YOUR FEEDBACK!
Call 1-866-345-6788 or visit www.churchs.com Phone number valid in U.S. only.

Other Passes

623 calories
32 g fat (8 g saturated, 3 g trans)
1,633 mg sodium

Premium Homestyle Sandwich

328 calories
21 g fat (8 g saturated, 2 g trans)
984 mg sodium

Tender Strips
(2) with honey mustard sauce

260 calories
11 g fat (4 g saturated, 2 g trans)
15 g sugars

Apple Pie

CiCi's Pizza

Did You Know?

● It takes 20 minutes for your brain to tell your body that it's full, which can be a perilous problem at free-for-all buffets like CiCi's. Give your brain a head start with these three rules: Begin with a salad, never place more than two slices on your plate, and wait 5 minutes between finishing what's on your plate and going back for more.

1,000

The total number of calories you'll slice from a 15-inch pizza if you order an Olé Pizza instead of the kid-friendly Macaroni & Cheese pie.

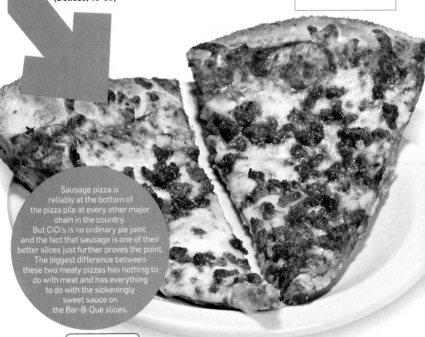

Eat This

Sausage Pizza

(2 slices, To-Go)

340 calories
14 g fat
(6 g saturated)
1,080 mg sodium

Sausage pizza is reliably at the bottom of the pizza pile at every other major chain in the country. But CiCi's is no ordinary pie joint, and the fact that sausage is one of their better slices just further proves the point. The biggest difference between these two meaty pizzas has nothing to do with meat and has everything to do with the sickeningly sweet sauce on the Bar-B-Que slices.

Other Picks

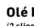

Olé Pizza
(2 slices, To-Go)

260 calories
10 g fat (4 g saturated)
820 mg sodium

Alfredo Pizza
(2 slices)

300 calories
12 g fat (5 g saturated)
720 mg sodium

480 calories
12 g fat
(6 g saturated)
1,420 mg sodium

Not That!

Bar-B-Que Pizza
(2 slices, To-Go)

CiCi's experiments with all sorts of untraditional pizza varieties, and their creations are evenly split between the nutritionally reasonable and the utterly dubious. The Tomato Alfredo and Olé are part of the former group, the Bar-B-Que and Macaroni & Cheese fall firmly in the latter.

MENU DECODER

● FLIP PIZZA:
A surprisingly decent CiCi's creation that folds a pizza over on itself so that the toppings are locked inside a jacket of crust.

HIDDEN DANGER

Zesty Veggie
(1 slice)

To be fair, the menus of America are littered with fat bombs far worse, but what irks us about this slice is that it's one of the few on CiCi's menu to harbor trans fat—and it's a vegetable pizza! The Pepperoni, Sausage, and Deep Dish pizzas don't have a trans-fat problem, but apparently CiCi's couldn't work it out with the Zesty Veggie. If it's a trans-fat-free meal you want, avoid pies with either "Zesty" or "Chicken" in their names.

130 calories
4 g fat
(1 g saturated,
1 g trans)
320 mg sodium

Other Passes

Cheese Pizza
(2 slices, To-Go)

380 calories
10 g fat (4 g saturated)
820 mg sodium

Ham and Pineapple Pizza
(2 slices, To-Go)

400 calories
12 g fat (5 g saturated)
1,000 mg sodium

Cold Stone Creamery

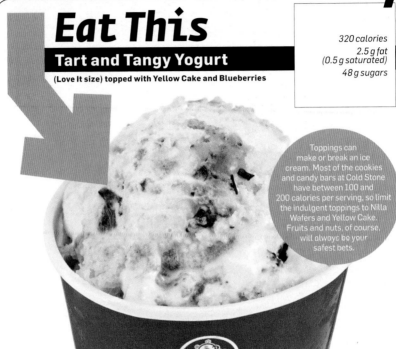

Eat This

Tart and Tangy Yogurt

(Love It size) topped with Yellow Cake and Blueberries

320 calories
2.5 g fat
(0.5 g saturated)
48 g sugars

Toppings can make or break an ice cream. Most of the cookies and candy bars at Cold Stone have between 100 and 200 calories per serving, so limit the indulgent toppings to Nilla Wafers and Yellow Cake. Fruits and nuts, of course, will always be your safest bets.

MENU MAGIC

Ordering an iced or blended coffee drink is a decent way to bypass the hazards of an otherwise bloated beverage menu, but only if you specify that you want yours made "Lite." It means you get skim milk instead of the high-fat proprietary blend that goes into each cup by default—a swap that saves you an average of 14 grams of fat per drink.

Other Picks

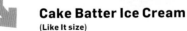

Cake Batter Ice Cream
(Like It size)

340 calories
19 g fat (12 g saturated, 0.5 g trans)
32 g sugars

Egg Nog Ice Cream
(Like It size)

260 calories
15 g fat (10 g saturated)
21 g sugars

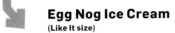

Vanilla Crème Latte
(Like It size)

280 calories
12 g fat (8 g saturated)
35 g sugars

Not That!
Blueberry Muffin Ice Cream
(Love It size)

530 calories
30 g fat
(20 g saturated,
1 g trans)
52 g sugars

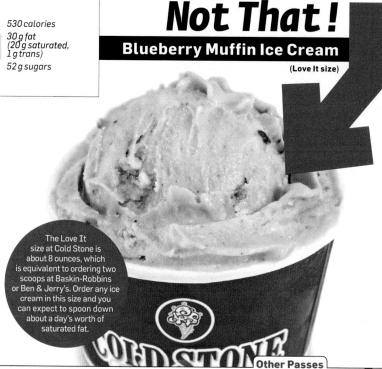

The Love It size at Cold Stone is about 8 ounces, which is equivalent to ordering two scoops at Baskin-Robbins or Ben & Jerry's. Order any ice cream in this size and you can expect to spoon down about a day's worth of saturated fat.

Other Passes

670 calories
7 g fat (2 g saturated)
57 g sugars

Sinless Cake 'n Shake Milkshake
(Like It size)

390 calories
24 g fat (13 g saturated)
35 g sugars

Nutter Butter Ice Cream
(Like It size)

1,320 calories
62 g fat (39 g saturated, 1.5 g trans)
134 g sugars

Lotta Caramel Latte Milkshake (Like It size)

WEAPON OF MASS DESTRUCTION
PB&C Shake
(Gotta Have It size)

2,010 calories
131 g fat (68 g saturated,
2.5 g trans) 153 g sugars

You could blend together four large orders of McDonald's French fries and still not reach this massive load of calories. But if, by chance, you did go the unfathomable fry route, at least you'd cut out 80 percent of the saturated fat. That's why we've dubbed this thing the Worst Drink in America.

STEALTH HEALTH FOOD
Roasted Almond Topping
(1 oz)

150 calories
14 g fat (1 g saturated)
85 mg sodium

Why not top your treat with a bona-fide health food? Almonds employ three mechanisms to help stabilize your blood glucose as you spoon down the sweet cream; monounsaturated fats, protein, and fiber. That makes them an effective weapon against both diabetes and cardiovascular disease.

Così

Did You Know?

● Così falls into the category of "Fast Casual Dining," joining the likes of Au Bon Pain, Chipotle, Panera, and Qdoba. The concept behind Fast Casual Dining is to provide more sophisticated food choices than fast-food restaurants, but with the same speed of delivery. Fast Casual places may give off virtuous vibes, but the potential for danger is every bit as rife as a drive-thru window.

GUILTY PLEASURE

S'mores with Oreos

350 calories
11 g fat
59 g carbohydrates

For what you get—chocolate, marshmallow, a giant Oreo—the caloric cost here is really reasonable, especially when you consider that it will save you 220 calories and 25 grams of fat when ordered instead of the Brownie Blondie.

124

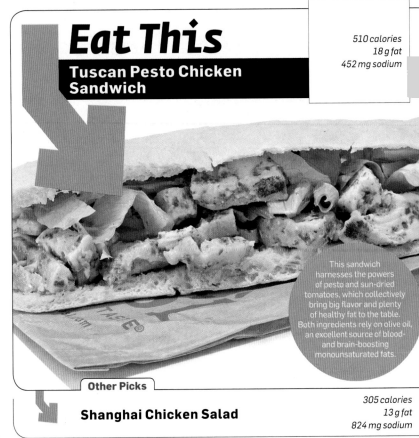

Eat This

Tuscan Pesto Chicken Sandwich

510 calories
18 g fat
452 mg sodium

This sandwich harnesses the powers of pesto and sun-dried tomatoes, which collectively bring big flavor and plenty of healthy fat to the table. Both ingredients rely on olive oil, an excellent source of blood- and brain-boosting monounsaturated fats.

Other Picks

Shanghai Chicken Salad

305 calories
13 g fat
824 mg sodium

Chocolate Croissant

324 calories
17 g fat
41 g carbohydrates

Apple Empanada

279 calories
15 g fat
32 g carbohydrates

722 calories
40 g fat
845 mg sodium

Not That!
Chicken TBM Sandwich

These two sandwiches are driven by all of the same flavors—tomatoes, basil, and chicken—but this version will saddle you with an extra 212 calories and more than double the fat of its pesto-paved relative.

MENU MAGIC

Look past the croissant and bagel-encased sandwiches and make Così's steel-cut oats the centerpiece of your breakfast. Ask them to sweeten it up with fresh strawberries and top it with pistachios, and then order a fruit salad and a cup of coffee on the side. All told, your damage will come in under 250 calories—that's about 400 fewer than any breakfast sandwich on the menu.

Other Passes

519 calories
34 g fat
1,347 mg sodium

Così Cobb Light Salad

510 calories
25 g fat
62 g carbohydrates

Banana Nut Muffin

964 calories
41 g fat
145 g carbohydrates

Cinnamon Apple Pie

Culver's

Did You Know?

● Culver's Butter-Burger is its claim to juicy-burger fame. But to native Midwesterners, it's standard fare. Some sandwich a butter pat between two hot beef burgers. Others add melted margarine to uncooked meat. Culver's recipe uses a traditional hamburger smeared with the full-fat spread. Shockingly, Culver's burgers still rank among the healthiest in the country.

Eat This

Mushroom & Swiss Burger

(single)

431 calories
20 g fat
(9 g saturated, 1 g trans)
551 mg sodium

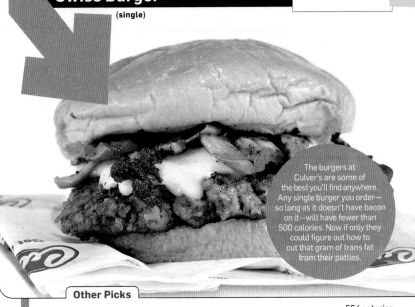

The burgers at Culver's are some of the best you'll find anywhere. Any single burger you order—so long as it doesn't have bacon on it—will have fewer than 500 calories. Now if only they could figure out how to cut that gram of trans fat from their patties.

Other Picks

Sourdough Melt
with mashed potatoes and gravy

554 calories
22 g fat (10 g saturated, 1 g trans)
994 mg sodium

Flame Roasted Chicken Sandwich
with small fries

584 calories
21 g fat (5 g saturated)
1,020 mg sodium

Vanilla Custard (1 scoop)
with pineapple and hot fudge

372 calories
19 g fat (12 g saturated, 1 g trans)
39 g sugars

663 calories
*41 g fat
(7 g saturated,
1 g trans)*
979 mg sodium

Not That!

North Atlantic Cod Fillet Sandwich

Here's a new rule to live by: Fish stops being seafood as soon as it gets battered and fried. After that, it's no better than the grease it was cooked in.

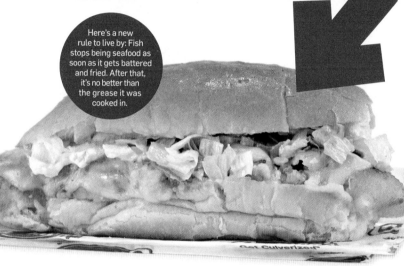

Got Culverized

Other Passes

881 calories
73 g fat (18 g saturated, 1 g trans)
1,691 mg sodium

Strawberry Fields Salad
with bleu cheese dressing

1,265 calories
67 g fat (16 g saturated)
2,336 mg sodium

Chicken Basket
(thigh, leg, and fries)

1,084 calories
64 g fat (28 g saturated, 1 g trans)
94 g sugars

Banana Split

Dairy Queen

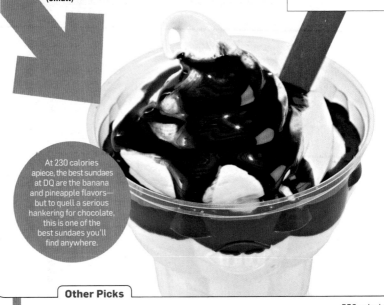

Did You Know?

● Surprise: Dairy Queen actually doesn't serve ice cream. Not in the traditional sense, anyway. Its soft serve is made with milk instead of cream and contains significantly less fat than regular frozen treats: 7 grams for a small vanilla cone, compared to 16 grams in Baskin Robbins' variety (which is also 20 percent smaller).

Eat This

Hot Fudge Sundae

(small)

300 calories
10 g fat
(7 g saturated)
37 g sugars

At 230 calories apiece, the best sundaes at DQ are the banana and pineapple flavors—but to quell a serious hankering for chocolate, this is one of the best sundaes you'll find anywhere.

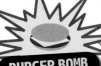

BURGER BOMB

½ lb Flame Thrower

1,060 calories
75 g fat (26 g saturated)
1,980 mg sodium

Laced with jalapeno bacon and Tabasco mayo, this novelty burger will torch any efforts at sustaining a health diet. If you want the heat, ask for the Flame Thrower treatment on a grilled chicken breast.

Other Picks

Original Hamburger and Grilled Chicken Wrap

550 calories
26 g fat (10 g saturated, 0.5 g trans)
1,130 mg sodium

Original Double Hamburger

540 calories
26 g fat (13 g saturated, 1 g trans)
740 mg sodium

Pancake Platter with Ham

380 calories
8 g fat (2 g saturated, 1 g trans)
1,510 mg sodium

700 calories
23 g fat
(16 g saturated,
1 g trans)
85 g sugars

Not That!

Hot Fudge Malt

(small)

Drinkable ice cream is nearly as bad of an idea as fried ice cream, but believe it or not, the former tends to be saddled with more sugar and more fat than the latter. You'd be wise to expunge shakes and malts from your list of acceptable desserts.

Other Passes

1,360 calories
63 g fat (11 g saturated, 1 g trans)
2,910 mg sodium

Chicken Strip Basket
(4 pieces) with country gravy

910 calories
54 g fat (25 g saturated, 1.5 g trans)
1,540 mg sodium

½ lb Classic GrillBurger

1,100 calories
64 g fat (15 g saturated, 8 g trans)
3,030 mg sodium

Country Platter with Ham

129

Del Taco

Did You Know?

● Del Taco is one of the few fast-food joints that actually cooks food on-site, rather than reheating prefab fare. The lard-free beans are made from scratch daily, the chicken is grilled fresh every hour, and the produce is fresh.

● As with Taco Bell, the salads on Del Taco's menu are among the worst things you can order. You're better off ordering almost any burrito, burger, or taco than you are ordering the Deluxe Taco Salad.

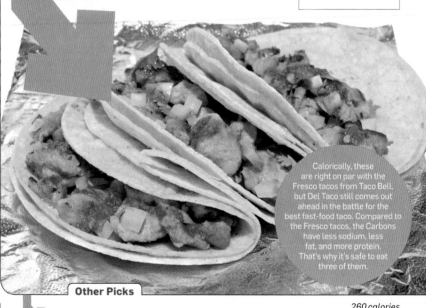

Eat This

Chicken Tacos Del Carbon

(3 tacos)

450 calories
15 g fat
(0 g saturated)
900 mg sodium

Calorically, these are right on par with the Fresco tacos from Taco Bell, but Del Taco still comes out ahead in the battle for the best fast-food taco. Compared to the Fresco tacos, the Carbons have less sodium, less fat, and more protein. That's why it's safe to eat three of them.

Other Picks

Tostada

260 calories
13 g fat (5 g saturated)
350 mg sodium

Breakfast Del Carbon Tacos (2)

280 calories
10 g fat (2 g saturated)
340 mg sodium

½ lb Green Burrito

430 calories
10 g fat (5 g saturated)
1,190 mg sodium

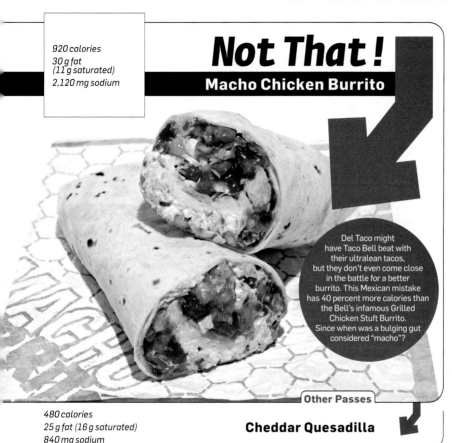

920 calories
30 g fat
(11 g saturated)
2,120 mg sodium

Not That!
Macho Chicken Burrito

Del Taco might have Taco Bell beat with their ultralean tacos, but they don't even come close in the battle for a better burrito. This Mexican mistake has 40 percent more calories than the Bell's infamous Grilled Chicken Stuft Burrito. Since when was a bulging gut considered "macho"?

Other Passes

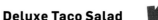

480 calories
25 g fat (16 g saturated)
840 mg sodium

Cheddar Quesadilla

520 calories
25 g fat (10 g saturated)
1,220 mg sodium

Steak & Egg Burrito

850 calories
46 g fat (18 g saturated)
1,690 mg sodium

Deluxe Taco Salad

Bacon & Egg Quesadilla

*430 calories
20 g fat (10 g saturated)
850 mg sodium*

A meal based around cheese and bacon rarely gets plaudits from us, but this quesadilla is an exception. If it weren't for the high saturated fat, it'd get a standing ovation. It has a couple grams of fiber, 20 grams of protein, and 35 percent of your day's calcium. Just be sure to go light on saturated fat for the rest of the day.

950

Number of calories in a Triple Del Cheeseburger.

MEET YOUR MATCH

Macho Nachos
(1,090 calories)
=
7.3 Fresco Crunchy Tacos from Taco Bell

131

Denny's

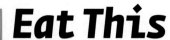

Did You Know?

● In July 2009, a New Jersey man filed a lawsuit against Denny's, alleging that the chain's heavy use of salt puts their customers at risk of high blood pressure, heart attack, and stroke. Credit Denny's for quickly revamping their menu, launching a new and improved section called Better For You.

ATTACK OF THE APPETIZER

Cheesy Three Pack

1,940 calories
125 g fat
(23 g saturated,
2 g trans)
3,850 mg sodium

Even split three ways, this trans-fatty triumvirate will cost you 650 calories, more than 1,000 milligrams of sodium, and 40 grams of fat...before dinner even arrives!

Eat This

Top Sirloin Steak & Fried Eggs

420 calories
21 g fat
(6 g saturated,
0.5 g trans)
920 mg sodium

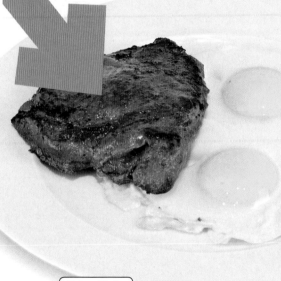

Believe it or not, this is actually a moderately healthy breakfast. Studies show that a protein-rich start to the day will supercharge your metabolism and prevent you from overeating later.

Other Picks

Fit Fare Grilled Chicken
with vegetables and tomatoes

380 calories
10 g fat (2 g saturated)
1,280 mg sodium

Bacon, Lettuce & Tomato Sandwich

570 calories
37 g fat (9 g saturated)
850 mg sodium

Hashed Browns

200 calories
12 g fat (3 g saturated)
560 mg sodium

1,150 calories
66 g fat
(20 g saturated,
0.5 g trans)
2,800 mg sodium

Not That!
Heartland Scramble

As used here, "heartland" must refer to the cardiac center at your nearest hospital. Between the moguls of cheese, bacon, and fried potatoes, this thing gobbles up a full day's worth of saturated fat and more than a day's worth of sodium.

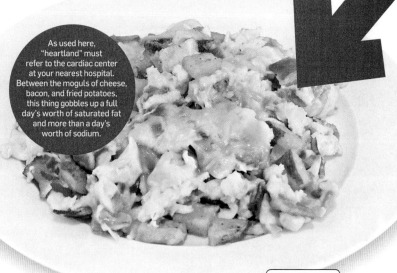

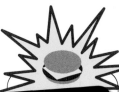

BURGER BOMB

Double Cheeseburger

1,540 calories
116 g fat
(52 g saturated, 7 g trans)
3,880 mg sodium

Care for a side of elevated blood pressure? That's basically what you're getting when you order this thing. It has more than 1½ days' worth of sodium, 2½ days' worth of saturated fat, and 3 days' worth of trans fat. Want to add Seasoned Fries? Tack on an extra 510 calories and 33 grams of fat. Hope you have good health care.

MENU MAGIC

A normal egg has about 5 or 6 grams of fat, but Denny's have a shocking 10 grams apiece—even more than a side of chicken sausage. Ask for egg whites, instead, to save a whopping 95 calories per egg. That adds up to close to 300 calories in a three-egg omelet.

Other Passes

600 calories
11 g fat (3 g saturated)
1,560 mg sodium

Fit Fare
Grilled Tilapia

970 calories
58 g fat (10 g saturated)
2,070 mg sodium

Grilled Chicken Sandwich

390 calories
28 g fat (6 g saturated)
560 mg sodium

Country-Fried Potatoes

Domino's

Did You Know?

● Four chains make up 71 percent of all pizza sales. Pizza Hut dominates with 32.7 percent, but Domino's comes in second with 19.4 percent of the pie market share.

● After a decline in sales in 2007, Domino's relaunched their "You Got 30 Minutes" slogan to play up their fast reputation. They also held a "world's fastest pizza maker" competition. The winner was Dennis Tran, an executive VP of operations for Domino's, who made three large pizzas in 46.4 seconds.

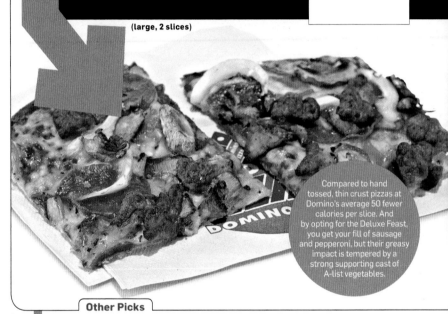

Eat This
Thin Crust Deluxe Feast

480 calories
29 g fat
(10 g saturated)
1,060 mg sodium

(large, 2 slices)

Compared to hand tossed, thin crust pizzas at Domino's average 50 fewer calories per slice. And by opting for the Deluxe Feast, you get your fill of sausage and pepperoni, but their greasy impact is tempered by a strong supporting cast of A-list vegetables.

Other Picks

Thin Crust Philly Cheese Steak Feast Pizza (medium, 2 slices)

360 calories
21 g fat (10 g saturated)
750 mg sodium

Hand Tossed Garlic and Green Olive Pizza (large, 2 slices)

510 calories
18 g fat (6 g saturated)
1,090 mg sodium

Hand Tossed Chicken and Bacon Pizza (medium, 2 slices)

410 calories
14 g fat (6 g saturated)
940 mg sodium

134

680 calories
32 g fat
(12 g saturated)
1,620 mg sodium

Not That!

Hand Tossed Sausage and Pepperoni

(large, 2 slices)

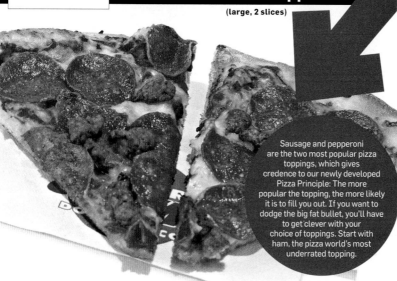

Sausage and pepperoni are the two most popular pizza toppings, which gives credence to our newly developed Pizza Principle: The more popular the topping, the more likely it is to fill you out. If you want to dodge the big fat bullet, you'll have to get clever with your choice of toppings. Start with ham, the pizza world's most underrated topping.

Other Passes

460 calories
31 g fat (11 g saturated)
1,210 mg sodium

Thin Crust ExtravaganZZa
(medium, 2 slices)

760 calories
38 g fat (15 g saturated)
1,640 mg sodium

Deep Dish Pacific Veggie Pizza
(large, 2 slices)

620 calories
35 g fat (12 g saturated)
1,250 mg sodium

Hand Tossed Cali Chicken Bacon Ranch Pizza **(medium, 2 slices)**

MEAT TOPPING TOTEM POLE
(per 2 medium slices)

HAM
8 calories, 0 g fat,
200 mg sodium

ANCHOVIES
8 calories, 0 g fat,
300 mg sodium

PHILLY MEAT
16 calories, 0 g fat,
120 mg sodium

CHICKEN
34 calories, 1 g fat,
180 mg sodium

BEEF
70 calories, 6 g fat,
140 mg sodium

PEPPERONI
70 calories, 6 g fat,
300 mg sodium

BACON
78 calories, 6 g fat,
200 mg sodium

SAUSAGE
88 calories, 7 g fat,
260 mg sodium

STEALTH HEALTH FOOD
Black Olives

You know all that hype about the healthy fats in olive oil? Well those fats, monounsaturates, are also found in olives, and they've been shown to reduce bad cholesterol and decrease the risk of heart disease and stroke. Olives are also a great source of vitamin E, an antioxidant that helps protect your skin.

Domino's (Continued)

Did You Know?

● Domino's partnered with Warner Bros. to promote the release of *The Dark Knight* in 2008. One promotional tactic was the creation of the new Gotham City Pizza, a large, hand-tossed pie with 50 percent more pepperoni than a standard portion. A pizza like that will leave you looking less like the Caped Crusader and more like Danny DeVito's Penguin from *Batman Returns*.

● People tend to consider pizza a guilty pleasure, and 8 in 10 respondents to a Mintel survey claimed to "not care if it's healthy or not." It would probably come as a surprise to them, then, that two slices of thin crust pizza with green peppers and sausage have only 340 calories and 12 grams of fat.

Eat This

Hand-Tossed Chicken, Bacon, and Tomato Pizza

(large, 2 slices)

600 calories
23 g fat
(8 g saturated)
1,420 mg sodium

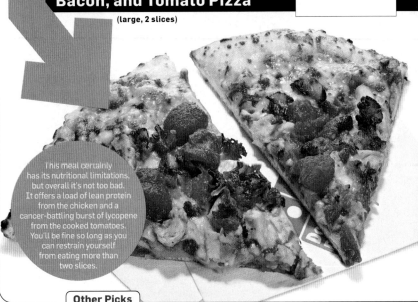

This meal certainly has its nutritional limitations, but overall it's not too bad. It offers a load of lean protein from the chicken and a cancer-battling burst of lycopene from the cooked tomatoes. You'll be fine so long as you can restrain yourself from eating more than two slices.

Other Picks

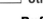

Buffalo Chicken Kickers
(6 pieces)

300 calories
13.5 g fat (1.5 g saturated)
840 mg sodium

Build Your Own Pasta with spinach, mushroom, pepperoni, and hearty marinara sauce

420 calories
11.5 g fat (3.5 g saturated)
1,160 mg sodium

Thin Crust Chicken and Green Pepper Pizza (medium, 2 slices)

300 calories
14 g fat (5 g saturated)
610 mg sodium

1,480 calories
56 g fat
(24 g saturated)
2,280 mg sodium

Not That!

Chicken Carbonara Bread Bowl Pasta

This one tops our list of Dumbest Ideas in Restaurant History. The bowl itself—before you fill in the pasta—carries 840 calories and a third of your day's saturated fat.

Domino's recently launched two new product lines: Bread Bowl Pastas, which average over 1,400 calories each, and Chocolate Lava Crunch Cakes, which ring in at 357 calories each. The most troubling thing, however, was their end-of-summer product promotion: Throughout August and September of 2009, any purchase of a Bread Bowl Pasta came with a free Chocolate Lava Crunch Cake, making for a cataclysmic carbohydrate load.

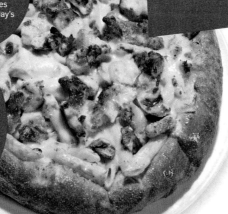

Other Passes

690 calories
42 g fat (10.5 g saturated)
1,230 mg sodium

Barbeque Buffalo Wings
(6 pieces)

770 calories
30 g fat (16 g saturated, 1 g trans)
2,130 mg sodium

Chicken Parm Oven Baked Sandwich

430 calories
33 g fat (9 g saturated)
1,070 mg sodium

Grilled Chicken Caesar Salad
with blue cheese

137

Dunkin' Donuts

Did You Know?

● Doughnut sales account for just 12 percent of Dunkin's revenue, but they've recently refocused their advertising to reverse that trend. The idea is that, since the average doughnut costs about 89 cents, money-conscious consumers will buy more of them.

● For 3 years in a row, Dunkin' Donuts has ranked first place for customer loyalty to their coffee, according to polls run by consulting firm Brand Keys.

● In 2008, Dunkin' ran an ad featuring Rachael Ray wearing a black and white scarf. Conservative bloggers quickly complained that the scarf looked like an Arab kaffiyah and somehow promoted jihad. DD caved and pulled the ad.

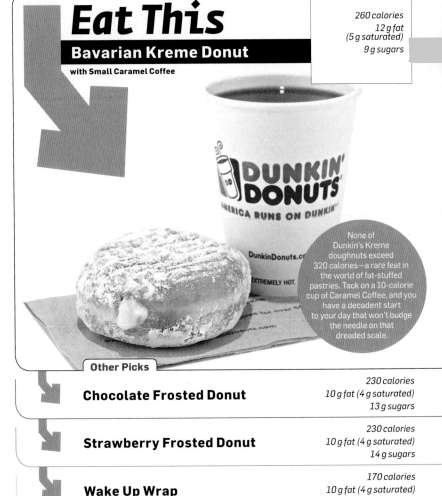

Eat This

Bavarian Kreme Donut

with Small Caramel Coffee

260 calories
12 g fat
(5 g saturated)
9 g sugars

None of Dunkin's Kreme doughnuts exceed 320 calories—a rare feat in the world of fat-stuffed pastries. Tack on a 10-calorie cup of Caramel Coffee, and you have a decadent start to your day that won't budge the needle on that dreaded scale.

Other Picks

Chocolate Frosted Donut

230 calories
10 g fat (4 g saturated)
13 g sugars

Strawberry Frosted Donut

230 calories
10 g fat (4 g saturated)
14 g sugars

Wake Up Wrap

170 calories
10 g fat (4 g saturated)
450 mg sodium

590 calories
20 g fat
(12 g saturated)
69 g sugars

Not That!

Apple Crumb Donut

with Small Coffee with Cream and Sugar

Fruity names aside, crumb doughnuts are the worst doughnut option. Just as bad is the normal coffee order. Cream and sugar add 115 calories to a small, so if you slug through two or three a day, expect to carry an extra 25 to 35 pounds.

Other Passes

380 calories
18 g fat (8 g saturated)
19 g sugars

Vanilla Frosted Coffee Roll

450 calories
10 g fat (1.5 g saturated)
45 g sugars

Reduced Fat Blueberry Muffin

450 calories
12 g fat (5.5 g saturated)
900 mg sodium

Wheat Bagel (with Reduced Fat Cream Cheese)

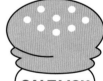

CONDIMENT CATASTROPHE

Plain Cream Cheese
(50 g)

150 calories
15 g fat (9 g saturated)
250 mg sodium

This spread stuffs your arteries with about half a day's worth of saturated fat. Your best bet is to switch to jelly, but if you're stuck on cream cheese, go for the unflavored, reduced-fat version. It still has 5 grams of saturated fat, though, so limit yourself to the thinnest layer you can stand.

SALT LICK

SALT BAGEL

3,540 mg sodium

The average U.S. adult already eats about 1,000 mg too much sodium each day. That's partially why heart disease is still the number one killer in this country. Unless it's a simple saltine, avoid any food with "salt" in its name.

Dunkin' Donuts (Continued)

Did You Know?

⬤ Dunkin' has made some major efforts to clean up their nutritional act in recent years, first by mostly eliminating trans fat from their menu in 2008 and then by introducing the DDSmart Menu. This new line is filled with low-calorie items like flatbread sandwiches, which contain fewer than 300 calories. When paired with a tea or coffee with Splenda, one makes the perfect breakfast.

75

Grams of sugar in the average medium Coolatta. That's the sugar equivalent of 12 Jelly Filled Donuts.

Eat This

Turkey Cheddar & Bacon Flatbread

390 calories
19 g fat
(7 g saturated)
1,090 mg sodium

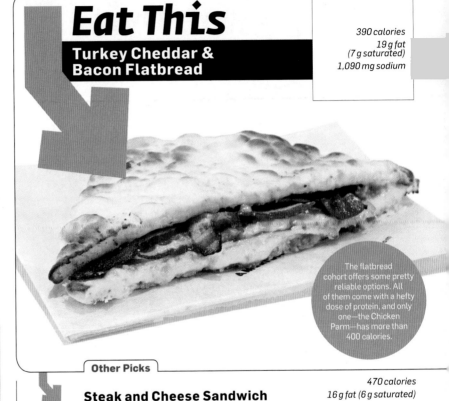

The flatbread cohort offers some pretty reliable options. All of them come with a hefty dose of protein, and only one—the Chicken Parm—has more than 400 calories.

Other Picks

Steak and Cheese Sandwich

470 calories
16 g fat (6 g saturated)
2,040 mg sodium

Ham, Supreme Omelet & Cheese
on English Muffin

390 calories
16 g fat (8 g saturated)
1,340 mg sodium

Vanilla Iced Latte Lite
(small, 16 fl oz)

90 calories
0 g fat
10 g sugars

Not That!

Chicken Parmesan Flatbread

480 calories
22 g fat
(7 g saturated)
1,220 mg sodium

What's the point of using low-calorie flatbread if you're just going to stuff it with fried chicken and cheese? Sadly, Dunkin's chicken sandwiches only get worse from here.

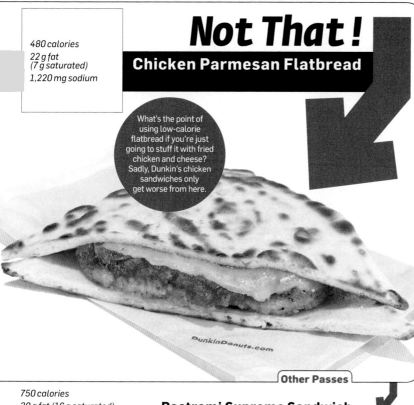

DunkinDonuts.com

Other Passes

750 calories
39 g fat (16 g saturated)
2,060 mg sodium

Pastrami Supreme Sandwich

510 calories
30 g fat (12 g saturated)
1,050 mg sodium

Ham, Egg & Cheese
on Croissant

430 calories
6 g fat (3.5 g saturated)
86 g sugars

Vanilla Bean Coolatta
(small, 16 fl oz)

MENU MISNOMER

Tuna (Albacore) Sandwich

660 calories
19 g fat (2.5 g saturated)
1,280 mg sodium

Let's set the record straight: There's a big difference between "tuna" and "tuna salad." Tuna is a lean fish loaded with protein, B vitamins, and other good stuff. Tuna salad, on the other hand, gets more of its calories from fatty mayonnaise than from the fish that's drowning in it. It is to tuna what French fries are to potatoes. With about a third of your day's calories, this sandwich falls decidedly in the "salad" category.

SMART SIDES

Chicken Noodle Soup
(8 oz)

130 calories
3 g fat (1 g saturated)
970 mg sodium

Broth-based soups are an ideal way to fill your stomach without adding a ton of extra calories to your diet. Pair this bowl with an Egg White Turkey Sausage Flatbread Sandwich for one of the leanest lunches on the menu: 410 calories and only 9 grams of fat. Just be careful to watch your sodium intake for the rest of the day: Soup is notoriously salty.

Einstein Bros./Noah's

Did You Know?

● In 2007, more than 63 percent of Einstein Bros.' sales were made during the breakfast rush. Breakfast sandwiches rank as the top menu item, as well as the fastest-growing menu item, which is unfortunate, considering that the average sandwich contains 636 calories and 28 g fat. The best on their menu is the 540-calorie Egg Way, Spinach Mushroom and Swiss Omelette Sandwich. Your best bet? Fruit and Yogurt Parfait.

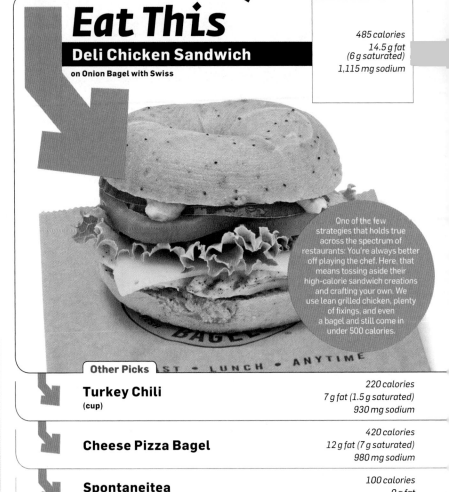

Eat This

Deli Chicken Sandwich

on Onion Bagel with Swiss

485 calories
14.5 g fat
(6 g saturated)
1,115 mg sodium

One of the few strategies that holds true across the spectrum of restaurants: You're always better off playing the chef. Here, that means tossing aside their high-calorie sandwich creations and crafting your own. We use lean grilled chicken, plenty of fixings, and even a bagel and still come in under 500 calories.

Other Picks

Turkey Chili
(cup)

220 calories
7 g fat (1.5 g saturated)
930 mg sodium

Cheese Pizza Bagel

420 calories
12 g fat (7 g saturated)
980 mg sodium

Spontaneitea
(large, 24 fl oz)

100 calories
0 g fat
25 g sugars

Not That!

Bros Bistro Salad

with Chicken

940 calories
71 g fat
(12 g saturated)
810 mg sodium

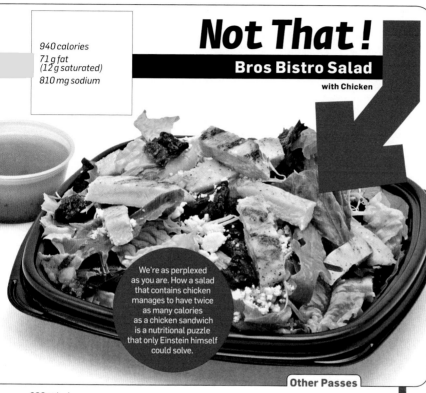

We're as perplexed as you are. How a salad that contains chicken manages to have twice as many calories as a chicken sandwich is a nutritional puzzle that only Einstein himself could solve.

Other Passes

290 calories
20 g fat (10 g saturated)
990 mg sodium

Vegetarian Broccoli Cheese Soup
(cup)

690 calories
41 g fat (9 g saturated, 1 g trans)
1510 mg sodium

Deli Turkey and Swiss

360 calories
3 g fat (2 g saturated)
105 g sugars

Chai Tea with 2% milk
(large, 20 oz)

CONDIMENT CATASTROPHE

Creamy Mustard Spread
(1.5 oz)

270 calories
29 g fat (4.5 g saturated)
220 mg sodium

This spread is actually mayonnaise masquerading as mustard. Mayo is the first ingredient listed, and the mixture contains less than 2 percent mustard. That's why every sandwich it touches has at least 690 calories. Ask them to switch yours to real, unadulterated mustard.

STEALTH HEALTH FOOD
Hummus
(1 oz)

70 calories
3 g fat
(0 g saturated)
150 mg sodium

A good bagel spread accomplishes two goals: It adds flavor and contributes healthy nutrients. Cream cheese might succeed on the first front, but it fails miserably on the second. Switch to Einstein's hummus, and you'll nail them both. Hummus is made from garbanzo beans, ground sesame seeds, and olive oil, so it packs the full gamut of healthy, hunger-fighting nutrients: fiber, protein, and healthy fats.

143

El Pollo Loco

Did You Know?

● El Pollo Loco, founded in Guasave, Mexico, in 1975 and moved to the United States in 1980, now considers itself to be at war with KFC. In one of a slew of recent attack ads, the El Pollo Loco president and CEO stands in a pasture with grazing cows and complains that KFC's new grilled chicken marinade contains beef ingredients. KFC has yet to respond.

Eat This

Chicken Caesar Bowl

490 calories
22 g fat
(4.5 g saturated)
1,200 mg sodium

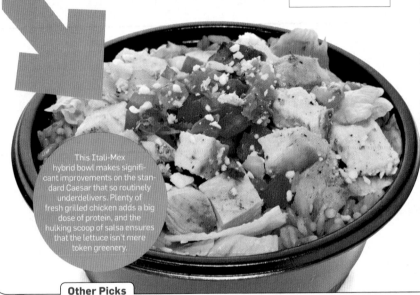

This Itali-Mex hybrid bowl makes significant improvements on the standard Caesar that so routinely underdelivers. Plenty of fresh grilled chicken adds a big dose of protein, and the hulking scoop of salsa ensures that the lettuce isn't mere token greenery.

Other Picks

Two BBQ Chicken Sliders

364 calories
10 g fat (2 g saturated)
954 mg sodium

Crunchy Chicken Tacos (2)

380 calories
16 g fat (5 g saturated)
960 mg sodium

Chicken Taquito with Avocado Salsa

230 calories
12 g fat (2.5 g saturated)
590 mg sodium

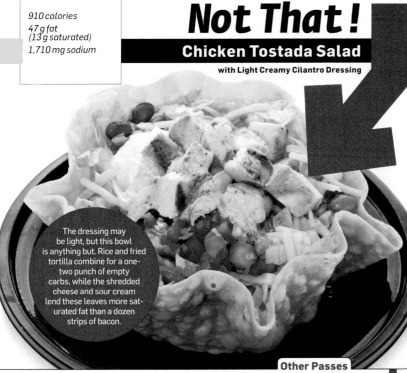

910 calories
47 g fat
(13 g saturated)
1,710 mg sodium

Not That!

Chicken Tostada Salad

with Light Creamy Cilantro Dressing

The dressing may be light, but this bowl is anything but. Rice and fried tortilla combine for a one-two punch of empty carbs, while the shredded cheese and sour cream lend these leaves more saturated fat than a dozen strips of bacon.

Other Passes

1,034 calories
64 g fat (12 g saturated)
1,942 mg sodium

Two Classic Chicken Sliders

710 calories
23 g fat (9 g saturated)
1,690 mg sodium

Ultimate Grilled Burrito

420 calories
23 g fat (13 g saturated)
810 mg sodium

Cheese Quesadilla

WEAPON OF MASS DESTRUCTION
Ultimate Pollo Bowl

1,050 calories
34 g fat (14 g saturated)
2,520 mg sodium

This thing is more like a Mexican buffet than a meal for one; by mass, it's bigger than six whole chicken legs. Unless you're looking for a meal to split, stick with one of the properly portioned, perfectly satisfying regular bowls, and avoid the Ultimate.

STEALTH HEALTH FOOD
Salsa Bar

Salsa is now America's most popular condiment (take that, ketchup!). Good thing El Pollo Loco lets you ladle on as much of the topping as you want. The restaurant offers four varieties, and only the Spicy Avocado surpasses 15 calories per a 1.5-ounce serving. The rest are tomato based, which means that they're loaded with vitamins C and A, as well as the antioxidant lycopene, a carotenoid that has been shown to fight many types of cancer, including breast, prostate, and lung.

145

Fazoli's

Eat This

Penne Rosa

with Savory Chicken

660 calories
16 g fat
(6 g saturated)
1,660 mg sodium

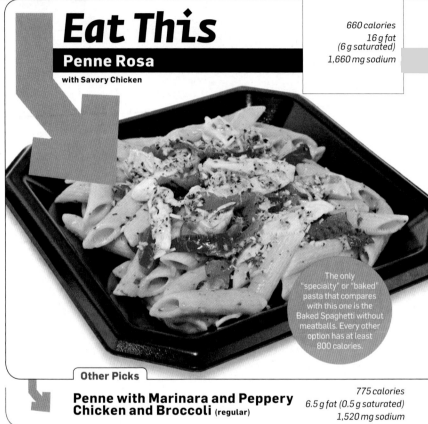

The only "specialty" or "baked" pasta that compares with this one is the Baked Spaghetti without meatballs. Every other option has at least 800 calories.

Other Picks

Penne with Marinara and Peppery Chicken and Broccoli (regular)

775 calories
6.5 g fat (0.5 g saturated)
1,520 mg sodium

Cheese Pizza (2 slices)

540 calories
22 g fat (10 g saturated, 1 g trans)
1,380 mg sodium

Grilled Chicken Artichoke Salad
with red wine vinaigrette

350 calories
14.5 g fat (4 g saturated)
1,320 mg sodium

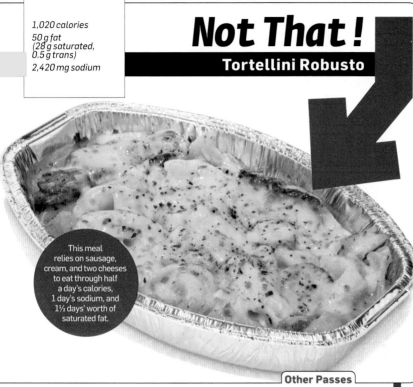

1,020 calories
50 g fat
(28 g saturated,
0.5 g trans)
2,420 mg sodium

Not That !

Tortellini Robusto

This meal relies on sausage, cream, and two cheeses to eat through half a day's calories, 1 day's sodium, and 1½ days' worth of saturated fat.

WEAPON OF MASS DESTRUCTION
Rigatoni Romano

880 calories
44 g fat
(20 g saturated, 1 g trans)
2,510 mg sodium

This baked pasta would be on the indulgent side even if split in half, so it's a mystery why Fazoli's would pile this much saturated fat and sodium onto one plate. Stick with sides of Seasoned Rice and Mashed Potatoes and Gravy.

HIDDEN DANGER

Garlic Breadstick

Casually nosh your way through a couple of these during the course of your meal, and you've just put yourself 300 calories deeper into caloric debt. If you haven't already worked out how you're going to pay it off, don't even bother eating it.

150 calories
7 g fat
(1.5 g saturated)
290 mg sodium

Other Passes

920 calories
42 g fat (24 g saturated, 0.5 g trans)
2,310 mg sodium

Chicken Broccoli Penne Bake

750 calories
37 g fat (10 g saturated)
2,550 mg sodium

Smoked Turkey Basil Submarino

570 calories
32 g fat (6 g saturated)
1,300 mg sodium

Cranberry & Walnut Chicken Salad with balsamic vinaigrette

147

Five Guys

Did You Know?

● Despite the high calorie counts of its burgers, Five Guys does boast two distinct firsts in the fast-food industry: First, they are the only burger chain without trans fat in their burgers, and second, they're the only chain to use 100 percent peanut oil for their fries.

● There are 512 different burger combinations available at Five Guys, but only one way to have it cooked: well done.

SMART SIDES

Raw onions

10 calories

Onions might be the best thing you could put on your burger. They're loaded with a trace mineral called chromium, which helps your body metabolize the influx of fat and protein that hits your stomach as you nosh your burger. Eating a few slices of onion might not wipe out the effects of a 700-calorie cheeseburger, but at least it's a step in the right direction.

Eat This

Little Bacon Burger

with Sautéed Mushrooms and A.1. Steak Sauce

575 calories
33 g fat
(14.5 g saturated)
920 mg sodium

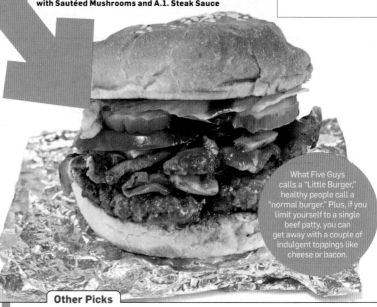

What Five Guys calls a "Little Burger," healthy people call a "normal burger." Plus, if you limit yourself to a single beef patty, you can get away with a couple of indulgent toppings like cheese or bacon.

Other Picks

Grilled Cheese Sandwich

430 calories
26 g fat (9 g saturated)
715 mg sodium

BLT
(4 slices of bacon, lettuce, tomato, and mustard)

433 calories
23 g fat (9.5 g saturated)
911 mg sodium

Little Hamburger
with mushrooms, green peppers, tomato, and ketchup

519 calories
26 g fat (11.5 g saturated)
674 mg sodium

900 calories
55 g fat
(22.5 g saturated)
1,450 mg sodium

Not That !

Cheeseburger

with BBQ Sauce

Even if you take the regular (i.e., bi-pattied) cheese-burger naked, you'll still be taking in more than 250 calories and 20 grams of fat extra over the seemingly decadent bacon and sautéed mush-room burger.

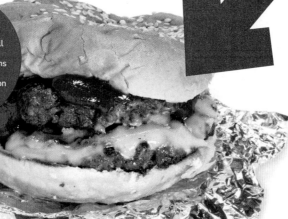

WEAPON OF MASS DESTRUCTION
Regular Fries

620 calories
30 g fat (6 g saturated)

We'd like to give these fries the green light—especially considering that they're the only side Five Guys offers. We can't, though. A regular serving has close to half the amount of fat you're supposed to eat in an entire day, and if you're eating them alongside a burger, you'll almost certainly exceed that allotment. Have a few complimentary peanuts instead.

Other Passes

615 calories
41 g fat (19 g saturated)
1,440 mg sodium

Cheese Dog

640 calories
42 g fat (18.5 g saturated)
1,580 mg sodium

Bacon Dog
with ketchup

690 calories
39 g fat (18 g saturated)
1,350 mg sodium

Little Bacon Cheeseburger
with BBQ Sauce

SAUCE SELECTOR
(Per Tbsp)

MUSTARD
0 calories, 0 g fat,
0 g sugars

A.1. STEAK SAUCE
15 calories, 0 g fat,
2 g sugars

KETCHUP
15 calories, 0 g fat,
4 g sugars

BBQ SAUCE
60 calories, 0 g fat,
10 g sugars

MAYONNAISE
100 calories, 11 g fat
(2 g saturated),
0 g sugars

Häagen-Dazs

Did You Know?

● Häagen-Dazs is not Scandinavian, as is commonly believed; it is simply two made-up words meant to "convey an aura of the old-world traditions," according to their Web site.

● In a recent industry survey, only 42 percent of consumers listed finding low-fat ice cream claims as very or somewhat important when choosing ice cream. Still, that was enough to rank it first among ice cream health concerns.

BAD BREED

SHAKES AND MALTS

Consider the milk shake: It liquefies a high-calorie, fast-digesting food to pack in even more calories and make it digest even faster. This is why Häagen-Dazs shakes and malts carry 850 to 1,170 calories apiece. Switch to Sorbet Sippers, instead, which run a more modest 300 to 470 calories each.

Eat This

Five Brown Sugar Ice Cream

(1 scoop)

230 calories
12 g fat
(7 g saturated)
23 g sugars

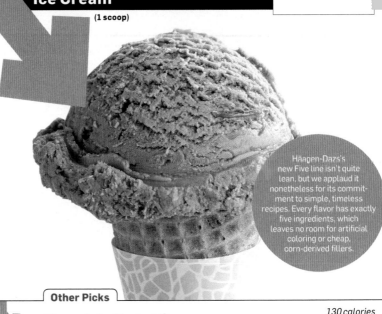

Häagen-Dazs's new Five line isn't quite lean, but we applaud it nonetheless for its commitment to simple, timeless recipes. Every flavor has exactly five ingredients, which leaves no room for artificial coloring or cheap, corn-derived fillers.

Other Picks

Chocolate Sorbet Cup
(1 scoop)

130 calories
0.5 g fat (0 g saturated)
20 g sugars

Brazilian Açai Sorbet Cup
(2 scoops)

240 calories
4 g fat (0 g saturated)
40 g sugars

Dulce de Leche Frozen Yogurt
in a cake cone (1 scoop)

207 calories
2.5 g fat (2 g saturated)
25 g sugars

360 calories
24 g fat
(11 g saturated)
24 g sugars

Not That!

Chocolate Peanut Butter Ice Cream

(1 scoop)

Still the single worst ice cream we've ever encountered. You'd have to chew your way through five Reese's Peanut Butter Cups to consume the amount of saturated fat in one scoop of this.

Other Passes

290 calories
19 g fat (11 g saturated, 0.5 g trans)
21 g sugars

Amazon Valley Chocolate Ice Cream Cup (1 scoop)

440 calories
22 g fat (12 g saturated)
48 g sugars

Five Passion Fruit Ice Cream Cup
(2 scoops)

340 calories
18 g fat (11 g saturated)
31 g sugars

Reserve Toasted Coconut Sesame Brittle Ice Cream in a sugar cone (1 scoop)

STEALTH HEALTH FOOD
Raspberry Sorbet

120 calories
0 g fat
26 g sugars

It's not necessarily the fact that you're eating sorbet that's healthy—it's the fact that you're avoiding other, less-wholesome ice creams. See, the more frequently you eat hyperpalatable foods—those stuffed full of fat and sugar—the more your body expects and demands them. Switching to more natural products will change your body's expectations over time. Real fruit is a great start.

GUILTY PLEASURE
Coffee Five
(1 scoop)

220 calories
12 g fat (7 g saturated)
21 g sugars

This is full-fat ice cream, no doubt about it. But what we love is that it's made with only five ingredients: skim milk, cream, sugar, egg yolks, and coffee. If you can limit yourself to just one scoop, go ahead and have a taste. You might be shocked to discover what real ice cream tastes like without all the sweeteners, dyes, and cheap fillers that we're used to.

Hardee's

Did You Know?

● Hardee's is the king of controversial marketing maneuvers. The most recent incident involved a "Name Our Holes" ad campaign, which asked consumers to come up with a new, better name for their sugary deep-fried biscuits. As a result, the Parents Television Council sent a letter to Hardee's saying the effort was "irresponsible advertising from any perspective."

● In another touchy advertising ploy, Hardee's sent four scantily clad French Maid mascots to concerts, sporting events, and festivals across the country as a way to promote their new French Dip Thickburger—an epic hamburger topped with roast beef and melted Swiss cheese, with a cup of au jus for dipping.

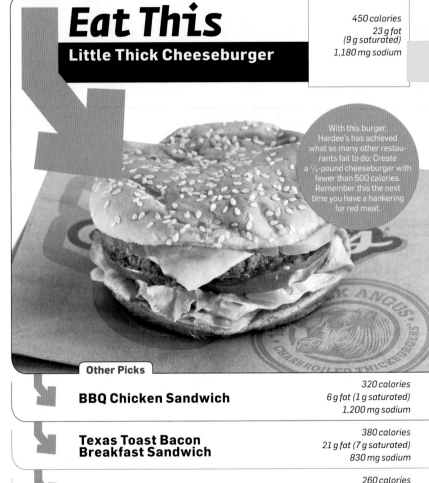

Eat This

Little Thick Cheeseburger

450 calories
23 g fat
(9 g saturated)
1,180 mg sodium

With this burger, Hardee's has achieved what so many other restaurants fail to do: Create a ¼-pound cheeseburger with fewer than 500 calories. Remember this the next time you have a hankering for red meat.

Other Picks

BBQ Chicken Sandwich
320 calories
6 g fat (1 g saturated)
1,200 mg sodium

Texas Toast Bacon Breakfast Sandwich
380 calories
21 g fat (7 g saturated)
830 mg sodium

Crispy Curls (small)
260 calories
13 g fat (3 g saturated)
660 mg sodium

560 calories
30 g fat
(8 g saturated)
1,430 mg sodium

Not That!

Charbroiled Chicken Club Sandwich

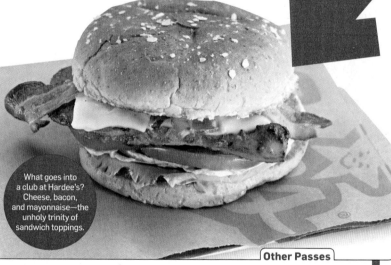

What goes into a club at Hardee's? Cheese, bacon, and mayonnaise—the unholy trinity of sandwich toppings.

Other Passes

630 calories
38 g fat (7 g saturated)
1,310 mg sodium

Fish Supreme

620 calories
50 g fat (21 g saturated)
1,380 mg sodium

Low Carb Breakfast Bowl

410 calories
24 g fat (4.5 g saturated)
470 mg sodium

Onion Rings

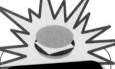

Hooters

Did You Know?

● On April Fool's Day, 1983, six friends (with no restaurant experience among them) decided to open a restaurant. Legend has it the first location (in Clearwater, Florida) didn't catch on until one of the six stood outside the doors in a chicken outfit to wave people inside. Sure, guys, it must have been the chicken outfit.

● Supposedly, the name "Hooters" was inspired by a popular Steve Martin sketch.

STEALTH HEALTH FOOD
Snow Crab Legs

370 calories

Look as hard as you like but you won't find legs leaner than these. Protein accounts for about 85 percent of the calories, and bound to that protein is a big dose of vitamin B_{12}. This vitamin is essential to your body's ability to produce DNA, nerve cells, and red blood cells.

Eat This

Philly Cheese Steak

600 calories*

* Hooters refuses to provide full nutritional information for all of its menu items.

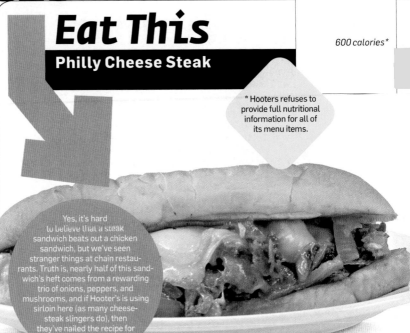

Yes, it's hard to believe that a steak sandwich beats out a chicken sandwich, but we've seen stranger things at chain restaurants. Truth is, nearly half of this sandwich's heft comes from a rewarding trio of onions, peppers, and mushrooms, and if Hooter's is using sirloin here (as many cheese-steak slingers do), then they've nailed the recipe for a solid sandwich.

Other Picks

Buffalo Shrimp
(10 pieces)

380 calories

Fried Pickles
(½ order)

305 calories

Garden Salad with Chicken (full size)

560 calories

800 calories*

Not That!

Smothered Chicken Sandwich

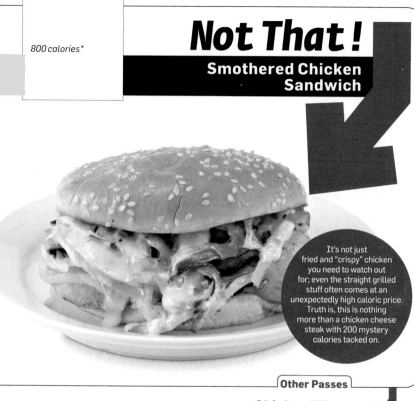

It's not just fried and "crispy" chicken you need to watch out for; even the straight grilled stuff often comes at an unexpectedly high caloric price. Truth is, this is nothing more than a chicken cheese steak with 200 mystery calories tacked on.

Other Passes

1,010 calories	**Chicken Wings** (10 pieces)
505 calories	**Onion Rings** (½ order)
800 calories	**Hooters Salad**

WEAPON OF MASS DESTRUCTION
20 Hooters Chicken Wings

(with blue cheese and Curley Q French Fries)

2,565 calories

The specialty at Hooters, aside from the serving staff, is the greasy selection of chicken wings, which means far too many patrons wind up with grisly meals like this one. Take a defensive approach by skipping the wing menu entirely and opting instead for a basket of fiery Buffalo Shrimp.

GUILTY PLEASURE

Grilled Cheese Platter

490 calories

Consider this the least-damaging indulgence on the menu. The reason? Portion. This grilled cheese is made on small, sandwich-size white bread just like the reasonable version you would make on your home stove. And that serving of curly fries that comes on the side? It's trivial enough to cap the calorie count before it hits the 500-calorie threshold. Add a few protein-packed shrimp to the beginning of the meal and escape mostly unscathed.

IHOP

Did You Know?

● IHOP has made an attempt to cater to those looking for more nutritious meals— their IHOP For Me menu items provide options that are low carb, low fat, and low calorie. The Garden Scramble is a great example— less than 15 grams of fat and under 450 calories, this vegetable-laden plate makes a decent breakfast.

Eat This

Spinach, Mushroom & Tomato Omelette

330 calories*
7 g fat (3 g saturated)
660 mg sodium

*IHOP refuses to offer full nutritional information for their menu items.

This is the only omelet on IHOP's menu that can guarantee you fewer than 1,000 calories. Therefore, it ought to be the only one you order.

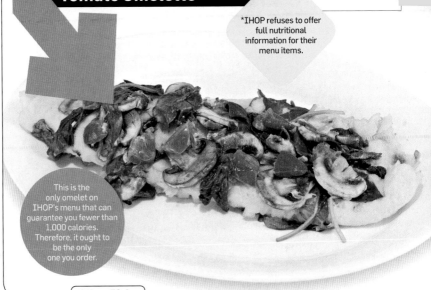

Other Picks

Two x Two x Two
(eggs, buttermilk pancakes, bacon strips)

616 calories
34 g fat (8 g saturated)
1,362 mg sodium

Buttermilk Pancakes
(short stack)

460 calories
7 g saturated fat
1,330 mg sodium

Chocolate Chip Pancakes

610 calories
6 g saturated fat
2,150 mg sodium

1,030 calories*
20.5 g saturated fat
1,230 mg sodium

Not That!

Garden Omelette

We'd hate to see the garden that produced this thorny sprout. IHOP manages to stuff a full day's worth of saturated fat and five glazed doughnuts' worth of calories into this oily envelope of eggs.

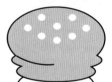

Other Passes

1,095 calories
22.5 g saturated fat
2,720 mg sodium

Ham & Egg Melt
with fresh fruit

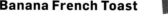

910 calories
9 g saturated fat
960 mg sodium

Strawberry Banana French Toast

990 calories
7 g saturated fat
2,250 mg sodium

Banana Pecan Pancakes

BAD BREED

HEARTY DINNER FAVORITES

"Hearty" at IHOP seems to be a euphemism for "stuffed with an unimaginable amount of calories." Really, the best-case scenario is that you choose your sides wisely and bag a Savory Pork Chop with only 680 calories. But it's more likely that you'll wind up taking in more than 1,000 calories and possibly even more than 2,000. You'd better rethink your dinner plans.

SALT LICK

PANCAKES

The Short Stack alone packs more than half a day's worth of sodium, and the flavored full-size plates all topple the 2,000-milligram barrier, meaning your sweet breakfast treat contains almost as much salt as six large orders of McDonald's fries.

IHOP (Continued)

(Continued)

Did You Know?

● Beware the IHOP "Classic Combo." Unless you ask for an order of three plain eggs, you'll be served a dish that has at least 980 calories (often much more) and 1,600 milligrams of sodium.

HIDDEN DANGER

Chicken, Spinach, and Apple Salad

There's no excuse for a salad to have 1½ days' worth of saturated fat or more calories than five McDonald's Cheeseburgers. The only purpose for the green on this plate is to fool you into thinking you're getting something remotely healthy. Other than that, this is just a big pile of bacon, fried chicken, and Cheddar cheese.

1,600 calories
30 g saturated fat
2,850 mg sodium

Eat This

Mediterranean Lemon Chicken

690 calories*
5 g saturated fat
1,440 mg sodium

*IHOP refuses to offer full nutritional information for their menu items.

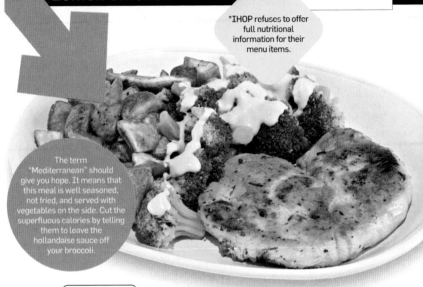

The term "Mediterranean" should give you hope. It means that this meal is well seasoned, not fried, and served with vegetables on the side. Cut the superfluous calories by telling them to leave the hollandaise sauce off your broccoli.

Other Picks

Chicken Florentine Crepes

880 calories
11 g saturated fat
1,970 mg sodium

Balsamic-Glazed Chicken

490 calories
3 g saturated fat
1,770 mg sodium

Tilapia Hollandaise For Me

400 calories
13 g fat (7 g saturated)
920 mg sodium

1,150 calories*
11 g saturated fat
2,020 mg sodium

Not That !

BBQ Chicken

An entrée is only as good as the sides that come with it, and this one hangs with some greasy characters. If you feel the need to order anything with this much sauce on it, go ahead and customize it by upgrading to some healthier sides.

Stuffed French Toast

560 calories
8 g saturated fat
315 mg sodium

The stuffing? Sweet cream cheese. The toast? Cinnamon raisin. Top it with strawberry and a small shot of whipped cream. One caveat: Don't make it a "combo." The eggs, hash browns, and bacon will ratchet it up to 1,210 calories.

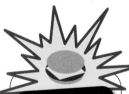

BURGER BOMB

Monster Cheeseburger

1,485 calories
40.5 g saturated fat
2,160 mg sodium

IHOP's iteration of Hardee's Monster Thickburger seems to have been cut from the same cloth: Both have more than 1,400 calories, both have more than 40 grams of saturated fat, and both have more than 2,000 milligrams of sodium. Beware the Monster, no matter where you are.

Other Passes

1,325 calories
30.5 g saturated fat
3,340 mg sodium

Grilled Turkey Super Stacker

1,100 calories
23.5 g saturated fat
2,935 mg sodium

Grilled Chicken Caesar Salad

1,795 calories
35.5 g saturated fat
3,695 mg sodium

Top Sirloin Steak

In-N-Out

Did You Know?

● Thanks to their customizable burger policy, the biggest burger anyone has ever ordered at In-N-Out consisted of a staggering 100 beef patties and 100 slices of cheese. A regular cheeseburger has 480 calories. The 100 x 100 weighed in at 19,490 calories!

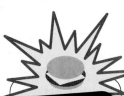

BURGER BOMB

4x4

1,190 calories
80 g fat (35 g saturated)
2,600 mg sodium

Four beef patties, four cheese slices. Sound like a lot? It is, but it only scratches the surface of In-N-Out's build-a-burger-as-big-as-you-like policy. Do yourself a favor and stick to singles and doubles—that way you can live to eat another day.

Eat This

Protein Style Double-Double

with grilled onion, ketchup, and mustard

440 calories
30 g fat
(16 g saturated)
1,080 mg sodium

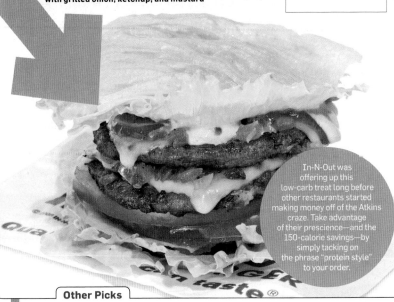

In-N-Out was offering up this low-carb treat long before other restaurants started making money off of the Atkins craze. Take advantage of their prescience—and the 150-calorie savings—by simply tacking on the phrase "protein style" to your order.

Other Picks

Double-Double
with mustard and ketchup instead of signature spread

590 calories
32 g fat (17 g saturated)
10 g sugars

Cheeseburger
with mustard and ketchup instead of signature spread

400 calories
18 g fat (9 g saturated)
1,080 mg sodium

Arnold Palmer
(half lemonade, half iced tea)

90 calories
0 g fat
19 g sugars

790 calories
37 g fat
(10 g saturated)
895 mg sodium

Not That!

Hamburger

with French fries

You're heading into dangerous territory whenever you add fries to your order. Sure they're trans-fat-free, but that won't protect you from the 400 greasy, gut-bloating calories they carry.

© 2008 IN-N-OUT BUR

Quality y

IN

Other Passes

678 calories
27 g fat (10 g saturated)
64 g sugars

Cheeseburger with Coca-Cola Classic

470 calories
28 g fat (12 g saturated)
1,260 mg sodium

Grilled Cheese

180 calories
0 g fat
38 g sugars

Lemonade

MENU MAGIC

In-N-Out may have the smallest menu in America, but the diner still has a good bit of freedom to carve out a reasonable meal. Start by ditching the spread in favor of ketchup and mustard to wipe out 80 calories and 9 grams of fat. Next, ask for extra tomatoes, pickles, and a pile of grilled onions—all of which won't add a cent to your bill or more than a few calories to your meal.

BAD BREED

ANIMAL STYLE
The most popular order of the "secret" menu is also the worst. Expect a Double-Double Animal Style to pack an extra 150 calories and 500 milligrams of sodium.

FOOD COURT

THE CRIME
Cheeseburger, Fries, and a Chocolate Shake
(1,570 calories)

THE PUNISHMENT
Jump on a trampoline for 6 hours and 23 minutes

Jack in the Box

Did You Know?

● Jack in the Box is still stubbornly refusing to give up their partially hydrogenated cooking oils. That means that their menu is littered with huge quantities of trans fat: The (small!) Fish and Chips, large Curly Fries, and Onion Rings all contain 10 grams—that's 5 days' worth. The restaurant's worst offenders are the Bacon Cheddar Potato Wedges, with 13 grams in an order.

Eat This
Chicken Teriyaki Bowl

580 calories
5 g fat
(1 g saturated)
1,460 mg sodium

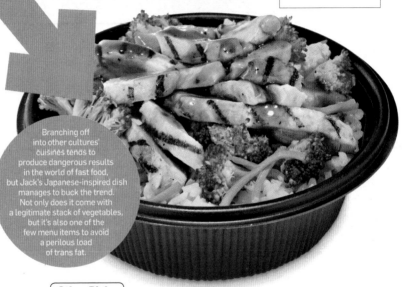

Branching off into other cultures' cuisines tends to produce dangerous results in the world of fast food, but Jack's Japanese-inspired dish manages to buck the trend. Not only does it come with a legitimate stack of vegetables, but it's also one of the few menu items to avoid a perilous load of trans fat.

Other Picks

Jumbo Jack
without sauce

470 calories
23 g fat (10 g saturated, 1 g trans)
770 mg sodium

Bacon Breakfast Jack

300 calories
14 g fat (5 g saturated, 0.5 g trans)
730 mg sodium

Cheesecake

310 calories
16 g fat (9 g saturated, 1 g trans)
23 g sugars

840 calories
58 g fat
(15 g saturated,
4.5 g trans)
1,980 mg sodium

Not That!

Crispy Chicken Club Salad

with Croutons and Ranch Dressing

The 2 ounces of ranch that top this salad contribute a third of the calories and half the fat. Switching to light ranch saves you 150 calories, but even if you eat your salad completely dressing-free, you're better off sticking with the Chicken Teriyaki Bowl.

Other Passes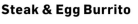

859 calories
53 g fat (14 g saturated, 2 g trans)
1,548 mg sodium

Sirloin Hamburger

790 calories
48 g fat (15 g saturated, 3.5 g trans)
1,320 mg sodium

Steak & Egg Burrito

1,290 calories
68 g fat (45 g saturated, 3 g trans)
118 g sugars

Vanilla Ice Cream Shake
(24 oz)

Jamba Juice

Did You Know?

● There are five servings of fruit in each of the Original-size all-fruit smoothies. Tacking on a Daily Vitamin Boost gives you 100 percent of your daily value of 18 different vitamins and minerals, including vitamins A, C, D, E, and K, as well as bone-booster calcium.

● In the summer of 2009, Jamba downsized their Original-size smoothie from 24 to 22 ounces. Only the juice gods know whether it was done to cut calories or cut costs.

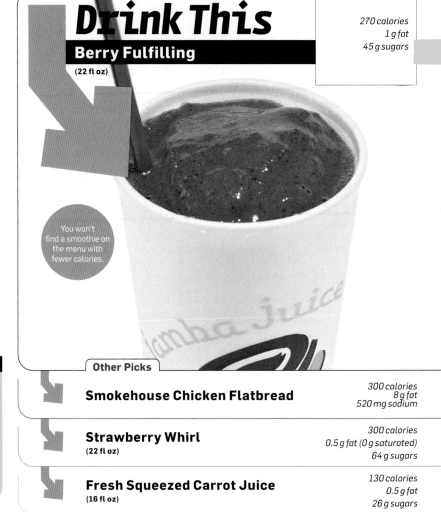

Drink This

Berry Fulfilling
(22 fl oz)

270 calories
1 g fat
45 g sugars

You won't find a smoothie on the menu with fewer calories.

Other Picks

Smokehouse Chicken Flatbread

300 calories
8 g fat
520 mg sodium

Strawberry Whirl
(22 fl oz)

300 calories
0.5 g fat (0 g saturated)
64 g sugars

Fresh Squeezed Carrot Juice
(16 fl oz)

130 calories
0.5 g fat
26 g sugars

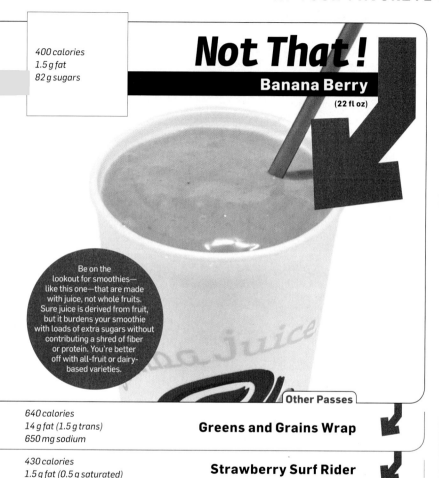

400 calories
1.5 g fat
82 g sugars

Not That!

Banana Berry
(22 fl oz)

Be on the lookout for smoothies—like this one—that are made with juice, not whole fruits. Sure juice is derived from fruit, but it burdens your smoothie with loads of extra sugars without contributing a shred of fiber or protein. You're better off with all-fruit or dairy-based varieties.

Other Passes

640 calories
14 g fat (1.5 g trans)
650 mg sodium

Greens and Grains Wrap

430 calories
1.5 g fat (0.5 g saturated)
93 g sugars

Strawberry Surf Rider
(22 fl oz)

220 calories
1 g fat
42 g sugars

Fresh Squeezed Orange Juice
(16 fl oz)

BOOST DECODER

● **3G CHARGER:** Combo of fiber, green tea extract, ginseng, and guarana

● **CALCIUM BOOST:** 100 percent of your day's calcium and vitamin D

● **ENERGY BOOST:** Taurine and B vitamins (often found in energy drinks)

● **FLAX AND FIBER:** Omega-3 fats from flaxseed, and fiber from inulin

● **HAPPY HEART:** Plant sterols and B vitamins

Jimmy John's

Did You Know?

● Jimmy John's rivals Quiznos for the honor of being America's unhealthiest sandwich chain. On the plus side, none of Jimmy's sandwiches top 1,000 calories (although the 984-calorie J.J. Gargantuan comes close). The bad news is that none of JJ's sandwiches have less than 500 calories—unless you count the sad roast beef or turkey breast "Plain Slims," both of which skip the produce altogether and simply slap a few slices of deli meat on bread.

● Jimmy John's does not offer soup or salads at their stores. The company claims that this is to maintain a focus on high-quality sandwiches, but this supposed focus leaves only chips, cookies, and pickle spears as sides.

Eat This

Big John

533 calories
24 g fat
(4 g saturated)
1,014 mg sodium

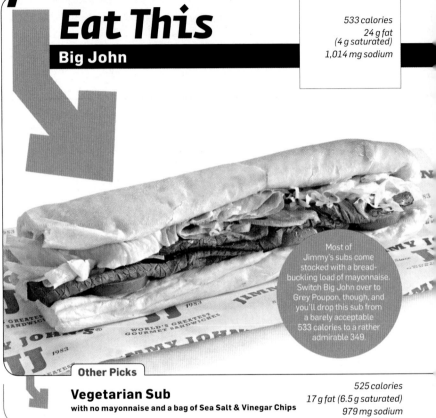

Most of Jimmy's subs come stocked with a bread-buckling load of mayonnaise. Switch Big John over to Grey Poupon, though, and you'll drop this sub from a barely acceptable 533 calories to a rather admirable 349.

Other Picks

Vegetarian Sub
with no mayonnaise and a bag of Sea Salt & Vinegar Chips

525 calories
17 g fat (6.5 g saturated)
979 mg sodium

Hunter's Club Unwich
without mayonnaise

277 calories
14 g fat (7 g saturated)
1,022 mg sodium

Turkey Tom with Avocado Spread

334 calories
1.5 g fat (1 g saturated)
982 mg sodium

951 calories
51 g fat
(12 g saturated)
2,166 mg sodium

Not That!
Italian Night Club

Most traditional cured Italian meats (think salami, pepperoni, and capicola) are utterly packed with fat and salt. Stick to the more common toppers—turkey, ham, chicken, and roast beef—and avoid exotic-sounding meats.

Other Passes

773 calories
38 g fat (12 g saturated)
1,235 mg sodium

Gourmet Veggie Club

615 calories
19 g fat (7 g saturated)
1,534 mg sodium

Hunter's Club
without mayonnaise on 7-Grain Wheat Bread

508 calories
10 g fat (5 g saturated)
1,244 mg sodium

Ham & Cheese Slim

MENU MAGIC

Stick with the French bread. The intuitive move would be to switch to Jimmy's 7-Grain Wheat, but the wheat bread, believe it or not, has 100 more calories than the French. The lesson here? If it's not "whole grain" bread, you just can't trust it.

2,314
Milligrams of sodium in one Whole Pickle Spear.

SMART SIDES

Skinny Chips
(1 bag, 28 g)

130 calories
5 g fat (1 g saturated)
105 mg sodium

Here's a novel idea: A potato chip that's neither dripping with oil nor riddled with salt. The skinny chips contain a third less fat than a regular sack; plus, each bag packs in a couple grams of fiber, making it the only side on Jimmy's menu that isn't a complete failure.

KFC

Did You Know?

● Kentucky Fried Chicken abbreviated its name to KFC in 1991. Some speculate that the Colonel made the switch to deemphasize the fact that most of the food on the chicken chain's menu was fried.

● KFC products are the most popular requests for death row inmates' last meals.

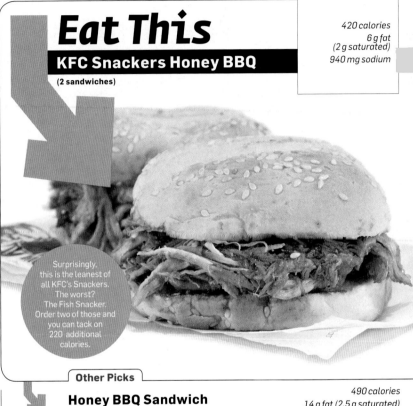

Eat This

KFC Snackers Honey BBQ

(2 sandwiches)

420 calories
6 g fat
(2 g saturated)
940 mg sodium

Surprisingly, this is the leanest of all KFC's Snackers. The worst? The Fish Snacker. Order two of those and you can tack on 220 additional calories.

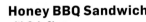

Other Picks

Honey BBQ Sandwich
with Cole Slaw

490 calories
14 g fat (2.5 g saturated)
1,080 mg sodium

Snack Bowl

320 calories
15 g fat (4.5 g saturated, 0.5 g trans)
990 mg sodium

Original Recipe Chicken Strips
(3) with Honey BBQ Dipping Sauce

350 calories
15 g fat (5 g saturated)
1,300 mg sodium

580 calories
30 g fat
(7 g saturated)
1,250 mg sodium

Not That!
Crispy Twister

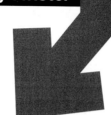

The crispy chicken is not the only problem here—there's also a heft of carbs in the tortilla and a load of fat in the "pepper mayo sauce" to worry about. Not even Original Recipe chicken can drop this thing below 500 calories.

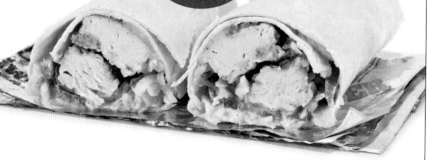

Other Passes

580 calories
30 g fat (7 g saturated)
1,270 mg sodium

Crispy Twister
with Crispy Strip

660 calories
38 g fat (7 g saturated, 0.5 g trans)
1,900 mg sodium

Popcorn Chicken Snack Box

720 calories
40 g fat (8 g saturated)
2,080 mg sodium

Boneless Honey BBQ Hot Wings (8)

WEAPON OF MASS DESTRUCTION
KFC Famous Bowls—Rice and Gravy

790 calories
28 g fat
(7 g saturated, 1 g trans)
2,690 mg sodium

To KFC's credit, no single food item on their menu breaks the 800-calorie barrier, but this greasy bowl comes precariously close. It also has more sodium than you should eat in an entire day. Stick with the piecemeal approach, instead—save more than 300 calories by pairing a Grilled Thigh and Drumstick with sides of Seasoned Rice and Mashed Potatoes and Gravy.

STEALTH HEALTH FOOD
Three Bean Salad

70 calories
170 mg sodium

A USDA study determined that kidney beans, which comprise this salad along with wax and green beans, have more free radical–savaging potential than cherries, apples, or even cranberries. That means the more you eat, the healthier you become.

KFC (Continued)

Did You Know?

● To celebrate KFC's new line of Kentucky Grilled Chicken, Oprah joined forces with the Colonel, offering coupons for a free two-piece meal on her Web site. The plan backfired, however, when franchises across the country experienced rabid demand and ran out of the grilled chicken long before the promotion was over. Hordes of angry customers nearly caused riots at a number of KFC locations.

DRUMSTICK TOTEM POLE

GRILLED
70 calories,
4 g fat (1 g saturated)

ORIGINAL RECIPE
110 calories,
7 g fat (1.5 g saturated)

EXTRA CRISPY
150 calories,
9 g fat (2 g saturated)

HOT & SPICY
160 calories,
10 g fat (2 g saturated)

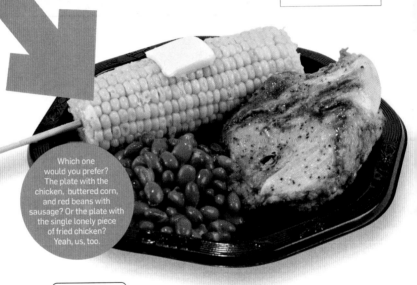

Eat This
Grilled Chicken Breast
with Red Beans and Corn on the Cob (3")

410 calories
7 g fat
(1.5 g saturated)
780 mg sodium

Which one would you prefer? The plate with the chicken, buttered corn, and red beans with sausage? Or the plate with the single lonely piece of fried chicken? Yeah, us, too.

Other Picks

Grilled Thigh and Drumstick
with mashed potatoes and gravy

340 calories
17.5 g fat (4.5 g saturated)
1,070 mg sodium

Roasted Chicken BLT Salad
with Fat-Free Ranch Dressing

235 calories
7 g fat (2 g saturated)
1,130 mg sodium

Cookie Dough Pie
(1 slice)

240 calories
12 g fat (7 g saturated)
21 g sugars

470 calories
28 g fat
(6 g saturated)
1,310 mg sodium

Not That!

Hot & Spicy Chicken Breast

The grilled chicken breast has less than half the calories you'll find in Extra Crispy, Original Recipe, or Hot & Spicy. Make sure to order accordingly.

Other Passes

490 calories
31 g fat (7 g saturated)
1,080 mg sodium

Extra Crispy Chicken Breast

520 calories
35 g fat (8 g saturated)
1,210 mg sodium

Roasted Chicken Caesar Salad
with croutons and Creamy Caesar Dressing

450 calories
22 g fat (8 g saturated)
22 g sugars

Sara Lee Pecan Pie
(1 slice)

173

The number of calories you save, on average, for every piece of chicken that you order grilled instead of Extra Crispy.

Krispy Kreme

Did You Know?

● In December 2004, a handful of North Carolina State University students decided to race the 2 miles from the campus bell tower to the local Krispy Kreme store, consume a dozen doughnuts, and then race back. In 2009, 5,519 participants lined up to race the 4 miles and consume the 2,400 calories' worth of doughnuts. The record currently belongs to Eric Mack, who ran the course in just over 28 minutes.

BAD BREED

KREME DOUGHNUTS

If the doughnut has the word "kreme" in its name, don't touch it. At best, you'll be consuming 340 calories and half your day's saturated fat—and that's for one doughnut. Turns out the namesake doughnuts are made with a liberal slathering of corn syrup, butter, and soybean oil.

Eat This

Cinnamon Apple Filled

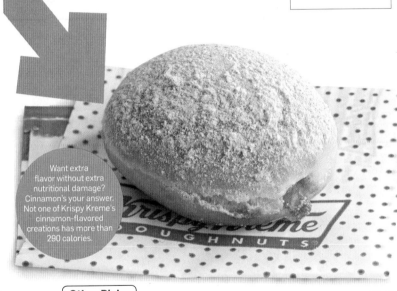

290 calories
16 g fat
(8 g saturated)
14 g sugars

Want extra flavor without extra nutritional damage? Cinnamon's your answer. Not one of Krispy Kreme's cinnamon-flavored creations has more than 290 calories.

Other Picks

Glazed Cinnamon Doughnut

210 calories
12 g fat (6 g saturated)
12 g sugars

Orange You Glad Chiller
(20 oz)

300 calories
0 g fat
71 g sugars

Glazed Chocolate Cake Doughnut Holes

210 calories
10 g fat (4.5 g saturated)
17 g sugars

380 calories
20 g fat
(10 g saturated)
24 g sugars

Not That!

Apple Fritter

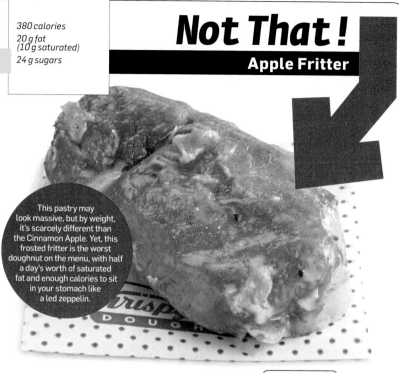

This pastry may look massive, but by weight, it's scarcely different than the Cinnamon Apple. Yet, this frosted fritter is the worst doughnut on the menu, with half a day's worth of saturated fat and enough calories to sit in your stomach like a led zeppelin.

WEAPON OF MASS DESTRUCTION
Lotta Latte Chiller
(20 oz)

1,050 calories
40 g fat (36 g saturated)
97 g sugars

A healthy diet calls for no more than about 20 grams of saturated fat per day. Order this drink and you'll annihilate that number in about 10 minutes—not to mention flood your bloodstream with as much sugar as you'll find in 10 Reese's Peanut Butter Cups.

Other Passes

300 calories
14 g fat (7 g saturated)
27 g sugars

Glazed Pumpkin Spice Doughnut

970 calories
40 g fat (36 g saturated)
115 g sugars

Oranges & Kreme Chiller
(20 oz)

300 calories
15 g fat (7 g saturated)
27 g sugars

Glazed Chocolate Cake Doughnut

DOUGHNUT DECODER

ORIGINAL AND SUGAR DOUGHNUT
200 calories, 12 g fat

CINNAMON DOUGHNUT
210 to 290 calories, as much as 16 g fat

CAKE DOUGHNUT
230 to 290 calories, as much as 14 g fat

ICED (BUT NOT FILLED) DOUGHNUT
240 to 280 calories, as much as 14 g fat

FILLED DOUGHNUT
290 to 350 calories, as much as 20 g fat

Little Caesars

Eat This

Ultimate Supreme Pizza

(1 slice) with Oven Roasted Caesar Wings (3)

460 calories
24.5 g fat
(9 g saturated)
1,090 mg sodium

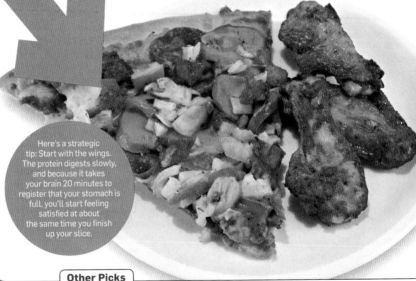

Here's a strategic tip: Start with the wings. The protein digests slowly, and because it takes your brain 20 minutes to register that your stomach is full, you'll start feeling satisfied at about the same time you finish up your slice.

Other Picks

Hula Hawaiian Pizza
(2 slices)

540 calories
18 g fat (9 g saturated)
1,200 mg sodium

Crazy Bread
(2) with Crazy Sauce

245 calories
3 g fat (0.5 g saturated)
410 mg sodium

Oven Roasted Caesar Wings
(6)

300 calories
21 g fat (6 g saturated)
900 mg sodium

720 calories
32 g fat
(12 g saturated)
1,220 mg sodium

Not That!

Pepperoni Deep Dish Pizza
(2 slices)

The crust is the biggest source of calories on a pizza, which is why deep-dish will never be a decent option. Eat one extra slice here, and you've just burned through half your day's calories and almost all of your saturated fat.

CAESAR DIP
(Per container, 43 g)

CRAZY SAUCE
45 calories, 0 g fat,
260 mg sodium

BUFFALO
140 calories,
14 g fat (2 g saturated),
940 mg sodium

CHEEZY
210 calories,
21 g fat (4 g saturated),
450 mg sodium

CHIPOTLE
220 calories,
24 g fat (3.5 g saturated),
560 mg sodium

BUFFALO RANCH
230 calories,
24 g fat (3.5 g saturated),
520 mg sodium

RANCH
250 calories,
26 g fat (4 g saturated),
380 mg sodium

BUTTERY GARLIC
380 calories,
42 g fat (9 g saturated),
420 mg sodium

BAD BREED

CHURROS

The Little Caesars menu is nearly trans-fat-free — it's just their poorly designed dessert that keeps them from being totally free of it. Both the Churros and the chocolate sauce that comes with them are loaded with harmful, cholesterol-spiking gunk.

Other Passes

700 calories
36 g fat (16 g saturated)
1,460 mg sodium

3 Meat Treat Pizza
(2 slices)

510 calories
37 g fat (10 g saturated)
1,010 mg sodium

Pepperoni Cheese Bread
(2 pieces) with Cheezy Caesar Dip

420 calories
24 g fat (6 g saturated)
1,320 mg sodium

Barbecue Caesar Wings
(6)

Long John Silver's

Did You Know?

In October 2008, LJS launched its Freshside Grille menu, which has entrées and sides with 10 grams of fat or less. Added bonuses to this genuinely healthier section include lower sodium content and almost no trans fat to speak of. Sadly, their other latest menu addition, the Baja Fish Taco, doesn't fare so well. For the low low price of 99 cents, you get 3.5 grams of trans fat.

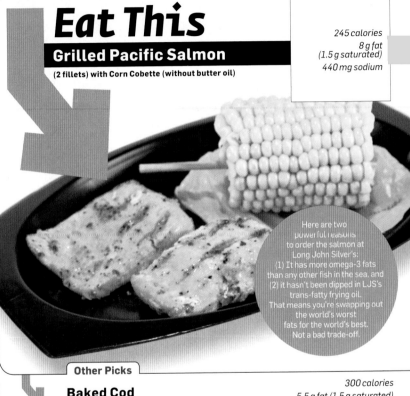

Eat This

Grilled Pacific Salmon

(2 fillets) with Corn Cobette (without butter oil)

245 calories
8 g fat
(1.5 g saturated)
440 mg sodium

Here are two powerful reasons to order the salmon at Long John Silver's: (1) It has more omega-3 fats than any other fish in the sea, and (2) it hasn't been dipped in LJS's trans-fatty frying oil. That means you're swapping out the world's worst fats for the world's best. Not a bad trade-off.

Other Picks

Baked Cod
with rice

300 calories
5.5 g fat (1.5 g saturated)
710 mg sodium

Lobster Stuffed Crab Cakes

170 calories
9 g fat (2 g saturated)
390 mg sodium

Shrimp Bowl with Sauce

380 calories
4.5 g fat (1.5 g saturated)
1,580 mg sodium

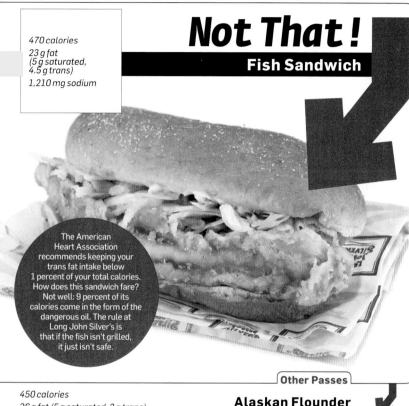

Not That!

Fish Sandwich

470 calories
23 g fat
(5 g saturated,
4.5 g trans)
1,210 mg sodium

The American Heart Association recommends keeping your trans fat intake below 1 percent of your total calories. How does this sandwich fare? Not well: 9 percent of its calories come in the form of the dangerous oil. The rule at Long John Silver's is that if the fish isn't grilled, it just isn't safe.

HIDDEN DANGER

Fish Combo Basket

Ordering deep-fried foods is dangerous when Long John Silver is the cook. The battered fish planks and fries that constitute this crunchy meal have both been subjected to the chain's infamously horrendous frying oil, which is how this simple and harmless-sounding basket manages to deliver 6 days' worth of trans fats.

750 calories
42 g fat
(10.5 g saturated,
12 g trans)
1,930 mg sodium

SAUCE DECODER
(Per 1 oz)

MALT VINEGAR
0 calories, 0 g fat,
70 mg sodium

COCKTAIL SAUCE
25 calories, 0 g fat,
250 mg sodium

GINGER TERIYAKI SAUCE
80 calories, 10 g sugars,
380 mg sodium

TARTAR SAUCE
100 calories,
9 g fat (1.5 g saturated),
250 mg sodium

Other Passes

Alaskan Flounder
with Cole Slaw

450 calories
26 g fat (5 g saturated, 3 g trans)
1,250 mg sodium

Buttered Lobster Bites

250 calories
9 g fat (3 g saturated, 3.5 g trans)
560 mg sodium

Baja Fish Tacos (2)

700 calories
44 g fat (10 g saturated, 7 g trans)
1,680 mg sodium

177

Manchu WOK

MENU MAGIC

There are no winners when you're choosing between noodles and rice—just different degrees of losers. Even the steamed rice—the best carb option—has more calories than nearly any entrée on the menu, and the source of those calories is fast-burning, blood-sugar–spiking starch. Instead, politely decline noodles or rice and order two entrées, instead. You'll save calories and get a boost of protein and nutrients.

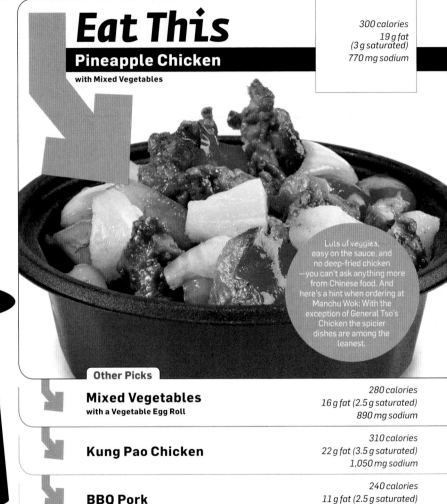

Eat This

Pineapple Chicken
with Mixed Vegetables

300 calories
19 g fat
(3 g saturated)
770 mg sodium

Lots of veggies, easy on the sauce, and no deep-fried chicken —you can't ask anything more from Chinese food. And here's a hint when ordering at Manchu Wok: With the exception of General Tso's Chicken the spicier dishes are among the leanest.

Other Picks

Mixed Vegetables
with a Vegetable Egg Roll

280 calories
16 g fat (2.5 g saturated)
890 mg sodium

Kung Pao Chicken

310 calories
22 g fat (3.5 g saturated)
1,050 mg sodium

BBQ Pork

240 calories
11 g fat (2.5 g saturated)
730 mg sodium

800 calories
21 g fat
(3.5 g saturated)
943 mg sodium

Not That!

Honey Garlic Chicken

with Steamed Rice

Switch to mixed vegetables instead of steamed rice, and you earn flavor and nutrients while eliminating 240 calories from your plate.

Other Passes

950 calories
37 g fat (6 g saturated)
3,290 mg sodium

Garden Plate
(Mixed Vegetables, Shanghai Noodles, and Fried Rice)

400 calories
21 g fat (3.5 g saturated)
700 mg sodium

Orange Chicken

360 calories
19 g fat (3.5 g saturated)
470 mg sodium

Sweet & Sour Pork

2,272

Milligrams of sodium in the average single-entrée meal with Shanghai noodles.

179

McDonald's

Did You Know?

● Since 2008, McDonald's has more than doubled their offerings of McCafés—their low-cost answer to Starbucks and Dunkin' Donuts. They sell a range of coffee items, from regular black coffees to fatty, high-calorie mochas.

MENU MAGIC

It's time to stop thinking of Value Meals as good bargains. You might save a few pennies on the fries and Coke, but you'll pay for the bigger pants you'll eventually have to buy to accommodate all the excess weight you put on from regularly ordering combos. Instead, bag a McMeal like this: Pair a regular hamburger with a 130-calorie Fruit 'n Yogurt Parfait. Even after adding granola on top, you're still facing a meal with only 410 calories and plenty of belly-filling protein.

Eat This

McDouble

390 calories
19 g fat
(8 g saturated,
1 g trans)
920 mg sodium

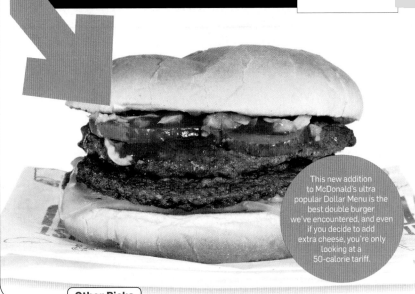

This new addition to McDonald's ultra popular Dollar Menu is the best double burger we've encountered, and even if you decide to add extra cheese, you're only looking at a 50-calorie tariff.

Other Picks

Big 'N Tasty
with cheese

510 calories
28 g fat (11 g saturated, 1.5 g trans)
960 mg sodium

Chicken McNuggets
(10 pieces) with sweet and sour sauce (0.5 oz)

510 calories
29 g fat (5 g saturated)
1,150 mg sodium

Bacon Ranch Salad
with Grilled Chicken and Creamy Southwest Dressing

360 calories
15 g fat (5 g saturated)
1,350 mg sodium

530 calories
17 g fat
(6 g saturated)
1,410 mg sodium

Not That!

Grilled Chicken Club Sandwich

Mayonnaise and bacon destroy any benefit you might have earned by ordering this sandwich grilled instead of crispy.

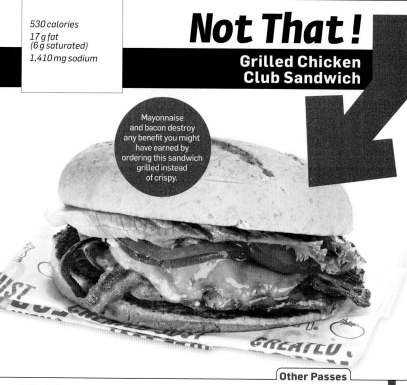

Other Passes

750 calories
39 g fat (16 g saturated, 2 g trans)
1,700 mg sodium

Angus Deluxe

710 calories
40 g fat (6 g saturated)
1,940 mg sodium

Chicken Selects
(5 pieces) with barbecue sauce

600 calories
35 g fat (6.5 g saturated)
1,450 mg sodium

Premium Southwest Salad
with Crispy Chicken and Ranch Dressing

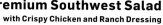

FOOD COURT

THE CRIME
Crispy Chicken Sandwich and medium Fries
(910 calories)

THE PUNISHMENT
Mow the lawn for 2 hours and 20 minutes

BAD BREED

ANGUS BURGERS

All three of Mickey D's Angus Burger iterations have between 750 and 790 calories. That's more than any other burger on the menu—including the infamous Double Quarter Pounder with Cheese.

DANGEROUS DESSERTS

Vanilla Triple Thick Shake
(large, 32 fl oz)

1,110 calories
26 g fat
(16 g saturated, 2 g trans)
145 g sugars

Tempted by the allure of a frosty finish to your meal? Here's what you're up against: Half a day's worth of calories and the same amount of sugar as in five whole Butterfinger bars in a single beverage. You'd be better off eating two Big Macs than downing this shady shake.

McDonald's (Continued)

Did You Know?

● No place better captures the affection of the kiddie crowd than the Golden Arches. A full 96 percent of American children recognize Ronald McDonald's face. Additionally, several studies reveal that children think that McDonald's-branded foods taste better than the same products served without any labels attached. That was true for burgers, French fries, chicken nuggets, and carrot sticks (which McDonald's doesn't even offer).

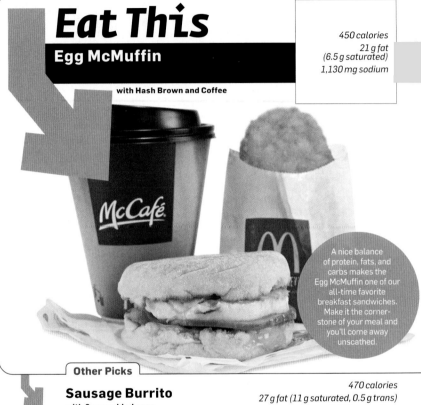

Eat This

Egg McMuffin

with Hash Brown and Coffee

450 calories
21 g fat (6.5 g saturated)
1,130 mg sodium

A nice balance of protein, fats, and carbs makes the Egg McMuffin one of our all-time favorite breakfast sandwiches. Make it the cornerstone of your meal and you'll come away unscathed.

Other Picks

Sausage Burrito
with 2 scrambled eggs

470 calories
27 g fat (11 g saturated, 0.5 g trans)
1,010 mg sodium

Southern Style Chicken Biscuit
(regular)

410 calories
20 g fat (8 g saturated)
49 g carbohydrates

Hot Fudge Sundae
(6 pieces)

330 calories
10 g fat (7 g saturated)
48 g sugars

Not That!

McSkillet Burrito with Sausage

610 calories
36 g fat
(14 g saturated)
1,390 mg sodium

Outside of the disastrous Deluxe Breakfasts, this is the single worst item on the morning menu. Start your day this way and you'll have just 6 grams of saturated fat and 1,000 milligrams of sodium to negotiate the rest of the day.

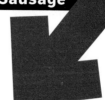

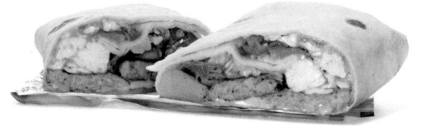

Other Passes

Sausage Biscuit
with egg (large)

570 calories
37 g fat (15 g saturated)
1,280 mg sodium

Hotcakes
with syrup and margarine

570 calories
13.5 g fat (3.5 g saturated)
105 g carbohydrates

McFlurry with M&M's
(small)

620 calories
20 g fat (12 g saturated, 1 g trans)
85 g sugars

183

Olive Garden

Did You Know?

● Six out of seven of the dinner options on Olive Garden's healthy-sounding Garden Fare menu contain more than half of your day's sodium allotment. The best option: Linguine alla Marinara, with 430 calories and 900 milligrams of sodium. Overall, the Garden serves one of America's saltiest menus.

ATTACK OF THE APPETIZER

Calamari
(with Parmesan Peppercorn Sauce)

1,190 calories
84 g fat
(10 g saturated)
2,680 mg sodium

Beware the wrath of the giant squid! Choose Marinara over Parmesan Peppercorn sauce and cut 230 calories from the tortured sea creature.

Eat This

Venetian Apricot Chicken

380 calories
4 g fat
(1.5 g saturated)
1,420 mg sodium

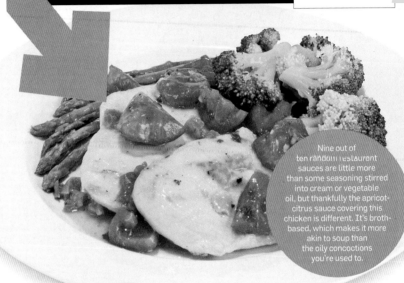

Nine out of ten random restaurant sauces are little more than some seasoning stirred into cream or vegetable oil, but thankfully the apricot-citrus sauce covering this chicken is different. It's broth-based, which makes it more akin to soup than the oily concoctions you're used to.

Other Picks

Lasagna Classico
(lunch portion)

580 calories
32 g fat (18 g saturated)
1,930 mg sodium

Grilled Chicken Spiedini

460 calories
13 g fat (2.5 g saturated)
1,180 mg sodium

Herb-Grilled Salmon

510 calories
26 g fat (6 g saturated)
760 mg sodium

184

960 calories
41 g fat
(18 g saturated)
2,180 mg sodium

Not That!

Garlic-Herb Chicken Con Broccoli

The flavor and fat both come from the garlic-infused cream sauce. Any time you order a meal that comes with white sauce, you can cut hundreds of calories by asking to have it prepared with marinara, instead.

WEAPON OF MASS DESTRUCTION
Tour of Italy

1,450 calories
74 g fat (33 g saturated)
3,830 mg sodium

Warning: Touring Italy via Olive Garden may be hazardous to your health. What you get with this dubious dinner is a slice of lasagna, a piece of chicken parmigiana, and a small serving of fettuccine Alfredo. You also get more calories and sodium than you would with any other entrée on the menu, save the Pork Milanese, and more than 1½ days' worth of saturated fat. Limit yourself to one entrée, and make it the lasagna. It will save you 600 calories.

Other Passes

820 calories
40 g fat (16 g saturated)
1,600 mg sodium

Spaghetti & Meatballs
(lunch portion)

1,020 calories
53 g fat (22 g saturated)
1,880 mg sodium

Chicken Scampi

900 calories
41 g fat (17 g saturated)
3,490 mg sodium

Grilled Shrimp Caprese

2,220

Milligrams of sodium in the average chicken dinner entrée. That's nearly a full day's worth of salt.

Olive Garden (Continued)

STEALTH HEALTH FOOD
Mussels di Napolia

180 calories
8 g fat (4 g saturated)
1,800 mg sodium

Mussels are stacked with protein and vitamin B$_{12}$, which is crucial to your body's ability to build new red blood cells, protect your nerves, and process proteins.

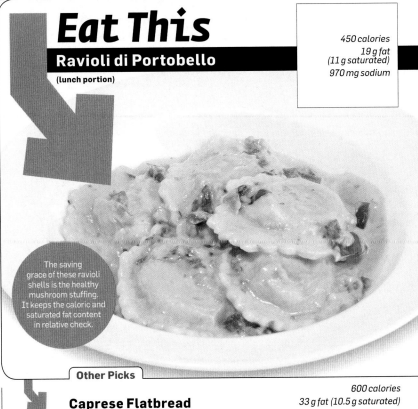

Eat This
Ravioli di Portobello
(lunch portion)

450 calories
19 g fat
(11 g saturated)
970 mg sodium

The saving grace of these ravioli shells is the healthy mushroom stuffing. It keeps the caloric and saturated fat content in relative check.

Other Picks

Caprese Flatbread

600 calories
33 g fat (10.5 g saturated)
1,520 mg sodium

Stuffed Mushrooms

410 calories
28 g fat (8 g saturated)
990 mg sodium

Tiramisu

510 calories
32 g fat (19 g saturated)
48 g carbohydrates

680 calories
33 g fat
(18 g saturated)
2,100 mg sodium

Not That !

Manicotti Formaggio

(lunch portion)

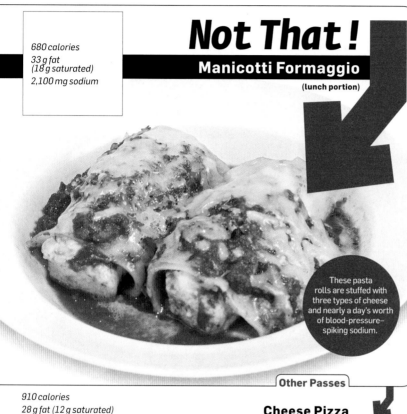

These pasta rolls are stuffed with three types of cheese and nearly a day's worth of blood-pressure–spiking sodium.

HIDDEN DANGER

Unlimited Salad

We've all seen the ads on TV, and many of us have taken the bait, tussling with endless baskets of breadsticks and a bottomless bowl of salad before even turning to the night's main course. But considering that a single bowl of Garden Fresh Salad with dressing packs 350 calories and 1,990 milligrams of sodium, there could be no worse prelude to a pasta feast. You're better off splitting almost any appetizer (save the dreaded calamari!) than saddling up to the bottomless bowl.

Per salad:
350 calories
26 g fat
(4.5 g saturated)
1,990 mg

Other Passes

910 calories
28 g fat (12 g saturated)
2,970 mg sodium

Cheese Pizza

960 calories
56.5 g fat (5.5 g saturated)
2,880 mg sodium

Calamari with Marinara Sauce

800 calories
51 g fat (29 g saturated)
75 g carbohydrates

Torta di Chocolate

SMART SIDES

Minestrone

*100 calories
1.5 g fat
1,090 mg sodium*

A mix of beans and vegetables lends 3 grams of fiber to each bowl, and that's just enough to cut through your hunger so that you're not ravenous when your meal arrives.

On the Border

Did You Know?

● On the Border is the Saltiest Restaurant in America. A tiny percentage of their entrée options, including the so-called "Border Smart" entrées, contain fewer than 2,000 milligrams of sodium. Blame it on their reliance on sodium-laden south-of-the-border standards like refried beans, tortillas, and salsa.

STEALTH HEALTH FOOD
Pico de gallo

15 calories
0.5 g fat
55 mg sodium

Consider this your portion of real food for the evening. Pico de gallo blends diced and uncooked tomatoes and onions, so it's loaded with immunity-boosting vitamins A and C. And thanks to the tomatoes, this topping is loaded with the anti-oxidant lycopene, which has been shown to improve cardiovascular health.

Eat This

Pico Shrimp Tacos
with black beans and grilled veggies

490 calories
5 g fat
(1 g saturated)
1,650 mg sodium

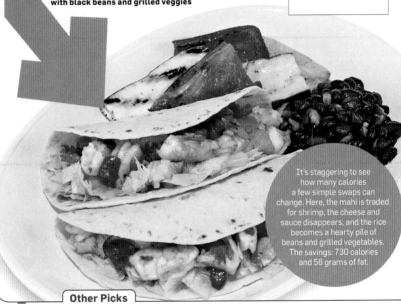

It's staggering to see how many calories a few simple swaps can change. Here, the mahi is traded for shrimp, the cheese and sauce disappears, and the rice becomes a hearty pile of beans and grilled vegetables. The savings: 730 calories and 56 grams of fat.

Other Picks

Grilled Fajita Chicken
with black beans and grilled veggies

570 calories
9 g fat (2 g saturated)
1,910 mg sodium

Beef Enchiladas
(2) with Chili Con Carne

420 calories
22 g fat (7 g saturated)
1,140 mg sodium

Citrus Chipotle Chicken Salad
with Mango Citrus Vinaigrette

290 calories
3.5 g fat (2 g saturated)
840 mg sodium

1,220 calories
61 g fat
(13 g saturated)
3,080 mg sodium

Not That!
Grilled Mahi Mahi Fish Tacos

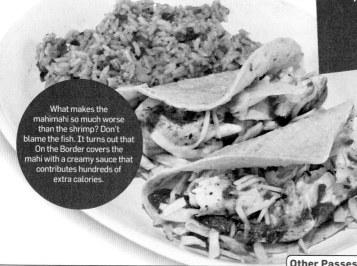

What makes the mahimahi so much worse than the shrimp? Don't blame the fish. It turns out that On the Border covers the mahi with a creamy sauce that contributes hundreds of extra calories.

WEAPON OF MASS DESTRUCTION
Dos XX Fish Tacos
with Creamy Red Chili Sauce

2,350 calories
152 g fat (31 g saturated)
4,060 mg sodium

To this day, there is no dish in America that evokes as much confusion, frustration, and ire as this plate of fish tacos. You'd be better off eating two pounds of sirloin steak, washed down with a half-dozen doughnuts.

LITTLE TRICK

Swap out the Mexican rice for grilled vegetables. You'll save yourself 220 calories and 660 milligrams of sodium.

BAD BREED

DESSERTS

All but one of On the Border's desserts (the 820-calorie Kahlúa Ice Cream Pie) have between 1,120 and 1,350 calories. Ask your server to bring the check before he has a chance to offer dessert.

Other Passes

1,680 calories
98 g fat (30.5 g saturated)
3,580 mg sodium

Beef Chimichanga
with ranchero sauce, refried beans, and rice

1,080 calories
78 g fat (30 g saturated)
2,080 mg sodium

Beef Empanada
with Chili Con Queso

1,070 calories
72 g fat (22 g saturated)
2,700 mg sodium

Chicken Fiesta Salad
with Chipotle Honey Mustard

Outback Steakhouse

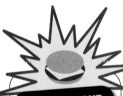

BURGER BOMB

The Bloomin' Burger (served with Aussie Fries)

1,880 calories
26 g saturated fat
2,930 mg sodium

Cheeseburgers already have a bad rap; they don't need gobs of greasy breading and oily Bloomin' Onion sauce to make matters worse. You could save 222 calories ordering two Wendy's Baconators, instead. But you don't want to do that, and you don't want to order a Bloomin' Burger, either.

Eat This

Teriyaki Marinated Sirloin

with Seasonal Veggies and mushrooms

699 calories
26 g fat
(11 g saturated)
2,034 mg sodium

The numbers are never great at Outback, so this is about as good a steak dinner as you can expect. Ask to have it prepared without butter to bring the saturated fat down to a more reasonable level.

Other Picks

Prime Rib
(8 oz) with au jus

537 calories
45 g fat (19 g saturated)
888 mg sodium

Grilled Chicken on the Barbie

444 calories
15 g fat (8.5 g saturated)
1,361 mg sodium

Outback Special
(12 oz)

559 calories
27 g fat (13 g saturated)
658 mg sodium

1,825 calories
149 g fat
(79 g saturated)
2,639 mg sodium

Not That!

New Zealand Rack of Lamb

with Garlic Mashed Potatoes and Seasonal Veggies

Don't even think of going into Outback without a clear plan of attack, or you risk winding up with one of many artery-clogging calorie bombs. This one looks harmless enough, but in reality has more saturated fat than 30 Twinkies!

WEAPON OF MASS DESTRUCTION
Baby Back Ribs

2,579 calories
68 g saturated fat
4,648 mg sodium

No, you're not seeing things. These ribs really do have 2 days' worth of sodium and more saturated fat than you should consume in 72 hours. That's a new low, even for Outback. As much as we'd like to tell you that these numbers are typos, it turns out that every dish that includes a stack of ribs suffers a similar fate.

MENU MAGIC

The Outback chefs rely on a systematic approach of reckless abandon as they pour torrents of butter over everything in the kitchen, so do yourself a favor and ask them to cook your food dry. This is especially important for meats and vegetables, where the absence of butter might be just enough to turn a lousy dish into a decent dinner.

Other Passes

811 calories
68 g fat (35 g saturated)
799 mg sodium

Victoria's Filet
(7 oz) with Blue Cheese Crumb Crust

585 calories
46 g fat (20 g saturated)
517 mg sodium

Atlantic Salmon

1,018 calories
81 g fat (36 g saturated)
1,123 mg sodium

Ribeye
(14 oz)

Outback (Continued)

Did You Know?

● In February 2009, Outback Steakhouse unveiled a new menu featuring 15 entrées under $15. But they may be pricier than you think. The Sweet Glazed Roasted Pork Tenderloin packs 1,114 calories and 31 grams of saturated fat, while the Ribs and Alice Springs Chicken combo platter is loaded with 1,880 calories and 9,279 milligrams of sodium.

DANGEROUS DESSERTS

Chocolate Thunder From Down Under

2,020 calories
88 g saturated fat
161 g carbohydrates

This natural disaster of a dessert has more calories than 9½ Hershey's chocolate bars. Even if you split it four ways, like Outback recommends, you'll still wind up with more than 500 calories and more than a day's worth of saturated fat.

Eat This

Grilled Chicken & Swiss Sandwich

696 calories
33 g fat
(10 g saturated)
1,323 mg sodium

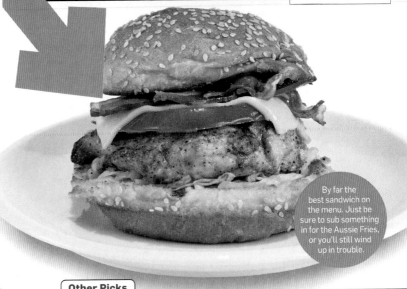

By far the best sandwich on the menu. Just be sure to sub something in for the Aussie Fries, or you'll still wind up in trouble.

Other Picks

Seared Ahi Tuna

526 calories
33 g fat (4 g saturated)
2,190 mg sodium

Fresh Seasonal Veggies

147 calories
11 g fat (7 g saturated)
202 mg sodium

Classic Roasted Filet Wedge Salad
with Blue Cheese Dressing and Balsamic Glaze

563 calories
30 g fat (10 g saturated)
1,982 mg sodium

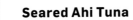

1,679 calories
115 g fat
(53 g saturated)
2,686 mg sodium

Not That!

Alice Springs Chicken

This meal ought to be called "find the chicken." The game would be to see if you could eat your way through all that cheese before your heart gives out under the strain of sodium and saturated fat.

ATTACK OF THE APPETIZER
Alice Springs Chicken Quesadilla

1,839 calories
53 g saturated fat
4,162 mg sodium

This monstrous starter is supposed to serve four. Even so, you'll each take in half a day's worth of sodium and saturated fat before the meal even arrives.

Other Passes

1,706 calories
129 g fat (59 g saturated)
3,464 mg sodium

Kookaburra Wings
(hot)

593 calories
21 g fat (11 g saturated)
200 mg sodium

Sweet Potato

908 calories
61 g fat (24 g saturated)
1,538 mg sodium

Chicken Caesar Salad

193

P.F. Chang's

Did You Know?

● P.F. Chang's recently introduced a comprehensive minidessert menu. The miniature version of the Great Wall of Chocolate shrinks the 1,440-calorie disaster down to just 150 calories and 5 grams of fat. The healthiest choices are the Mini Apple Pie with 127 calories and 5 grams of fat (1 gram saturated) and the Mini Lemon Dream, with 164 calories and 6 grams of fat (2 grams saturated).

MENU MAGIC

With the exception of the Lunch Bowls, all the items on Chang's menu are portioned for splitting. Plan on ordering no more than half as many entrées as there are people at your table, and then pass the plates among the group.

Eat This

Sweet & Sour Chicken

828 calories
39 g fat
(6 g saturated)
840 mg sodium

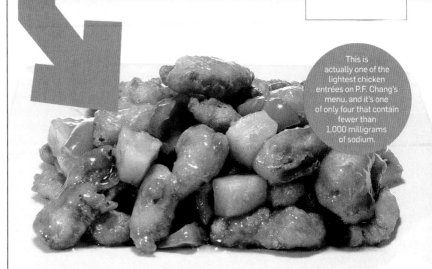

This is actually one of the lightest chicken entrées on P.F. Chang's menu, and it's one of only four that contain fewer than 1,000 milligrams of sodium.

Other Picks

Asian Marinated New York Strip

558 calories
30 g fat (12 g saturated)
864 mg sodium

Pan-Fried Peking Dumplings

372 calories
20 g fat (4 g saturated)
860 mg sodium

Lemon Pepper Shrimp
(large)

454 calories
20 g fat (4 g saturated)
2,450 mg sodium

2,016 calories
60 g fat
(12 g saturated)
750 mg sodium

Not That!

Crispy Honey Chicken

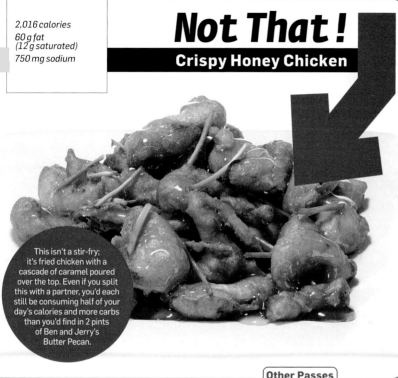

This isn't a stir-fry; it's fried chicken with a cascade of caramel poured over the top. Even if you split this with a partner, you'd each still be consuming half of your day's calories and more carbs than you'd find in 2 pints of Ben and Jerry's Butter Pecan.

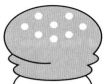

SALT LICK

EGG DROP SOUP BOWL

6,731 mg sodium

With nearly 3 days' worth of sodium, this is easily the saltiest bowl of soup in America. It's a wonder it doesn't pickle the bowl that it's served in. Now we understand why P.F. Chang's was reluctant to disclose its odious sodium information.

DANGEROUS DESSERT

The Great Wall of Chocolate

*1,440 calories
61 g fat (20 g saturated)
231 g carbohydrates*

This massive hunk of cake packs in more saturated fat than five large orders of McDonald's French fries, and—believe it or not—it has more sodium than three orders of those same fries! Unless you plan to split it 6 ways, don't even think about it.

Other Passes

942 calories
39 g fat (9 g saturated)
5,592 mg sodium

Pepper Steak

1,288 calories
24 g fat (4 g saturated)
1,388 mg sodium

Chang's Chicken Lettuce Wrap

1,216 calories
88 g fat (20 g saturated)
2,856 mg sodium

Lemongrass Prawns
with Garlic Noodles

195

Panda Express

Did You Know?

● Panda Express attempts to market its fare as "gourmet" Chinese food in a fast-food environment. Unfortunately, that means that each plate comes with two or three entrées. Alone, these entrées average about 230 calories, but those calories can add up quickly, especially when considering the fact that combo meals come with either a side of rice or chow mein, which tacks on at least 400 calories to your meal.

FOOD COURT

THE CRIME
Two-Entrée Plate with Kung Pao Chicken, Beijing Beef, and Steamed Rice
(1,380 calories)

THE PUNISHMENT
Climb the 1,665 stairs of the Eifffel Tower 3 times

Eat This

Pineapple Chicken and Broccoli Beef

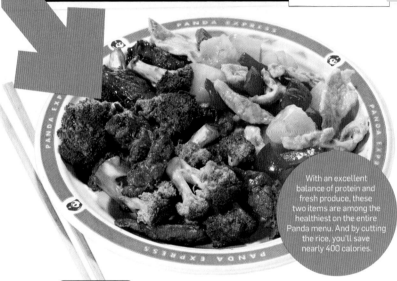

380 calories
16 g fat
(3.5 g saturated)
1,430 mg sodium

With an excellent balance of protein and fresh produce, these two items are among the healthiest on the entire Panda menu. And by cutting the rice, you'll save nearly 400 calories.

Other Picks

Tangy Shrimp

140 calories
4.5 g fat (1 g saturated)
660 mg sodium

Mongolian Beef

200 calories
9 g fat (2 g saturated)
830 mg sodium

Black Pepper Chicken

200 calories
11 g fat (2.5 g saturated)
740 mg sodium

820 calories
20 g fat
(3.5 g saturated)
640 mg sodium

Not That!

Orange Chicken

with Steamed Rice

This dish and the Sweet & Sour Chicken are the worst choices at Panda Express. The chicken alone—before adding rice—has more calories than the combined load of the Pineapple Chicken and Broccoli Beef.

Other Passes

230 calores
14 g fat (2.5 g saturated)
850 mg sodium

Kung Pao Shrimp

660 calories
41 g fat (7 g saturated)
860 mg sodium

Beijing Beef

310 calories
24 g fat (3 g saturated)
680 mg sodium

Eggplant & Tofu

SIDE SELECTOR

● **MIXED VEGETABLES:**
190 calories,
13 g fat (2 g saturated),
440 mg sodium

● **CHOW MEIN:**
400 calories,
12 g fat (2 g saturated),
1,060 mg sodium

● **STEAMED RICE:**
420 calories, 0 g fat

● **FRIED RICE:**
570 calories,
18 g fat (4 g saturated),
900 mg sodium

SMART SIDES

Egg Flower Soup

90 calories
2 g fat
810 mg sodium

Think of Panda's soup as an easy way to fill your belly without adding a significant load of extra calories to your meal. In fact, if you pair this or the Hot & Sour Soup with the right Panda Bowl (Mixed Vegetables and Broccoli Beef, for instance), then you'll manage to escape with a full stomach for fewer than 350 calories. That's a calorie bargain no matter where you eat.

Panera Bread

Did You Know?

● In 2009, *Health* magazine named Panera America's healthiest fast-food chain for its selection of whole grain bread, fruit, and half-size menu items. But with sandwiches like the Sierra Turkey, which contains more calories than a Wendy's Baconator and the sodium content of five large orders of fries, this title is suspect at best.

Eat This

Chicken Bacon Dijon on French Bread

half, with Summer Corn Chowder

650 calories
24 g fat (11 g saturated)
1,140 mg sodium

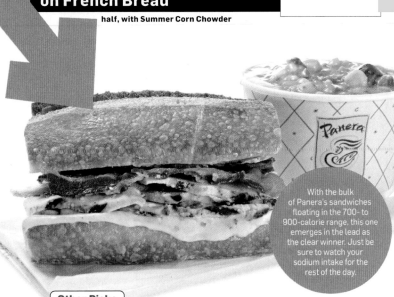

With the bulk of Panera's sandwiches floating in the 700- to 900-calorie range, this one emerges in the lead as the clear winner. Just be sure to watch your sodium intake for the rest of the day.

Other Picks

You Pick Two: Half Mediterranean Veggie on Tomato Basil Bread
with Low-Fat Chicken Noodle Soup

410 calories
9 g fat (1.5 g saturated)
1,840 mg sodium

Strawberry Poppyseed Salad
with Cherry Balsamic Vinaigrette

300 calories
18 g fat (2 g saturated)
470 mg sodium

Egg and Cheese Grilled Breakfast Sandwich

380 calories
14 g fat (6 g saturated)
620 mg sodium

Not That!

Chipotlé Chicken on Artisan French Bread

1,020 calories
57 g fat
(20.5 g saturated,
1.5 g trans)
1,900 mg sodium

Panera's Signature Sandwich menu houses some of the biggest gutbombs in the entire restaurant, so minimize the damage by sticking to the Café Sandwiches.

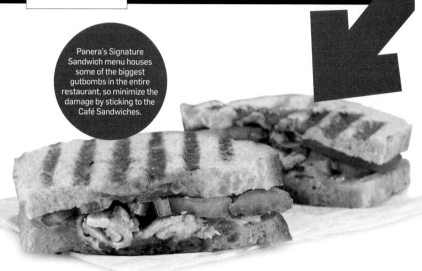

MEET YOUR MATCH

Spinach & Bacon Egg Souffle
(20 g saturated fat)
=
20 strips of Oscar Mayer bacon

SOUP SELECTOR
(12 oz)

● **CHICKEN NOODLE:**
140 calories, 2.5 g fat, 1,350 mg sodium

● **VEGETARIAN BLACK BEAN:**
170 calories, 4 g fat, 1,590 mg sodium

● **FOREST MUSHROOM:**
250 calories, 18 g fat, 1,150 mg sodium

● **BROCCOLI CHEDDAR:**
290 calories, 16 g fat, 1,540 mg sodium

● **NEW ENGLND CLAM CHOWDER:**
450 calories, 34 g fat, 1,190 mg sodium

Other Passes

870 calories
43 g fat (14 g saturated, 0.5 g trans)
1,650 mg sodium

You Pick Two: Half Chicken Caesar on Focaccia
with Half Tomato and Mozzarella Salad

920 calories
47 g fat (19 g saturated, 1.5 g trans)
1,750 mg sodium

Tomato & Mozzarella Salad
with Fat-Free Raspberry Dressing

520 calories
14.5 g fat (6 g saturated)
620 mg sodium

Whole Wheat Bagel
with Reduced Fat Honey Walnut Cream Cheese

Papa John's

Did You Know?

● In 1983, John Schnatter sold his '71 Camaro to earn enough money to open a pizza restaurant (which later grew into the Papa John's chain). In August 2009, he offered a $250,000 reward to anyone who could track down his original ride. A Kentucky man who had bought the car in 2004 claimed the prize.

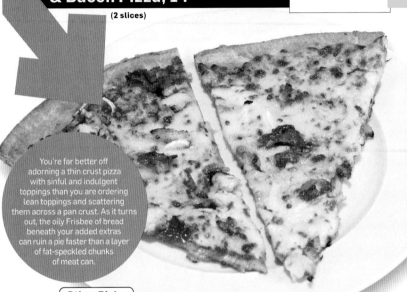

Eat This

Thin Crust BBQ Chicken & Bacon Pizza, 14"

(2 slices)

540 calories
26 g fat
(7 g saturated)
1,500 mg sodium

You're far better off adorning a thin crust pizza with sinful and indulgent toppings than you are ordering lean toppings and scattering them across a pan crust. As it turns out, the oily Frisbee of bread beneath your added extras can ruin a pie faster than a layer of fat-speckled chunks of meat can.

Other Picks

Original Crust Spinach Alfredo Pizza, 12" (2 slices)

420 calories
16 g fat (6 g saturated)
900 mg sodium

Thin Crust The Works Pizza, 14"
(2 slices)

520 calories
26 g fat (12 g saturated)
1,360 mg sodium

Chickenstrips
(2) with Cheese Sauce

200 calories
11.5 g fat (3 g saturated)
510 mg sodium

880 calories
44 g fat
(14 g saturated)
1,880 mg sodium

Not That!

Pan Crust Hawaiian BBQ Chicken Pizza, 12"

(2 slices)

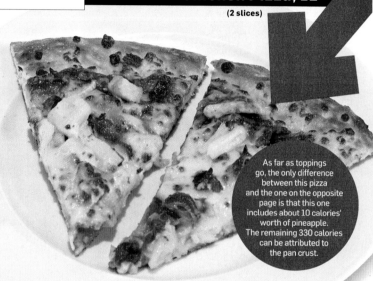

As far as toppings go, the only difference between this pizza and the one on the opposite page is that this one includes about 10 calories' worth of pineapple. The remaining 330 calories can be attributed to the pan crust.

Other Passes

Pan Crust Cheese Pizza, 12"
(2 slices)

820 calories
46 g fat (14 g saturated)
1,500 mg sodium

Thin Crust Spicy Italian, 14"
(2 slices)

620 calories
26 g fat (22 g saturated)
720 mg sodium

Garlic Parmesan Breadsticks
(2)

330 calories
10 g fat (1.5 g saturated)
720 mg sodium

DANGEROUS DESSERTS

Cinnapie
(4 sticks)

560 calories
19 g fat (6 g saturated)
39 g sugars

Each sticky rectangle of dough weighs less than 1.5 ounces, yet packs in 140 calories, close to 5 grams of fat, and as much sugar as a single Twix bar. If you don't think you have the will to limit yourself to just one, forget them entirely.

SAUCE SELECTOR
(1 packet)

● **BUFFALO:** 15 calories, 890 mg sodium

● **PIZZA:** 20 calories, 140 mg sodium

● **BBQ:** 40 calories, 240 mg sodium

● **BLUE CHEESE:** 50 calories, 70 mg sodium

● **CHEESE:** 70 calories, 150 mg sodium

● **HONEY MUSTARD:** 150 calories, 120 mg sodium

● **GARLIC:** 150 calories, 310 mg sodium

Pizza Hut

Did You Know?

● Pizza Hut was founded in 1958, making it America's first national pizza chain.

● In April 2008, Pizza Hut sent out mailers claiming that they served "pasta so good we've changed our name to Pasta Hut." Thankfully, it was an April Fools' gimmick. The truth is, if you do order pasta here, the joke's on you: Every single option contains more than half a day's worth of sodium and saturated fat.

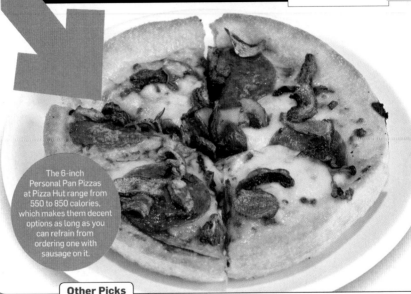

Eat This

Pepperoni & Mushroom Personal Pan Pizza

570 calories
23 g fat
(9 g saturated)
1,260 mg sodium

The 6-inch Personal Pan Pizzas at Pizza Hut range from 550 to 850 calories, which makes them decent options as long as you can refrain from ordering one with sausage on it.

Other Picks

Thin 'N Crispy Ham & Pineapple Pizza, 12" (2 slices)

360 calories
12 g fat (5 g saturated)
1,060 mg sodium

All Natural Pepperoni Pizza Mia, 12" (2 slices)

400 calories
16 g fat (7 g saturated)
1,020 mg sodium

Thin 'N Crispy Supreme Pizza, 14" (2 slices)

640 calories
32 g fat (14 g saturated)
1,800 mg sodium

740 calories
36 g fat
(14 g saturated)
1,700 mg sodium

Not That!

Pan Crust All Natural Pepperoni, 14"

(2 slices)

Order any large pan pizza and you're facing a minimum of 320 calories per slice. That's nearly as bad as the infamous Stuffed Crust Pizza.

GUILTY PLEASURE

Hand Tossed Spicy Sicilian Pizza, 12"
(2 slices)

500 calories
22 g fat (10 g saturated)
1,460 mg sodium

Beef and sausage are far from the leanest pie toppers, but the Spicy Sicilian recipe employs both meats alongside sweet red onions and spicy jalapeños. Surprisingly, the outcome is leaner than any other multimeat pie on the Pizza Hut menu. That's not to say that this should be your everyday pie, just that it earns its place as an occasional indulgence.

Other Passes

500 calories
20 g fat (8 g saturated)
1,200 mg sodium

Pan Crust Hawaiian Luau Pizza, 12" (2 slices)

460 calories
18 g fat (8 g saturated)
1,060 mg sodium

The Natural All Natural Pepperoni Pizza, 12" (2 slices)

900 calories
56 g fat (22 g saturated)
2,480 mg sodium

The Edge Meaty Pizza, 14"
(2 slices)

Pizza Hut (Continued)

Did You Know?

● In May 2009, Pizza Hut unveiled the Viva Lasagna Pizza: This monstrous culinary creation is half pizza, half pasta, piled high with three cheeses and meat sauce. No nutrition information has been posted yet, but in our experience, this type of carb-on-carb crime comes with a hefty nutritional toll.

● In 2007, Pizza Hut guaranteed Reese Witherspoon's son a future position as a delivery boy after a British newspaper reported that it was his dream job.

Eat This

All American Traditional Wings
(6)

240 calories
15 g fat
(4.5 g saturated)
960 mg sodium

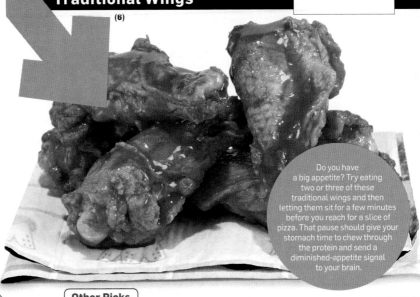

Do you have a big appetite? Try eating two or three of these traditional wings and then letting them sit for a few minutes before you reach for a slice of pizza. That pause should give your stomach time to chew through the protein and send a diminished-appetite signal to your brain.

Other Picks

Ham, Red Onion & Mushroom Fit 'n Delicious Pizza, 12" (2 slices)

320 calories
9 g fat (3 g saturated)
1,100 mg sodium

Bacon Mac 'n Cheese Pasta, 12" (¼ of a full pan)

520 calories
22 g fat (12 g saturated, 0.5 g trans)
1,170 mg sodium

Stuffed Pizza Rolls
(¼ order) with marinara

520 calories
22 g fat (10 g saturated)
1,620 mg sodium

840 calories
60 g fat
(12 g saturated)
2,430 mg sodium

Not That!

Garlic Parmesan Bone-Out Wings

(6)

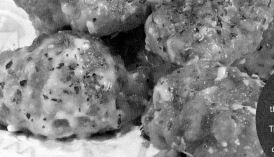

In the hierarchy of wings at Pizza Hut, "Bone Out" ranks even worse than the decadent-sounding Crispy Wings. Stick to the Traditional recipe, and you'll save hundreds of calories on every flavor-to-flavor matchup.

Other Passes

---

440 calories
16 g fat (8 g saturated)
1,100 mg sodium

The Natural Cheese Pizza, 12" (2 slices)

---

640 calories
33 g fat (11g saturated, 0.5 g trans)
1,190 mg sodium

All Natural Chicken Alfredo Pasta (¼ of a full pan)

---

690 calories
23 g fat (11 g saturated, 0.5 g trans)
1,920 mg sodium

Classic P'Zone Pizza
(½ order) with marinara

SALT LICK

MEATY P'ZONE

3,680 mg sodium
1,480 calories
66 g fat
(30 g saturated)

This calamitous calzonelike concoction packs more salt than seven large McDonald's fries.

MENU MISHAP

Stuffed Crust Pizza

When you start stuffing cheese into the crust, food stops being about sustenance and starts being about novelty, and that novelty will cost anywhere from 330 to 480 calories per single slice. Even with the best, least caloric toppings, you're still looking at a third of your day's saturated fat. Going for slice number two? You might have just burned through the whole thing. It may taste delicious, but you'd better find a healthier way to get your kicks.

205

Popeyes

Did You Know?

● To ditch its reputation as a fried chicken joint, Popeyes introduced the Big Easy Chicken bowl—a Cajun-style dish with pulled chicken and red beans and rice. That may sound healthy, but don't be fooled: It still has more calories than five Popeyes fried spicy chicken legs.

Chicken Sausage Jambalaya

220 calories
11 g fat (3 g saturated)
760 mg sodium

Nothing says Southern cooking like jambalaya, but usually there's an overload of sodium and sausage to give it a nutritional profile like, well, traditional Southern cooking. Thankfully, this bowl was made with a prudent hand. It bucks the excessive-fat tradition by subbing chicken sausage in place of pork or beef, and the sodium level is entirely reasonable. Just don't forget the hot sauce.

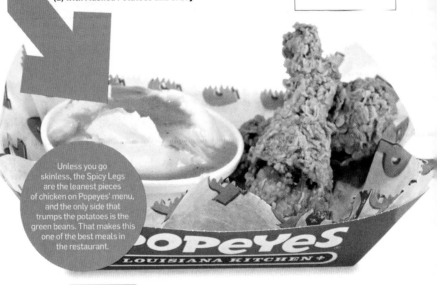

Eat This

Spicy Chicken Legs

(2) with Mashed Potatoes and Gravy

320 calories
14 g fat
(6 g saturated)
1,030 mg sodium

Unless you go skinless, the Spicy Legs are the leanest pieces of chicken on Popeyes' menu, and the only side that trumps the potatoes is the green beans. That makes this one of the best meals in the restaurant.

Other Picks

Smothered Chicken
with Mashed Potatoes and Gravy

330 calories
12 g fat (4 g saturated)
1,313 mg sodium

Po Boy Sandwich

330 calories
17 g fat (3 g saturated)
560 mg sodium

Chicken Etouffee

160 calories
10 g fat (3 g saturated)
870 mg sodium

620 calories
43 g fat
(14 g saturated,
0.5 g trans)
1,200 mg sodium

Not That!

Spicy Chicken Thigh

with Red Beans and Rice

A scoop of Red Beans and Rice on your plate will set you back 320 calories. Switch to Cajun Rice and you'll cut that number nearly in half.

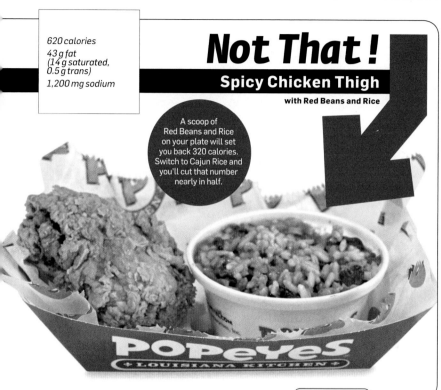

POPeyeS
LOUISIANA KITCHEN

Other Passes

570 calories
29 g fat (10 g saturated, 1 g trans)
1,600 mg sodium

Chicken Bowl

560 calories
23 g fat (8 g saturated, 1 g trans)
1,690 mg sodium

Crispy Chicken Sandwich

400 calories
17 g fat (6 g saturated)
1,100 mg sodium

Loaded Chicken Wrap

WEAPON OF MASS DESTRUCTION
Cajun Wing Segments
(6)

595 calories
43 g fat
(15 g saturated, 1.5 g trans)
1,274 mg sodium

What's a "wing segment"? We have no idea, and we don't have any desire to find out. The bottom line is this: No item on the Popeyes' menu has more saturated or trans fat than these crispy Cajun oil bombs. That's an impressive feat, considering the fact that Popeyes' fare is notoriously heavy with these artery-clogging fats. Want something with flavor that won't put you in danger of a health mishap? Opt instead for a couple of the Spicy Chicken Legs.

FOOD COURT

THE CRIME
Create Your Own Combo Meal with Grilled Salmon and Sirloin
(1,170 calories)

THE PUNISHMENT
4 hours and 45 minutes vacuuming

Quiznos

Did You Know?

● In early 2009, Quiznos announced a "1,000,000 free subs" promotion—and franchisees were up in arms. Store owners had to foot the bill, while the corporation made money on the ingredients for the free sandwiches.

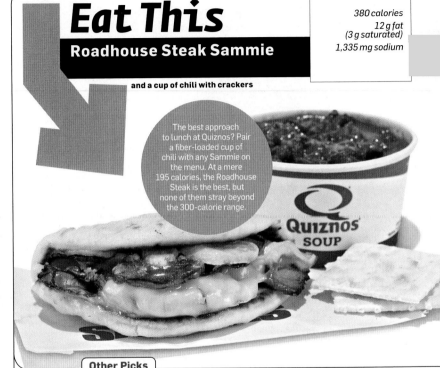

Eat This
Roadhouse Steak Sammie

380 calories
12 g fat
(3 g saturated)
1,335 mg sodium

and a cup of chili with crackers

The best approach to lunch at Quiznos? Pair a fiber-loaded cup of chili with any Sammie on the menu. At a mere 195 calories, the Roadhouse Steak is the best, but none of them stray beyond the 300-calorie range.

Other Picks

Honey Bourbon Chicken (regular)

540 calories
7 g fat (1.5 g saturated)
1,540 mg sodium

Black Angus Steak and Cheddar Breakfast Sandwich

390 calories
17.5 g fat (9 g saturated)
1,040 mg sodium

Honey Mustard Chicken Bacon Sub (small)

530 calories
26 g fat (5.5 g saturated)
1,085 mg sodium

Not That!

Prime Rib Cheesesteak Sub

(small)

670 calories
41 g fat (10 g saturated, 1 g trans)
1,085 mg sodium

Quiznos relies heavily on bottled sauces, which creates a wide discrepancy between the best and worst subs on their sandwich menu. This fat-laden faux-Philly sub is officially the worst on offer. The best? The 320-calorie small Honey Bourbon Chicken.

Other Passes

Classic Club with Bacon
(regular)

920 calories
54 g fat (15 g saturated)
2,340 mg sodium

Bacon, Egg, and Cheddar Breakfast Sandwich

440 calories
25.5 g fat (12 g saturated)
1,120 mg sodium

Chicken Salad with Honey Mustard

1,070 calories
71 g fat (13.5 g saturated)
1,770 mg sodium

BAD BREED

FLATBREAD CHOPPED SALADS

Quiznos would like you to believe that these salads were made with an eye to nutrition, but the numbers tell a different story. Only one has fewer than 800 calories, and two swell above the 1,000-calorie threshold. The flatbread itself adds a head-scratching 330 calories.

2,570

The amount of sodium, in milligrams, in a large Prime Rib and Peppercorn Sub.

GUILTY PLEASURE

Small Primo Meatball

480 calories
22 g fat (8 g saturated)
1,500 mg sodium

Meatball subs are among the worst options on a sub shop's menu, but this one fares better than most of the sandwiches in the Quiznos repertoire. The saturated fat and sodium are a little heavy, though, so don't make it a regular order.

209

Red Lobster

Did You Know?

● Red Lobster only began offering up nutritional information for their menu items in 2008. Thankfully, the numbers they released were among the best we've seen, prompting us to change their Restaurant Report Card grade from an F to an A- and making Red Lobster America's healthiest sit-down restaurant.

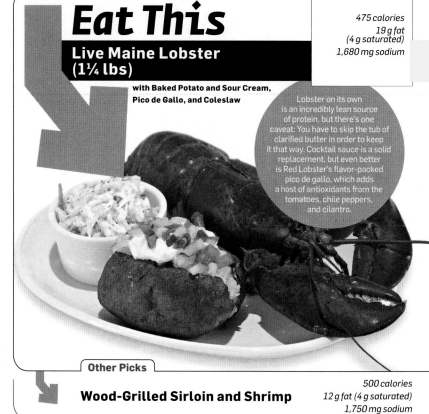

Eat This

Live Maine Lobster (1¼ lbs)

with Baked Potato and Sour Cream, Pico de Gallo, and Coleslaw

475 calories
19 g fat
(4 g saturated)
1,680 mg sodium

Lobster on its own is an incredibly lean source of protein, but there's one caveat: You have to skip the tub of clarified butter in order to keep it that way. Cocktail sauce is a solid replacement, but even better is Red Lobster's flavor-packed pico de gallo, which adds a host of antioxidants from the tomatoes, chile peppers, and cilantro.

Other Picks

Wood-Grilled Sirloin and Shrimp

500 calories
12 g fat (4 g saturated)
1,750 mg sodium

Create Your Own Feast: Garlic Shrimp Scampi with Seafood-Stuffed Flounder

355 calories
19.5 g fat (4 g saturated)
2,728 mg sodium

Broiled Seafood Platter

280 calories
8 g fat (2 g saturated)
1,660 mg sodium

Not That!

Chef's Signature Lobster and Shrimp Pasta

1,020 calories
50 g fat
(22 g saturated)
2,180 mg sodium

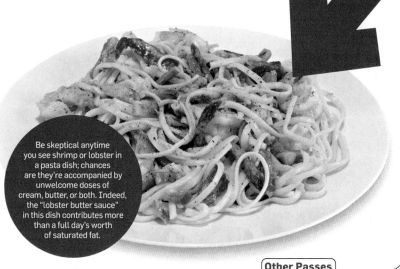

Be skeptical anytime you see shrimp or lobster in a pasta dish; chances are they're accompanied by unwelcome doses of cream, butter, or both. Indeed, the "lobster butter sauce" in this dish contributes more than a full day's worth of saturated fat.

Other Passes

990 calories
60 g fat (26 g saturated)
2,410 mg sodium

Steak Lobster-and-Shrimp Oscar

1,056 calories
58.5 g fat (5.5 g saturated)
2,738 mg sodium

Create Your Own Feast: Walt's Favorite Shrimp with Fried Oysters

1,090 calories
62 g fat (6.5 g saturated)
2,830 mg sodium

Classic Fried Seafood Platter

211

Red Lobster (Continued)

Did You Know?

● Former Red Lobster CEO Edna Morris "left" the company in 2003 after a financially devasting all-you-can-eat snow crab promotion. Crab prices peaked and diners proved hungrier than the execs anticipated, resulting in a loss of millions of dollars. They now limit the endless eating to shrimp.

ATTACK OF THE APPETIZER

Crispy Calamari and Vegetables

1,520 calories
98 g fat
(12 g saturated)
3,060 mg sodium

This app is a beige sea of deep-fried foods—calamari, broccoli, and bell peppers. There's nothing remotely healthy about breaded and fried vegetables.

Eat This

Pan-Seared Crab Cakes

360 calories
22 g fat
(3.5 g saturated)
1,200 mg sodium

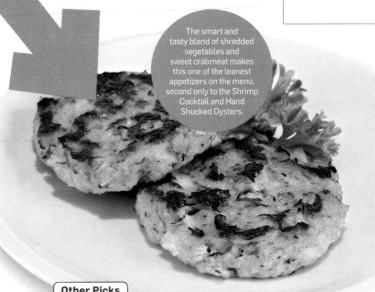

The smart and tasty blend of shredded vegetables and sweet crabmeat makes this one of the leanest appetizers on the menu, second only to the Shrimp Cocktail and Hand Shucked Oysters.

Other Picks

Chilled Jumbo Shrimp Cocktail

120 calories
1 g fat (0 g saturated)
590 mg sodium

Manhattan Clam Chowder
(bowl)

160 calories
2 g fat (1 g saturated)
1,380 mg sodium

New York–Style Cheesecake
with Strawberries

520 calories
36 g fat (21 g saturated)
39 g carbohydrates

870 calories
51 g fat
(13 g saturated)
1,430 mg sodium

Not That!
Southwestern Lobster Rolls

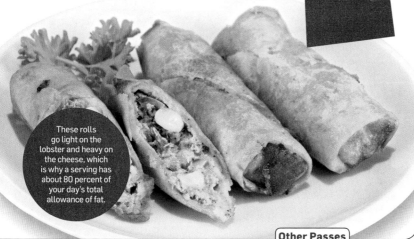

These rolls go light on the lobster and heavy on the cheese, which is why a serving has about 80 percent of your day's total allowance of fat.

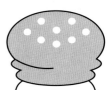
MENU MAGIC

Order a regular dessert at Red Lobster and you're looking at a caloric price tag that could climb to 1,490 calories. A better way to satisfy your sweet tooth: Order off the kids' menu. The Surf's Up Sundae offers a reasonable portion of ice cream with chocolate syrup for a mere 170 calories. Too childish? Choose an after-dinner adult beverage, instead—an Irish Coffee will cost you only 90 calories.

Other Passes

1,200 calories
74 g fat (20 g saturated)
1,950 mg sodium

Lobster, Artichoke, and Seafood Dip
with tortilla chips and pico de gallo

480 calories
33 g fat (19 g saturated)
1,360 mg sodium

New England Clam Chowder
(bowl)

1,070 calories
51 g fat (23 g saturated)
142 g carbohydrates

Warm Chocolate Chip Lava Cookie

Red Robin

Did You Know?

● In 1994, Red Robin started offering diners Bottomless Steak Fries. But with 434 calories and 18 grams of fat per order, define "bottomless" as half a basket.

● 2009 Red Robin Kids' Cook-Off winner Charlie Beckett's Holy-Peño burger is far from child's play. It's piled high with jalapeños, pepper Jack cheese, and caramelized onions. It packs nearly 1,000 calories and more than a day's worth of fat.

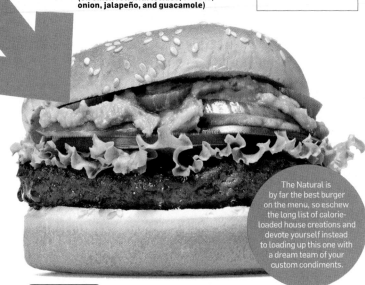

Eat This

Natural Burger

(on onion roll with lettuce, tomato, onion, jalapeño, and guacamole)

613 calories
27 g fat
914 mg sodium

The Natural is by far the best burger on the menu, so eschew the long list of calorie-loaded house creations and devote yourself instead to loading up this one with a dream team of your custom condiments.

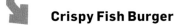

Other Picks

Crispy Fish Burger

605 calories
30 g fat
1,892 mg sodium

BLTA Croissant without mayonnaise

609 calories
29 g fat
1,581 mg sodium

Asian Chicken Salad with Asian Dressing

600 calories
15 g fat
1,945 mg sodium

946 calories
57 g fat
2,002 mg sodium

Not That!

California Chicken Burger

Think chicken burgers grant you amnesty from the calorie conundrum presented by the rest of RR's burger lineup? Not quite. Two-thirds of these birds have more than 900 calories apiece.

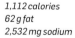

Other Passes

856 calories
50 g fat
1,244 mg sodium

Salmon Burger

1,112 calories
62 g fat
2,532 mg sodium

Whiskey River BBQ Chicken Wrap

1,010 calories
64 g fat
1,319 mg sodium

Mighty Salmon Caesar Salad
with Caesar Dressing

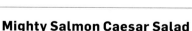

DANGEROUS DESSERTS

Mountain High Mudd Pie

1,373 calories
63 g fat
184 g carbohydrates

In case the restaurant's Towering Onion Rings didn't make it clear, Red Robin uses size to impress—a cheap, reckless restaurant tactic. This Mountain High Mudd Pie has more calories than Hardee's ⅔ Lb Double Bacon Cheese Thickburger. If you must have a dessert, tell your server it's your birthday. Oddly enough, the 378-calorie Birthday Sundae (it's the same as the Kid's Sundae) is the only sane option available.

ATTACK OF THE APPETIZER

Towering Onion Rings

1,819 calories
122 g fat
3,789 mg sodium

Most people who order this appetizer realize that they're merely indulging their bigger-is-better sensibility, but do they also realize that they're dropping 2 days' worth of fat on their table?

215

Romano's Macaroni Gr

Did You Know?

● Romano's Macaroni Grill wins our award for America's Most Improved Restaurant. Their new CEO, Brad Blum, oversaw a sweeping (and desperately needed) menu revise. Long-standing calamities like their Spaghetti and Meatballs were shrunk by more than 1,000 calories per serving, and a new Italian Mediterranean menu was added. It's filled with solid and tasty options, like the 290-calorie Jumbo Shrimp Spiedini.

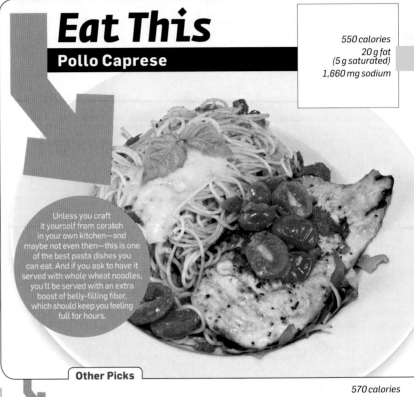

Eat This

Pollo Caprese

550 calories
20 g fat
(5 g saturated)
1,660 mg sodium

Unless you craft it yourself from scratch in your own kitchen—and maybe not even then—this is one of the best pasta dishes you can eat. And if you ask to have it served with whole wheat noodles, you'll be served with an extra boost of belly-filling fiber, which should keep you feeling full for hours.

Other Picks

Spaghetti Bolognese

570 calories
6 g saturated fat
1480 mg sodium

Simple Salmon

420 calories
22 g fat (5 g saturated)
770 mg sodium

Simple Lemon Pound Cake with a cup of coffee

250 calories
6 g saturated
35 carbohydrates

1,020 calories
76 g fat
(17 g saturated)
2,830 mg sodium

Not That!

Chicken Florentine

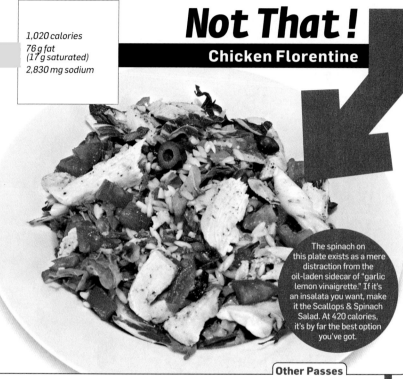

The spinach on this plate exists as a mere distraction from the oil-laden sidecar of "garlic lemon vinaigrette." If it's an insalata you want, make it the Scallops & Spinach Salad. At 420 calories, it's by far the best option you've got.

Other Passes

1,200 calories
38 g saturated fat
1,870 mg sodium

Pollo Limone Rustica

750 calories
35 g fat (8 g saturated)
550 mg sodium

Grilled Salmon

1,120 calories
48 g saturated
88 g carbohydrates

Tiramisu

WEAPON OF MASS DESTRUCTION
Pesto Chicken Pizza

1,550 calories
24 g saturated fat
3,710 mg sodium

This pie is intended to feed just one person, yet it has more calories than an entire Medium Pepperoni & Mushroom Thin 'N Crispy Pizza from Pizza Hut. If you must have a pizza, make it the Margherita Pizza; it will save you nearly 600 calories.

SMART SIDES

Scallops & Spinach Salad

420 calories
4 g saturated fat
1,510 mg sodium

What a makeover! The old version of this salad contained almost 1,200 calories and 3,000 milligrams of sodium. Now, in its new trimmed-down iteration, it proves to be one of Macaroni Grill's best dishes. The wilted spinach delivers a massive load of immune-boosting vitamin A and disease-fighting antioxidants, and the scallops are loaded with protein and mood-boosting omega-3 fats.

Ruby Tuesday

Eat This

Turkey Burger Wrap

551 calories
19 g fat
44 g carbohydrates

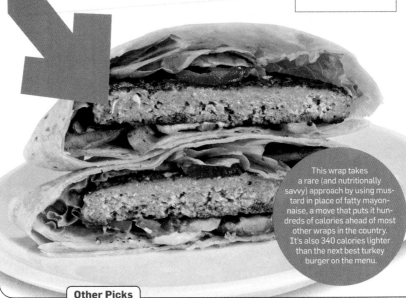

This wrap takes a rare (and nutritionally savvy) approach by using mustard in place of fatty mayonnaise, a move that puts it hundreds of calories ahead of most other wraps in the country. It's also 340 calories lighter than the next best turkey burger on the menu.

ATTACK OF THE APPETIZER

Fresh Guacamole Dip

1,388 calories
92 g fat

We love a well-made guac as much as anyone, and usually it serves as a great source of heart-healthy fats, but you would have to eat 6 whole avocados just to match the sky-high calorie counts here.

Other Picks

Bayou Sirloin
with green beans and white cheddar mashed potatoes

602 calories
28 g fat
25 g carbohydrates

Chicken Bella

387 calories
17 g fat
6 g carbohydrates

Louisiana Fried Shrimp

423 calories
17 g fat
48 g carbohydrates

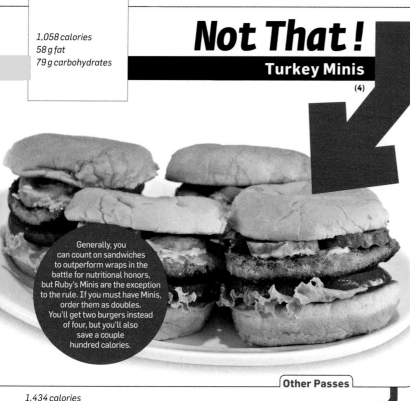

Not That!
Turkey Minis
(4)

1,058 calories
58 g fat
79 g carbohydrates

Generally, you can count on sandwiches to outperform wraps in the battle for nutritional honors, but Ruby's Minis are the exception to the rule. If you must have Minis, order them as doubles. You'll get two burgers instead of four, but you'll also save a couple hundred calories.

Other Passes

1,434 calories
97 g fat
84 g carbohydrates

Smokehouse Burger

1,145 calories
67 g fat
77 g carbohydrates

Chicken BLT

1,048 calories
72 g fat
48 g carbohydrates

Thai Phoon Chicken Strips

HIDDEN DANGER

Veggie Burger

The menu promotes this burger as a blend of all-natural vegetables mixed with rice and black beans. Sure, there's a slice of Swiss cheese on top, but that doesn't account for the 53 grams of fat. The culprit? There's a torrent of oil helping to soften and hold this burger together. You're better off pairing a lean piece of chicken or fish with a couple of healthy sides.

952 calories
53 g fat
95 mg sodium

SMART SIDES

White Cheddar Mashed Potatoes

130 calories
7 g fat
15 g carbohydrates

Indulgent as it sounds, these spuds are actually one of the lightest sides on the menu. And for as much as potatoes get bashed, they are proven to be sources of antioxidant concentrations that can rival even the most vaunted vegetables.

219

Sbarro

SMART SIDES

String Bean & Cherry Tomato Salad

100 calories
7 g fat

When you see a salad called "Garden Fresh," chances are it's little more than a flavorless pile of iceberg lettuce with a few shards of grated carrot on top. But add a couple high-quality ingredients, as this one does, and you'll be able to use less dressing without sacrificing flavor.

MEET YOUR MATCH

Two slices of Gourmet Cheese Pizza
(1,320 mg sodium)
=
22 slices of Kraft Velveeta Cheese

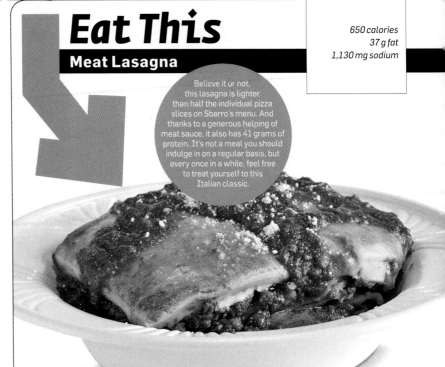

Eat This

Meat Lasagna

650 calories
37 g fat
1,130 mg sodium

Believe it or not, this lasagna is lighter than half the individual pizza slices on Sbarro's menu. And thanks to a generous helping of meat sauce, it also has 41 grams of protein. It's not a meal you should indulge in on a regular basis, but every once in a while, feel free to treat yourself to this Italian classic.

Other Picks

Eggplant Rollatini with cheese	580 calories 38 g fat 900 mg sodium
New York Thin-Crust Cheese Pizza (1 slice)	460 calories 13 g fat 1,078 mg sodium
Chicken Parmigiana	520 calories 22 g fat 750 mg sodium

960 calories
42 g fat
3,198 mg sodium

Not That!

Stuffed Pepperoni Pizza

(1 slice)

Two large slices of Stuffed Pepperoni Pizza at Pizza Hut will cost you 200 fewer calories than one slice from the same pie at Sbarro. What's more, this pizza has more calories than any pasta dish on the menu. No surprise, then, that it is the worst single slice in America.

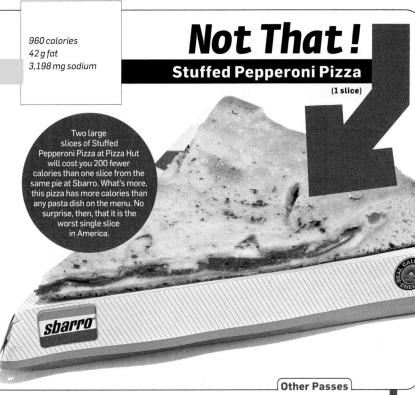

sbarro

HIDDEN DANGER

Garlic Roll

Think 170 calories are no big deal? Maybe not for some, but if you can bring yourself to cut this much off every meal, you'll lose more than a pound of fat per week. The problem is that chains like Sbarro like to sneak them onto your plate, and once they're there, you'll eat them without giving it a second thought.

170 calories
4.5 g fat
370 mg sodium

BAD BREED

GOURMET PIZZAS

Be careful how you use the word "gourmet" at Sbarro. If the word happens to slip out of your mouth while you're standing at the order counter, you might wind up with one of the chain's high-fat, oversize pan-crust pizzas. Maybe all you really want is a slice of cheese pizza, but if you order it gourmet, you're looking at 200 extra calories. Stick to New York Thin Crust if it's your ambition to stay thin.

Other Passes

780 calories
28 g fat
1,540 mg sodium

Pan Crust Gourmet Broccoli & Spinach Pizza (1 slice)

570 calories
23 g fat
1,150 mg sodium

New York Thin-Crust White Pizza
(1 slice)

930 calories
36 g fat
950 mg sodium

Chicken Parmigiana
with Spaghetti

Schlotzsky's

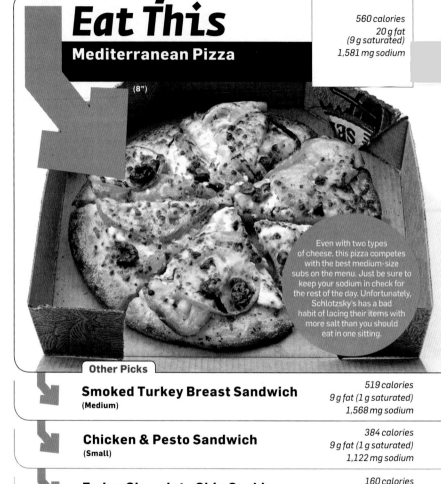

Eat This

Mediterranean Pizza

560 calories
20 g fat
(9 g saturated)
1,581 mg sodium

(8")

Even with two types of cheese, this pizza competes with the best medium-size subs on the menu. Just be sure to keep your sodium in check for the rest of the day. Unfortunately, Schlotzsky's has a bad habit of lacing their items with more salt than you should eat in one sitting.

Did You Know?

● Schlotzsky's began in 1971 as a mom-and-pop shop serving only a single sandwich: The Original, which is still their most popular sandwich today. Made with ham, two types of salami, and three cheeses, it's also one of the least-healthy items on the menu.

● Schlotzsky's recently launched three new massive gastronomic disasters in the form of sandwiches: The Bacon Smokecheezy Threezy line. They now offer Turkey & Bacon Smokecheezy, the Ribeye Steak & Bacon Smokecheezy, and the Chicken & Bacon Smokecheezy. All feature either turkey, rib eye, or chicken with smoked Cheddar cheese, bacon strips, fresh lettuce, tomatoes, red onions, and chipotle mayo.

Other Picks

Smoked Turkey Breast Sandwich
(Medium)

519 calories
9 g fat (1 g saturated)
1,568 mg sodium

Chicken & Pesto Sandwich
(Small)

384 calories
9 g fat (1 g saturated)
1,122 mg sodium

Fudge Chocolate Chip Cookie
(bowl)

160 calories
8 g fat (5 g saturated)
14 g sugars

AT YOUR FAVORITE RESTAURANTS

831 calories
35 g fat
(14 g saturated,
1 g trans)
2,529 mg sodium

Not That!

Original-Style Turkey Sandwich

(Medium)

Half the medium subs on the menu break the 700-calorie barrier, and few sound as harmless as this one. The problem is the salami and three types of cheese. Eat a Smoked Turkey Breast Sandwich, instead. It has no secrets.

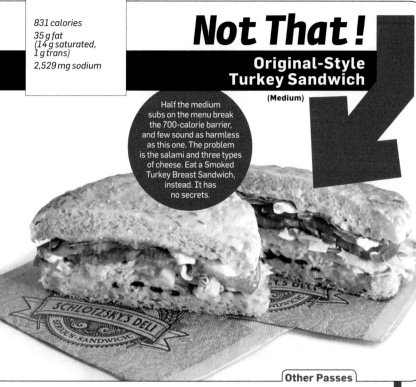

Other Passes

974 calories
51 g fat (16 g saturated, 1 g trans)
2,609 mg sodium

Albuquerque Turkey Sandwich (Medium)

689 calories
36 g fat (10 g saturated)
1,404 mg sodium

Grilled Chicken and Guacamole Wrap

417 calories
22 g fat (9 g saturated)
39 g sugars

Brownie

GUILTY PLEASURE

Double Cheese Pizza

597 calories
21 g fat
(10 g saturated, 1 g trans)
1,374 mg sodium

Sometimes you just want to eat like a kid, and this is a pretty safe way to do it. The "double cheese" refers to a mix of mozzarella and Parmesan, not the layer of grease that covers other extra-cheese pies. Better yet: It's topped with a tasty layer of sun-dried tomato pesto.

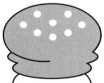

SALT LICK

DELUXE ORIGINAL-STYLE SUB

4,084 mg sodium
956 calories
46 g fat
(18 g saturated,
1 g trans)

You'll have to look hard for a salt reprieve, since the average sub at Schlotzsky's packs 2,168 milligrams of sodium. Still, this one stands out as particularly heinous.

Smoothie King

Did You Know?

● Smoothie King claims to have pioneered the nutritional fruit- and function-based, fresh-blended smoothie. They offer a comprehensive package of enhancers and supplements with their drinks—but they may be more hype than help. For example, "Energy" enhancers contain ginkgo biloba and Siberian ginseng; however, ginseng has never been shown to actually boost energy.

9

Percentage of Americans who eat the daily recommended five to seven servings of fruits and vegetables.

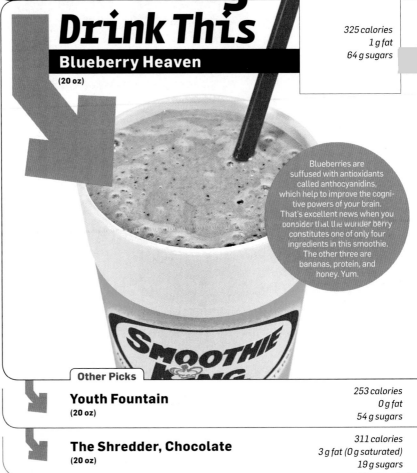

Drink This

Blueberry Heaven
(20 oz)

325 calories
1 g fat
64 g sugars

Blueberries are suffused with antioxidants called anthocyanidins, which help to improve the cognitive powers of your brain. That's excellent news when you consider that the wonder berry constitutes one of only four ingredients in this smoothie. The other three are bananas, protein, and honey. Yum.

Other Picks

Youth Fountain
(20 oz)

253 calories
0 g fat
54 g sugars

The Shredder, Chocolate
(20 oz)

311 calories
3 g fat (0 g saturated)
19 g sugars

Banana Berry Treat
(20 oz)

364 calories
0 g fat
75 g sugars

Not That!

Skinny Cranberry Supreme

(20 oz)

454 calories
1 g fat
73 g sugars

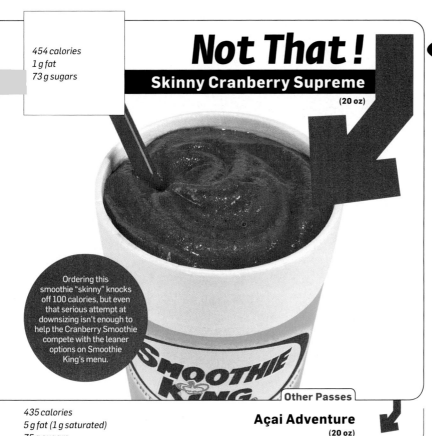

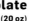

Ordering this smoothie "skinny" knocks off 100 calories, but even that serious attempt at downsizing isn't enough to help the Cranberry Smoothie compete with the leaner options on Smoothie King's menu.

Other Passes

435 calories
5 g fat (1 g saturated)
75 g sugars

Açai Adventure
(20 oz)

717 calories
27 g fat (4 g saturated)
63 g sugars

Peanut Power Plus Chocolate
(20 oz)

524 calories
12 g fat (6 g saturated)
77 g sugars

Banana Boat
(20 oz)

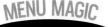

MENU MAGIC

One phrase will cut about 25 grams of sugar out of your smoothie: "Make it skinny." This tells your Smoothie King specialist that you want yours without the sugary base that goes into almost every cup.

BAD BREED

HULK SMOOTHIES

Arnold Schwarzenegger circa 1972 probably had the metabolism to burn off one of these shakes. For the rest of us, the average 928 calories is far too many to tussle with. If you want muscle mass, try a healthy diet and lots of lean protein.

GUILTY PLEASURE

Coffee Smoothie Mocha
(20 oz)

260 calories
2 g fat
36 g sugars

The mocha flavor comes from a blend of iced coffee and chocolate protein powder, so it adds great taste as well as 17 grams of belly-filling protein. It's also 140 calories lighter than a same-size Iced Mocha from Starbucks.

Sonic

Did You Know?

● In 2006, *New York Times* food critic Frank Bruni traveled across the country to sample and compare as many fast-food restaurants as he possibly could. He deemed Sonic's tots "the sultans of spuds," waxing poetic about their "exterior crackle." Don't mistake Bruni for a nutritionist, though; a large order of the touted tots will run you 530 calories, 34 grams of fat, and 1,140 milligrams of sodium.

FOOD COURT

THE CRIME
California Cheeseburger with small fries and a medium Grape Slush
(1,450 calories)

THE PUNISHMENT
Use a stair-stepping machine for 3 hours and 20 minutes

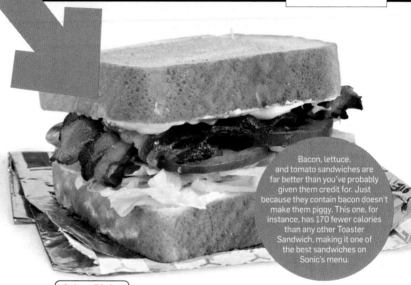

Eat This
BLT Toaster Sandwich

500 calories
29 g fat
(7 g saturated,
1 g trans)
950 mg sodium

Bacon, lettuce, and tomato sandwiches are far better than you've probably given them credit for. Just because they contain bacon doesn't make them piggy. This one, for instance, has 170 fewer calories than any other Toaster Sandwich, making it one of the best sandwiches on Sonic's menu.

Other Picks

Burrito Deluxe

420 calories
22 g fat (7 g saturated, 0.5 g trans)
640 mg sodium

Bacon, Egg & Cheese Breakfast Burrito

450 calories
27 g fat (10 g saturated, 0.5 g trans)
1,290 mg sodium

Ched 'r' Bites (12)

280 calories
15 g fat (6 g saturated)
740 mg sodium

740 calories
46 g fat
(11 g saturated,
0.5 g trans)
1,740 mg sodium

Not That!

Chicken Club Toaster Sandwich

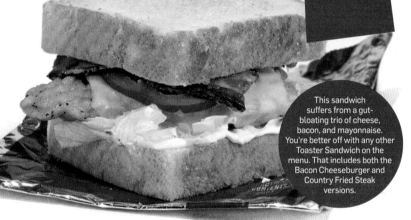

This sandwich suffers from a gut-bloating trio of cheese, bacon, and mayonnaise. You're better off with any other Toaster Sandwich on the menu. That includes both the Bacon Cheeseburger and Country Fried Steak versions.

Other Passes

670 calories
39 g fat (13 g saturated, 0.5 g trans)
1,420 mg sodium

Fritos Chili Cheese Wrap

600 calories
46 g fat (18 g saturated, 1 g trans)
1,000 mg sodium

Sausage, Egg & Cheese CroisSonic Breakfast Sandwich

440 calories
22 g fat (9 g saturated, 0.5 g trans)
1,050 mg sodium

Mozzarella Sticks

MENU MAGIC

Craft your own burger masterpiece, starting with a Jr. Burger and piling on a few of Sonic's "Upgrades." The worst condiments are cheese and bacon, but you can still earn big flavor by topping with chili, coleslaw, jalapeños, green chiles, and grilled onions. Feeling like a Jr. Burger with green chiles and slaw? That's only 360 calories and 18 grams of fat.

MENU MISHAP

Strawberry Fruit Smoothie
(regular)

540 calories
0 g fat
99 g sugars

A regular 14-ounce cup of this stuff will net you a quarter of your day's calories. By comparison, the 16-ounce All Fruit smoothies at Jamba Juice have between 190 and 220. So what's the problem here? Lots and lots of added sugars—enough to contaminate this drink with as much sweetness as 10 Krispy Kreme original glazed doughnuts. A better name would be "Blended Strawberry Shortcake."

Starbucks

Did You Know?

● Is it the beginning of the end of the $4 latte? The recession hit Starbucks hard—the coffee giant closed at least 600 stores and eliminated 6,700 jobs in 2009. To combat the slump, some Starbucks locations offer $2 cold drinks in the afternoon if the customer shows a receipt from earlier that day. If you're planning to double up, better stick to low-calorie options like regular joe or Americanos.

FOOD COURT

THE CRIME
Double Iced Cinnamon Roll and a Grande 2% Gingersnap Latte with whipped cream
(830 calories)

THE PUNISHMENT
Run nearly 7 miles at a moderate pace

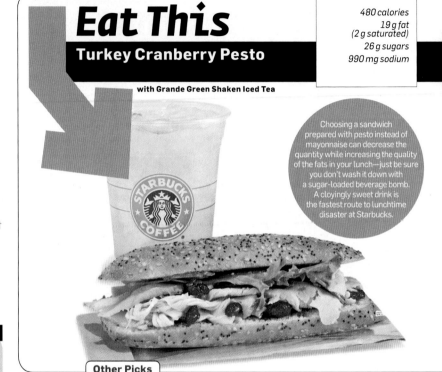

Eat This

Turkey Cranberry Pesto

with Grande Green Shaken Iced Tea

480 calories
19 g fat
(2 g saturated)
26 g sugars
990 mg sodium

Choosing a sandwich prepared with pesto instead of mayonnaise can decrease the quantity while increasing the quality of the fats in your lunch—just be sure you don't wash it down with a sugar-loaded beverage bomb. A cloyingly sweet drink is the fastest route to lunchtime disaster at Starbucks.

Other Picks

Pumpkin Loaf
320 calories
12 g fat (2 g saturated)
32 g sugars

Ham, Egg Frittata, Cheddar Cheese on Artisan Roll
370 calories
16 g fat (6 g saturated)
730 mg sodium

Blueberry Oat Bar
250 calories
10 g fat (6 g saturated)
15 g sugars

740 calories
12 g fat
(2 g saturated)
73 g sugars
1,335 mg sodium

Not That!

Tarragon Chicken Salad Sandwich

with Grande Berry Chai Infusion

We applaud Starbucks for using light mayo in their chicken salad, but it's not enough to keep this sandwich from being the worst lunch option on the menu. What's worse is the Berry Chai Infusion: It has more sugar than three Twinkies.

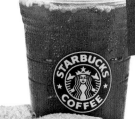

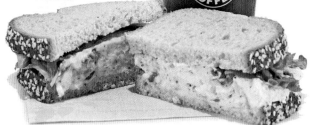

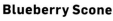
Other Passes

480 calories
19 g fat (2.5 g saturated)
44 g sugars

Banana Nut Bread

460 calories
22 g fat (12 g saturated)
420 mg sodium

Blueberry Scone

490 calories
21 g fat (8 g saturated)
32 g sugars

Maple Oat Nut Scone

WEAPON OF MASS DESTRUCTION
Salted Caramel Signature Hot Chocolate
(Venti)

720 calories
32 g fat (20 g saturated)
85 g sugars

Salted caramel desserts were one of the biggest food trends in 2009. Too bad this iteration is officially the worst item on the entire Starbucks menu. Even with nonfat milk, it packs in as much saturated fat as 20 strips of bacon and more sugar than 16 Chewy Chips Ahoy! cookies.

STEALTH HEALTH FOOD
Perfect Oatmeal with Sweetened Fruit and Nuts

340 calories
11.5 g fat
(1.5 g saturated)
21 g sugars

Ordinarily we warn against sweetened fruit, but here it's not too bad. What's different? This fruit is eaten alongside whole grain oats, almonds, walnuts, and pecans, which together lend this bowl 7 grams of hunger-thwarting fiber and a nice blend of mind-sharpening fats.

Starbucks (Continued)

Did You Know?

● Starbucks revamped its breakfast menu in late 2008, focusing on lowering the calorie counts. As with other chains, avoid pastries—including muffins—and stick with the egg-based breakfast sandwiches, ideally on English muffins instead of on higher-calorie Artisan Bread.

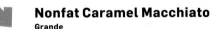

MENU MAGIC

Grab that cinnamon shaker to add flavor with a health kick. Repeated studies have shown that a flavonoid called MHCP, which is found in cinnamon, makes fat cells more responsive to insulin, thus helping to keep your blood sugar in the healthy range. That might not cut calories from your latte or pastry, but it will help minimize the damage caused by all those sugars.

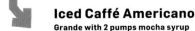

Drink This

Strawberry Banana Vivanno

280 calories
1.5 g fat
(1 g saturated)
41 g sugars

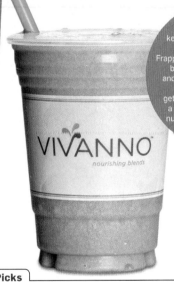

The Vivanno beverages offer two key elements that put them leagues ahead of any Frappuccino: real fruit (one whole banana in each smoothie) and a shot of whey protein and fiber. That means you get a kick of antioxidants with a helping of slow-digesting nutrients to keep your blood sugar stable.

VIVANNO™
nourishing blends

Other Picks

Nonfat Caramel Macchiato
Grande

190 calories
1 g fat (0.5 g saturated)
32 g sugars

Iced Caffé Americano
Grande with 2 pumps mocha syrup

65 calories
1 g fat
9 g sugars

Nonfat Cinnamon Dolce Crème
Tall without whip

170 calories
0 g fat
31 g sugars

470 calories
3.5 g fat
(1.5 g saturated)
75 g sugars

Not That!

Strawberries & Creme
Frappuccino Blended Crème

without whipped cream

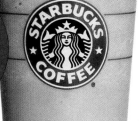

Frappuccinos are easily the worst beverages on offer at Starbucks, so if you must have one, make it a Frappuccino Light. Even if you order a Grande, you still have a good chance of landing one under 200 calories.

Other Passes

420 calories
13 g fat (9 g saturated)
60 g sugars

Nonfat White Chocolate Mocha
Grande

200 calories
6 g fat (2.5 g saturated)
26 g sugars

Iced Caffé Mocha
Grande with 2% milk (no whip)

350 calories
9 g fat (5 g saturated)
57 g sugars

Nonfat Hazelnut Signature
Hot Chocolate Tall without whip

SMART SIDES

Protein Plate with Peanut Butter

370 calories
17 g fat
(5 g saturated)
600 mg sodium

Some people resort to bloated muffins and fattening pastries just to avoid dumping acidic coffee and caffeine into an empty stomach. If you're one of those people, consider this your new fix. The combined forces of a whole wheat bagel, hard-boiled eggs, apples, and grapes lend this little plate 5 grams of fiber and 17 grams of protein. Those are numbers no muffin or scone will ever live up to.

GUILTY PLEASURE

Espresso Frappuccino Blended Coffee
(Grande)

190 calories
2.5 g fat (1.5 g saturated)
31 g sugars

The Espresso Frappuccino deviates from the traditional Frappuccino recipe in two ways:
(1) It removes a couple ounces of the sugary base to make room for the espresso shot, and
(2) it doesn't include whipped cream on top. That makes it the least damaging Frappuccino on the menu.

Subway

Did You Know?

● Subway gained a reputation for being healthy when Jared Fogle lost 245 pounds on a diet of mainly Subway sandwiches and exercise. Jared's diet was first spotlighted in a 1999 *Men's Health* article titled "Crazy Diets That Work." A decade later Subway is now the largest chain eatery in the world, surpassing even McDonald's in total stores.

BAD BREED

WRAPS

Wraps have an unearned reputation for being good for your health, but look at this thing: It has 50 more calories than the worst bread on Subway's menu. And what's worse is that it has more surface area, increasing the potential to lock in more oil and dressing than bread, thus mutating your lean sandwich into a greasy sack of meat and vegetables. Stick with the 9-Grain Wheat Bread.

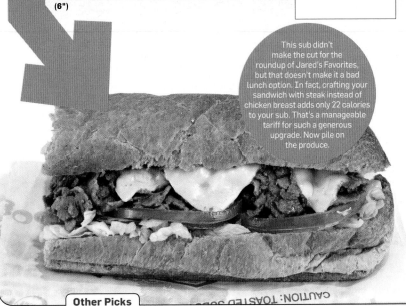

Eat This

Steak and Cheese

(6")

390 calories
10 g fat
(4.5 g saturated)
1,670 mg sodium

This sub didn't make the cut for the roundup of Jared's Favorites, but that doesn't make it a bad lunch option. In fact, crafting your sandwich with steak instead of chicken breast adds only 22 calories to your sub. That's a manageable tariff for such a generous upgrade. Now pile on the produce.

CAUTION: TOASTED

Other Picks

Roast Beef on 9-grain wheat (6")

320 calories
4.5 g fat (1.5 g saturated)
980 mg sodium

Subway Melt on 9-grain wheat (6")

390 calories
11 g fat (5 g saturated, 0.5 g trans)
1,670 mg sodium

BLT on 9-grain wheat (6")

360 calories
13 g fat (6 g saturated)
990 mg sodium

580 calories
23 g fat
(9 g saturated,
1 g trans)
1,660 mg sodium

Not That!

Meatball Marinara
(6")

Subway's fat-loaded meatballs make this the biggest blemish on the restaurant's menu. Go for a footlong, and you're facing more than half your day's calories, nearly the entire day's saturated fat, and well over a day's worth of sodium.

DELI MEAT DECODER
(Amount on a 6" sub)

● **TURKEY:**
50 calories,
500 mg sodium

● **HAM:** 60 calories,
790 mg sodium

● **ROAST BEEF:**
80 calories,
430 mg sodium

● **GRILLED CHICKEN:** 90 calories, 330 mg sodium

● **SUBWAY CLUB MEATS:** 90 calories, 750 mg sodium

● **STEAK:**
112 calories,
560 mg sodium

● **COLD CUT COMBO MEATS:**
140 calories,
830 mg sodium

● **ITALIAN BMT MEATS:** 180 calories, 1,120 mg sodium

● **TUNA:** 260 calories, 310 mg sodium

● **MEATBALLS:**
310 calories,
910 mg sodium

Other Passes

410 calories
8 g fat (1.5 g saturated)
1,220 mg sodium

Sweet Onion Chicken Teriyaki on Flatbread (6")

520 calories
28 g fat (11 g saturated, 0.5 g trans)
1,960 mg sodium

Spicy Italian on 9-grain wheat (6")

630 calories
29 g fat (10 g saturated, 0.5 g trans)
1,350 mg sodium

Chicken & Bacon Ranch on Honey Oat (6")

233

Subway (Continued)

Did You Know?

● A study from Cornell University found that subjects ate 350 calories more at Subway than they did at McDonald's. Researchers call it the "health halo": the tendency to overeat when they believe they're eating at a healthy restaurant. Stick to 6-inch subs and zero-calorie drinks and you'll escape the allure of the halo.

MENU MAGIC

Feeling like a snack or a light meal? Forget the nutritionally void bags of chips and cookies around the register and opt instead for the underappreciated mini 4-inch sub, which Subway will make any sandwich on. Most of your favorite combos will weigh in around 200 calories, mostly from lean protein—an ideal snack in every regard.

Eat This

Black Forest Ham & Cheese Breakfast Sandwich

450 calories
19 g fat
(7 g saturated)
1,450 mg sodium

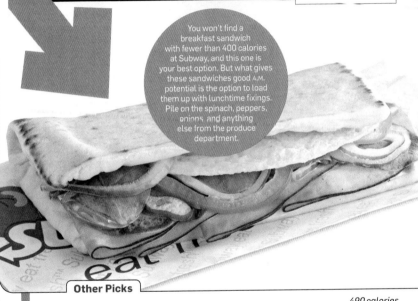

You won't find a breakfast sandwich with fewer than 400 calories at Subway, and this one is your best option. But what gives these sandwiches good A.M. potential is the option to load them up with lunchtime fixings. Pile on the spinach, peppers, onions, and anything else from the produce department.

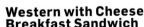

Other Picks

Western with Cheese Breakfast Sandwich

490 calories
22 g fat (8 g saturated)
1,560 mg sodium

Rosemary Chicken & Dumpling Soup (10 oz)

90 calories
1.5 g fat (0.5 g saturated)
810 mg sodium

Turkey Breast & Black Forest Ham Sub on Parmesan Oregano Bread (6")

310 calories
5 g fat (1.5 g saturated)
1,350 mg sodium

740 calories
25 g fat
(11 g saturated)
1,210 mg sodium

Not That!

Sausage & Cheese Flatbread Breakfast Sandwich

So you really love sausage? Okay, fine, but are you willing to gain 13 pounds a year over it? That's exactly what you're looking at if you make a choice like this three times a week. We'll take the ham and pocket the calories every time.

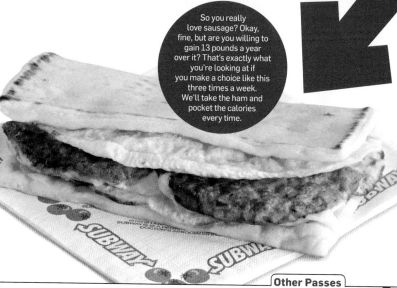

Other Passes

720 calories
45 g fat (18 g saturated)
1,580 mg sodium

Mega Breakfast Flatbread Sandwich

170 calories
5 g fat (2 g saturated)
810 mg sodium

Chicken & Dumpling Soup

390 calories
10.5 g fat (3 g saturated)
1,540 mg sodium

Black Forest Ham Wrap

235

T.G.I. Friday's

Did You Know?

● T.G.I. Friday's was founded in 1965 by a perfume salesman who wanted to meet women. He bought a broken-down beer joint in his neighborhood, jazzed it up, and called it "the T.G.I.F." in hopes of attracting a career crowd. The restaurant was a hit and made $1 million in its first year (quite a bit of cash back then).

ATTACK OF THE APPETIZER

Loaded Potato Skins

2,270 calories

What's not to loathe about potato skins? The deep-fried potatoes? The bacon? Cheese? Sour cream? Come to think of it, this thing provides more than a day's worth of calories without a shred of nutritional redemption!

Eat This

Cobb Salad

590 calories*

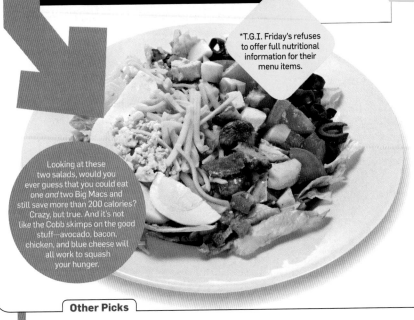

*T.G.I. Friday's refuses to offer full nutritional information for their menu items.

Looking at these two salads, would you ever guess that you could eat one *and* two Big Macs and still save more than 200 calories? Crazy, but true. And it's not like the Cobb skimps on the good stuff—avocado, bacon, chicken, and blue cheese will all work to squash your hunger.

Other Picks

Shrimp Key West *370 calories*

Buffalo Chicken Sandwich *576 calories*

Classic Sirloin
with **Mashed Potatoes** *540 calories*

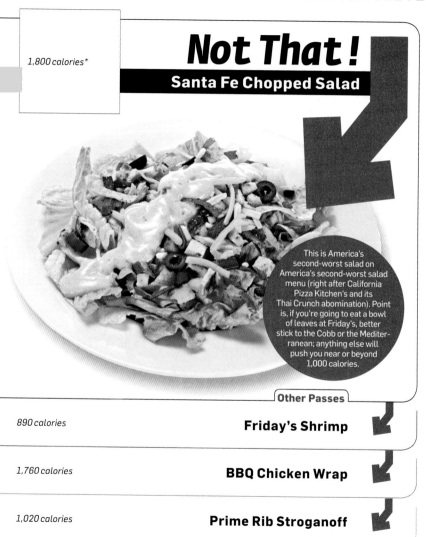

1,800 calories*

Not That!
Santa Fe Chopped Salad

This is America's second-worst salad on America's second-worst salad menu (right after California Pizza Kitchen's and its Thai Crunch abomination). Point is, if you're going to eat a bowl of leaves at Friday's, better stick to the Cobb or the Mediterranean; anything else will push you near or beyond 1,000 calories.

Petite Sirloin

How does Friday's manage to load more than 1,000 calories onto a "petite" piece of an already-lean meat? Especially considering that they sell it off the Right Portion, Right Price menu? The real villain here is actually the side. You wouldn't know it by the name, but this meal is served with an order of Mac N' Cheese. Either tell them to leave the mac off the plate, or stick with a regular-size sirloin and a vegetable side.

1,120 calories

Other Passes

890 calories	**Friday's Shrimp**
1,760 calories	**BBQ Chicken Wrap**
1,020 calories	**Prime Rib Stroganoff**

1,321

The number of calories in the average hamburger at T.G.I. Friday's. Not a single one has fewer than 1,000.

T.G.I. Friday's (Continued)

(Continued)

Did You Know?

● In general, value meals are never worth the pennies saved. But Friday's offers a real deal: In 2007, they introduced the Right Portion, Right Price menu, which offered standard entrées with portion sizes reduced by 30 percent at lower prices. Guest traffic increased by 1.4 percent as a result.

BAD BREED

JACK DANIELS GRILL

Do you really want your meal to be inspired by a man whose name is synonymous with belligerence and bar fights? It's hard to imagine the man would know a whole lot about nutrition. Perhaps that's why every meaty dish bearing the JD seal of approval packs in more than 1,000 calories. They average nearly 1,500. Jack's Glazed Ribs? 1,720 calories. His Pulled Pork Sandwich? 1,380 calories. Apparently Jack could use a lesson in prudence. Until then, search elsewhere.

Eat This

Blackened Chicken Alfredo

610 calories

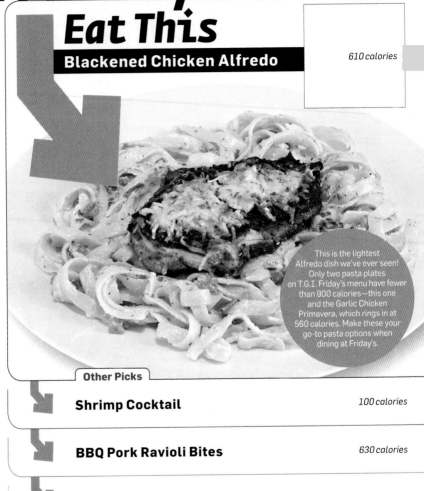

This is the lightest Alfredo dish we've ever seen! Only two pasta plates on T.G.I. Friday's menu have fewer than 900 calories—this one and the Garlic Chicken Primavera, which rings in at 560 calories. Make these your go-to pasta options when dining at Friday's.

Other Picks

Shrimp Cocktail — 100 calories

BBQ Pork Ravioli Bites — 630 calories

Chocolate Angel Swirl Cake — 330 calories

1,420 calories

Not That!
Cajun Shrimp & Chicken Pasta

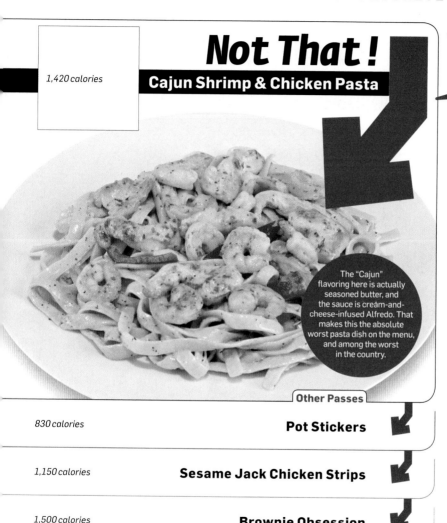

The "Cajun" flavoring here is actually seasoned butter, and the sauce is cream-and-cheese-infused Alfredo. That makes this the absolute worst pasta dish on the menu, and among the worst in the country.

Other Passes

830 calories	**Pot Stickers**
1,150 calories	**Sesame Jack Chicken Strips**
1,500 calories	**Brownie Obsession**

BURGER BOMB

Triple Stacked Burger

1,680 calories

The trio of ham, bacon, and cheese that adorns this burger might make a decent sandwich on its own, but when it plays garnish to a hunk of beef, it helps create a fusillade of artery-clogging fat. Don't come here for ground beef—not one of Friday's burgers has fewer than 1,000 calories and their steak entrées don't fare much better.

GUILTY PLEASURE

Flat Iron Steak with Wild Mushroom Sauce

540 calories

Forget guilt, you should feel a tinge of pride for locating one of the healthiest dishes on the menu. The flat iron cut doesn't show up in many restaurants, but here it proves even leaner than the sirloin. Topped with a melange of mushrooms, it makes for a satisfying sub-600 calorie meal (and will save you 500 calories over the Jack Daniels Flat Iron).

239

Taco Bell

Did You Know?

● The Taco Bell Fresco line (so named to evoke the image of freshness) was introduced in 2008 and contains nine items with 8 grams of fat or less. Even more impressive, however, is that the items also come with relatively few calories. If you order anything at Taco Bell, make it a Fresco order.

Eat This

Fresco Crunchy Beef Tacos

(3)

450 calories
21 g fat
(7.5 g saturated)
750 mg sodium

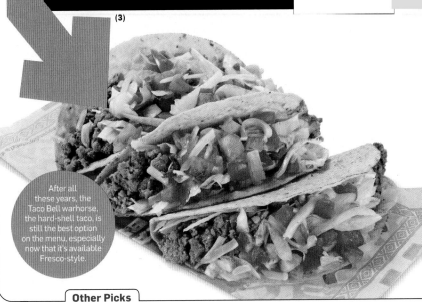

After all these years, the Taco Bell warhorse, the hard-shell taco, is still the best option on the menu, especially now that it's available Fresco-style.

Other Picks

Fresco Ranchero Chicken Soft Tacos (2)

340 calories
8 g fat (3 g saturated)
1,480 mg sodium

½ lb Beef Combo Burrito

450 calories
17 g fat (7 g saturated, 1 g trans)
1,610 mg sodium

Steak Gordita Supreme

290 calories
13 g fat (4 g saturated)
550 mg sodium

950 calories
59 g fat
(11 g saturated,
1 g trans)
1,760 mg sodium

Not That!

Chipotle Steak Fully Loaded Salad

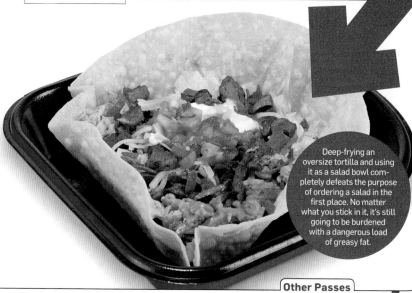

Deep-frying an oversize tortilla and using it as a salad bowl completely defeats the purpose of ordering a salad in the first place. No matter what you stick in it, it's still going to be burdened with a dangerous load of greasy fat.

WEAPON OF MASS DESTRUCTION
Volcano Box
with Large Sprite

1,755 calories
76 g fat
(20.5 g saturated, 1 g trans)
2,925 mg sodium

For about 7 bucks, you can get a Volcano Taco, Volcano Burrito, Crunchy Taco, order of Cinnamon Twists, and a large beverage. Sounds like an excellent deal, except for the terrifying fact that this explosive order is meant to feed just one person! Good for your wallet, perhaps, but it's certainly no bargain for your waistline—or your heart. This box harbors more sodium and saturated fat than you should eat in an entire day. Excessive intake of either has been linked to cardiovascular disease via high blood pressure and clogged arteries.

Other Passes

800 calories
42 g fat (12 g saturated, 1 g trans)
2,010 mg sodium

Volcano Burrito

690 calories
30 g fat (10 g saturated, 1 g trans)
2,110 mg sodium

Grilled Stuft Burrito

380 calories
23 g fat (4 g saturated)
690 mg sodium

Baja Steak Chalupa

FOOD COURT

THE CRIME
Crunchwrap
Supreme
(540 calories)

THE PUNISHMENT
Shovel snow
for 75 minutes

241

Taco Bell (Continued)

Did You Know?

● Gidget, the Chihuahua star of the chain's memorable 90's commercials, was euthanized this year at the age of 15 after a massive stroke. The "Yo quiero Taco Bell" commercials were an instant hit, though a pair of cartoonists later sued the company for breach of contract (they claimed the idea for a talking dog character was theirs) and won $40 million.

GUILTY PLEASURE

Chili Cheese Burrito

370 calories
16 g fat
(8 g saturated, 0.5 g trans)
1,080 mg sodium

Out with the beef and chicken; in with the chili. Generally we rebuke this sort of over-the-top food pileup, but as far as indulgences go, this one is relatively low-consequence. It has less fat than a Beef Gordita Baja and as much protein as a Grilled Chicken Burrito.

Eat This

Nacho Cheese Chicken Gordita and a Soft Chicken Taco

500 calories
22 g fat
(6 g saturated)
1,440 mg sodium

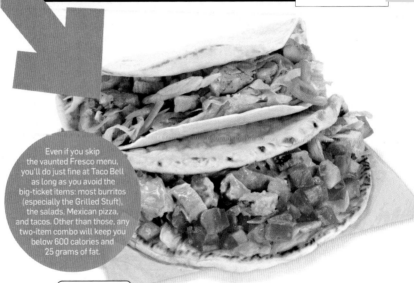

Even if you skip the vaunted Fresco menu, you'll do just fine at Taco Bell as long as you avoid the big-ticket items: most burritos (especially the Grilled Stuft), the salads, Mexican pizza, and tacos. Other than those, any two-item combo will keep you below 600 calories and 25 grams of fat.

Other Picks

Fresco Ranchero Chicken Soft Tacos (2)

340 calories
8 g fat (3 g saturated)
1,480 mg sodium

Chicken Taquitos

320 calories
11 g fat (4.5 g saturated)
1,000 mg sodium

Pintos 'n Cheese

180 calories
7 g fat (3 g saturated)
720 mg sodium

Not That!

Grilled Chicken Burrito and Ranchero Chicken Soft Taco

710 calories
34 g fat
(9 g saturated)
2,100 mg sodium

With 100 calories more than the Triple Layer Nachos, the Grilled Chicken Burrito is the worst item on the Why Pay More! Value Menu. Order this meal Fresco, however, and you'll shave off an easy 200 calories.

Other Passes

420 calories
22 g fat (6 g saturated, 0.5 g trans)
1,030 mg sodium
Big Taste Taco

520 calories
28 g fat (12 g saturated, 0.5 g trans)
1,490 mg sodium
Chicken Quesadilla

270 calories
16 g fat (2.5 g saturated)
840 mg sodium
Cheesy Fiesta Potatoes

SMART SIDES

Guacamole
(42 g)

70 calories
6 g fat
(0 g saturated)
170 mg sodium

Want to boost the nutrient profile of your take-out lunch? Ask for a side of delicious guacamole. The avocado-based spread is loaded with heart-healthy fats, fiber, and vitamin C. What's more, avocados are replete with potassium, which will help to counter-act the sodium overload in nearly every item on TB's menu. The problem with high sodium is that it throws your potassium-sodium balance out of whack—a healthy diet calls for a 1:1 ratio and this super spread can help achieve that.

BAD BREED

NACHOS
Here's the premise of a nacho plate: A meal constructed of deep-fried tortilla chips layered with taco meat and covered in nacho cheese sauce. Sound healthy? Of course not. Especially when you learn that—unless it's in New York—Taco Bell's cheese sauce earns its viscosity through a decidedly unhealthy load of partially hydrogenated oil. The wrong nacho plate will net you 3 grams of trans fat and 760 calories.

Tim Hortons

Did You Know?

● Tim Hortons, Canada's mega doughnut purveyor, has begun to invade the United States. Over a single weekend in July 2009, a dozen Dunkin' Donuts locations in New York City were completely remodeled and opened on Monday as the first 12 Tim Hortons to hit Manhattan. In total, more than 3,200 locations are in the northern United States.

DONUT DECODER

● **YEAST DONUT:** Traditional yeast-leavened doughnut that's soft and puffy

● **CAKE DONUT:** Denser, spongier bread with more fat and calories

● **TIMBIT:** The Tim Hortons version of a doughnut hole

Eat This

Croissant

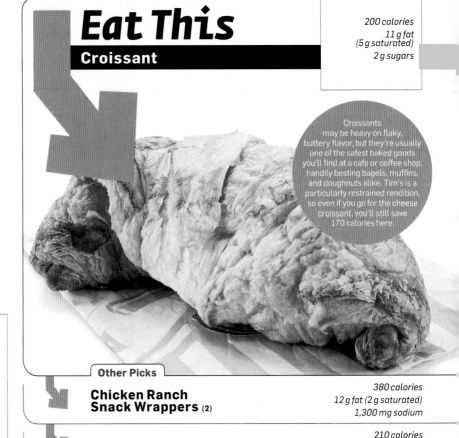

200 calories
11 g fat
(5 g saturated)
2 g sugars

Croissants may be heavy on flaky, buttery flavor, but they're usually one of the safest baked goods you'll find at a cafe or coffee shop, handily besting bagels, muffins, and doughnuts alike. Tim's is a particularly restrained rendition, so even if you go for the cheese croissant, you'll still save 170 calories here.

Other Picks

Chicken Ranch Snack Wrappers (2)
380 calories
12 g fat (2 g saturated)
1,300 mg sodium

Chocolate Chip Donut
210 calories
8 g fat (3.5 g saturated)
9 g sugars

Cafe mocha
180 calories
8 g fat (6 g saturated)
24 g sugars

400 calories
19 g fat
(2.5 g saturated)
26 g sugars

Not That!

Wheat Carrot Muffin

These are the types of numbers you'd expect from a hunk of coffee cake, not a wheat muffin. Truth is, the two are more similar than you'd think. After all, this carrot top is teeming with more sugar than you'd find in a pack of Reese's Peanut Butter Cups.

Other Passes

450 calories
18 g fat (5 g saturated)
850 mg sodium

BLT Sandwich

320 calories
19 g fat (9 g saturated)
22 g sugars

Old Fashioned Glazed Donut

260 calories
10 g fat (9 g saturated, 0.5 g trans)
28 g sugars

Hot smoothee

Uno Chicago Grill

Did You Know?

● Uno's displays its nutritional information online, but make sure to read the fine print—in the top right corner of each nutrition chart, it tells how many servings each dish contains. In an effort to appear less gluttonous, Uno's divides each dish by two, three, four, and sometimes even five.

ATTACK OF THE APPETIZER
Pizza Skins

2,400 calories
155 g fat
(45 g saturated)
3,600 mg sodium

Would you order a medium Deep Dish Beef and Pepperoni Pizza from Domino's as an appetizer? Probably not, but that's how many calories you're getting when you order these pizza skins.

Eat This

Filet Mignon
(7 oz) with Shrimp Skewer

520 calories
26 g fat
(6 g saturated)
1,340 mg sodium

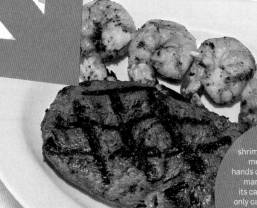

Filet mignon and shrimp are two of the leanest meats you can get your hands on, which is how this meal manages to earn fully half its calories from protein. The only caveat: Watch your sodium intake for the rest of the day. Most of Uno's dishes are stuffed with salt, which can wreak havoc on your blood pressure.

Other Picks

Mediterranean Flatbread Pizza
(½ pizza)

420 calories
22.5 g fat (7.5 g saturated)
1,170 mg sodium

Grilled Chicken
with Mango Salsa and Roasted Vegetables

310 calories
10.5 g fat (0 g saturated)
1,220 mg sodium

Crispy Cheese Dippers
(½ order)

420 calories
24 g fat (9 g saturated)
1,245 mg sodium

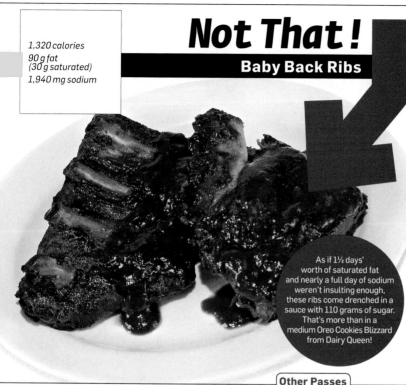

Not That!

Baby Back Ribs

1,320 calories
90 g fat
(30 g saturated)
1,940 mg sodium

As if 1½ days' worth of saturated fat and nearly a full day of sodium weren't insulting enough, these ribs come drenched in a sauce with 110 grams of sugar. That's more than in a medium Oreo Cookies Blizzard from Dairy Queen!

Other Passes

Spinoccoli Deep Dish Pizza
(½ pizza)

930 calories
67.5 g fat (16.5 g saturated)
1,245 mg sodium

Chicken & Broccoli Fettuccine

1,300 calories
74 g fat (28 g saturated)
2,020 mg sodium

Onion Strings
(½ order)

900 calories
63 g fat (10.5 g saturated)
945 mg sodium

HIDDEN DANGER

Uno Breadstick

Far too many entrées at Uno come with one of these soggy loaves hanging off the side of the plate, and the extra calories are just enough to push an otherwise decent meal into the blubber zone. The reason the restaurant gives them away is that the flour, fat, and salt from which they're made are among the cheapest ingredients in the world. Never trust a food handout.

210 calories
13 g fat
(4 g saturated)
460 mg sodium

SMART SIDES

Brown Rice with Cranberry & Mango

180 calories
5 g fat
(0.5 g saturated)
85 mg sodium

Brown rice is superior to white because it retains the bran and germ—the more nutritious and fibrous parts of the original grain. Even better: it's flavored with fruit, carrots, and olive oil. You won't find a healthier side on the menu.

247

Wendy's

Did You Know?

● Wendy's is responsible for two popular innovations that have increased the amount of fast food we consume: the drive-thru window in 1970 and the Value Menu in 1989. Today, 70 percent of Americans eat behind the wheel. Let's hope Wendy's policy of posting nutrition facts in all stores catches on, too.

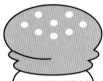

SALT LICK

BUFFALO BONELESS WINGS

2,630 mg sodium
520 calories

In theory, nixing the bone should make these healthier, but instead you get more sodium than you'll find in any other fast-food entrée in America.

Eat This

Spicy Chicken Fillet Sandwich

440 calories
16 g fat
(3 g saturated)
1,200 mg sodium

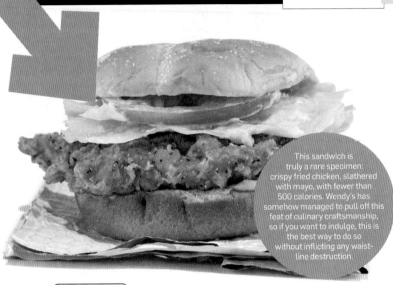

This sandwich is truly a rare specimen: crispy fried chicken, slathered with mayo, with fewer than 500 calories. Wendy's has somehow managed to pull off this feat of culinary craftsmanship, so if you want to indulge, this is the best way to do so without inflicting any waistline destruction.

Other Picks

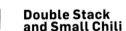

Double Stack and Small Chili

570 calories
22 g fat (10.5 g saturated, 0.5 g trans)
1,640 mg sodium

Crispy Chicken Sandwich

360 calories
18 g fat (3.5 g saturated)
710 mg sodium

Chicken Nuggets
(10 piece) with Barbecue Sauce

515 calories
32 g fat (7 g saturated)
1,120 mg sodium

550 calories
26 g fat
(8 g saturated)
1,290 mg sodium

Not That!
Chicken Club Sandwich

The three strips of bacon, Swiss cheese, and a load of mayo are basically three types of fat on top of a piece of chicken that's already been fried in hot fat. Any other chicken sandwich or wrap on the menu will save you at least 100 calories.

BURGER BOMB

½ lb. Triple with Everything and Cheese

970 calories
60 g fat
(27 g saturated, 3.5 g trans)
2,010 mg sodium

No more than 10 percent of the calories you eat should come from saturated fats. This precarious burger carries a caloric load that's 25 percent from saturated fats. If you value your heart, you'll leave this burger behind the counter, where it belongs.

| Other Passes |

700 calories
40 g fat (17 g saturated, 2 g trans)
1,440 mg sodium

Double Cheeseburger
with everything

440 calories
16 g fat (3 g saturated)
1,050 mg sodium

Homestyle Chicken Fillet Sandwich

695 calories
36 g fat (7.5 g saturated)
1,020 mg sodium

Chicken Nuggets (5 piece)
with Barbecue Sauce and medium French Fries

SMART SIDES

Baked Potato with Sour Cream & Chives

320 calories
3.5 g fat
(2 g saturated)
50 mg sodium

This baked spud has less fat and sodium than an order of fries, and it also packs in twice as much protein and fiber—two nutrients that'll quash your hunger. Order it with a Jr. Hamburger, and you have a decent meal.

249

Wendy's (Continued)

Did You Know?

● Wendy's ranked number one Mega-Chain in three categories in restaurant guide *Zagat's* 2009 Fast Food Survey: Food, Facilities, and Top Overall. Founder Dave Thomas would be proud.

CONDIMENT CATASTROPHE

Honey Mustard Nugget Sauce
(1 oz)

130 calories
12 g fat (2 g saturated)
5 g sugars

In essence, nuggets are chicken chunks wrapped in tiny jackets of flour that are made crunchy by replacing water with fat. So doesn't it seem like a bad idea to run them through a bath of even more fat? Basically, that's what this sauce is—the honey and mustard are both secondary to oil. Want a safe dunking experience? Limit yourself to Barbecue Nugget Sauce, Sweet & Sour Nugget Sauce, or regular old ketchup. Everything else carries a load of extra calories.

Eat This

Single with Everything
and Side Salad with Balsamic Vinaigrette

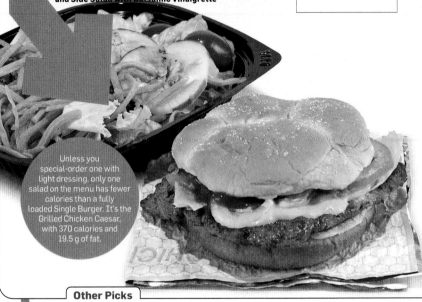

555 calories
26 g fat
(8 g saturated, 1 g trans)
1,275 mg sodium

Unless you special-order one with light dressing, only one salad on the menu has fewer calories than a fully loaded Single Burger. It's the Grilled Chicken Caesar, with 370 calories and 19.5 g of fat.

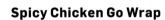

Other Picks

Spicy Chicken Go Wrap

320 calories
15 g fat (4 g saturated)
880 mg sodium

Jr. Bacon Cheeseburger

310 calories
16 g fat (6 g saturated)
670 mg sodium

Frosty-cino
small

390 calories
10 g fat (6 g saturated, 0.5 g trans)
52 g sugars

790 calories
53.5 g fat
(13.5 g saturated,
0.5 g trans)
1,665 mg sodium

Not That!

Chicken BLT Salad

with Croutons and Honey Dijon Dressing

Your salad is only as healthy as its dressing. Honey mustard is the worst dressing on the menu. The best? Fat-free French. Make the swap and you'll save 170 calories. Unless labeled "fat free," avoid creamy dressings.

MENU MAGIC

Your perfect burger is just a few strategic modifications away. Here's an example: A ¼-lb. Single, as served, contains 430 calories. But if you eliminate the mayo, swap out the cheese for a junior cheese serving, and tell them to serve it on a regular-size burger bun—the one typically reserved for Jr. Burgers—you'll cut it down to 320 calories.

Other Passes

550 calories
18 g fat (3.5 g saturated)
2,530 mg sodium

Sweet & Spicy Asian Chicken Boneless Wings

420 calories
20 g fat (4 g saturated)
380 mg sodium

French Fries
medium

550 calories
21 g fat (15 g saturated, 0.5 g trans)
68 g sugars

Chocolate Coffee Toffee Twisted Frosty

BAD BREED

FROSTIES

It's been only a few years since the Frosty was a modest answer to the typical fast-food milk shake, but those days now seem as ancient as 10-ounce bottles of Coca-Cola Classic. Today's Frosty is a mere starting point for a line of indulgent shakes layered with fudge swirls, cookie dough, whipped cream, and candy pieces. The average caloric cost of one of these beefed-up shakes? Around 489 calories for a small cup—which is about 170 calories more than the classic Frosty of yesteryear.

Whataburger

Did You Know?

● Whataburger offers breakfast items throughout the day. That's not necessarily a good thing: The 690-calorie Biscuit Sandwich with Sausage, Egg, and Cheese isn't good for you no matter what time of day you eat it. If you're really feeling the need for breakfast at dinner-time, choose the Breakfast on a Bun with bacon and save 330 calories and more than 700 milligrams of sodium.

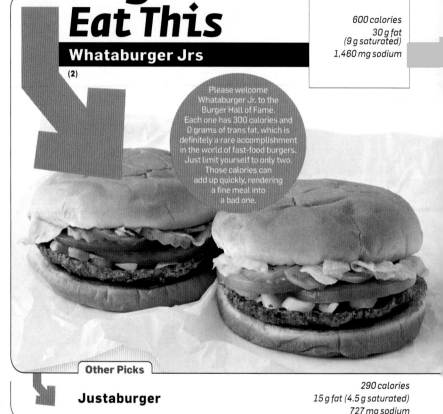

Eat This

Whataburger Jrs

(2)

600 calories
30 g fat
(9 g saturated)
1,460 mg sodium

Please welcome Whataburger Jr. to the Burger Hall of Fame. Each one has 300 calories and 0 grams of trans fat, which is definitely a rare accomplishment in the world of fast-food burgers. Just limit yourself to only two. Those calories can add up quickly, rendering a fine meal into a bad one.

Other Picks

Justaburger

290 calories
15 g fat (4.5 g saturated)
727 mg sodium

Whatachick'n Sandwich

550 calories
20 g fat (3.5 g saturated, 1 g trans)
1,408 mg sodium

Taquitos with Bacon and Egg

380 calories
21 g fat (7 g saturated)
932 mg sodium

Not That!
Double Meat Whataburger

870 calories
49 g fat
(18 g saturated,
1 g trans)
1,510 mg sodium

You can save nearly 300 calories by ordering two of the smaller burgers, instead of one burger with double-stacked beef patties. Make a swap like this once a day for 6 months and you could lose 14 pounds of body fat.

Whatacatch Dinner
(2 pieces)

One might think that a fish dinner would be a vast nutritional improvement over the burger bombs populating most of Whataburger's menu. Unfortunately, reason is no match for a deep fryer. This meal consists of two fish patties drenched in partially hydrogenated oil and served alongside a medium order of fries, and it's easily the trans-fattiest meal on the menu.

1,580 calories
92 g fat
(19 g saturated,
11 g trans)
1,916 mg sodium

Other Passes

420 calories 28 g fat (13 g saturated) 494 mg sodium	**Onion Rings** medium
700 calories 59 g fat (9.5 g saturated, 0.5 g trans) 1,346 mg sodium	**Grilled Chicken Salad** with Ranch
630 calories 12 g fat (3 g saturated) 2,373 mg sodium	**Pancakes with Bacon**

MEET YOUR MATCH

Large Strawberry Malt
(250 g sugars)

=

19 McDonald's Hot Apple Pies

White Castle

Did You Know?

⚫ Meat rationing during World War II forced White Castle to switch from burgers to hot dogs and eggs. When sliders made it back to the menu, they were priced at 5 cents each.

100 billion

The number of calories in all White Castle burgers sold each year.

MENU MAGIC

Order your sandwiches sans meat—get just plain cheese. Then ask for a container of marinara. Each cheese slider will cost you only 100 calories, and the marinara is a mere 15.

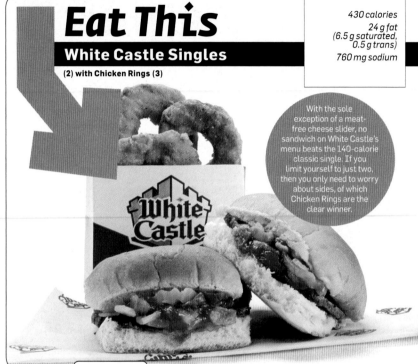

Eat This

White Castle Singles

(2) with Chicken Rings (3)

430 calories
24 g fat
(6.5 g saturated,
0.5 g trans)
760 mg sodium

With the sole exception of a meat-free cheese slider, no sandwich on White Castle's menu beats the 140-calorie classic single. If you limit yourself to just two, then you only need to worry about sides, of which Chicken Rings are the clear winner.

Other Picks

Bacon, Egg, and Cheese Sandwiches (2)
460 calories
28 g fat (10 g saturated)
1,080 mg sodium

Chicken Rings (3)
150 calories
10 g fat (2 g saturated)
340 mg sodium

Jalapeño Cheeseburgers (2)
360 calories
20 g fat (9 g saturated, 1 g trans)
760 mg sodium

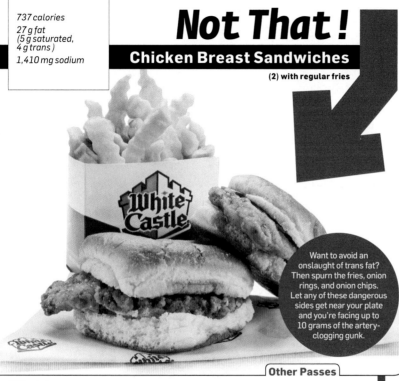

737 calories
27 g fat
(5 g saturated,
4 g trans)
1,410 mg sodium

Not That!

Chicken Breast Sandwiches

(2) with regular fries

Want to avoid an onslaught of trans fat? Then spurn the fries, onion rings, and onion chips. Let any of these dangerous sides get near your plate and you're facing up to 10 grams of the artery-clogging gunk.

Other Passes

680 calories
50 g fat (18 g saturated)
1,320 mg sodium

Sausage, Egg, and Cheese Sandwiches (2)

480 calories
23 g fat (4 g saturated, 5 g trans)
670 mg sodium

Onion Chips
regular

400 calories
22 g fat (10 g saturated, 1 g trans)
960 mg sodium

Bacon Cheeseburgers (2)

WEAPON OF MASS DESTRUCTION
Onion Chips
(sack)

980 calories
47 g fat
(8 g saturated, 10 g trans)
1,350 mg sodium

Wow, these chips just earned a new spot on our list of trans-fattiest foods in America. Most health experts agree that people should top out at around 2 grams per day. The breading on these onions, to be clear, has soaked up enough dangerous oil to fill your quota for 5 days.

GUILTY PLEASURE

Surf & Turf Sandwich

340 calories
18 g fat (6 g saturated)
420 mg sodium

This ain't your average gourmet dinner. It's a burger comprising two beef patties and a fish patty all sandwiched into a single bun, an idea that's only worth considering because of White Castle's miniature portions. Just be sure you limit yourself to one. That's all it takes to feel the thrill.

4

MENU DECODER

Roll on down the strip in our town and you'll see what looks at first like a smorgasbord of dining options. You can opt for seafood at Red Lobster, Italian food at Olive Garden, or red meat at Long-Horn Steakhouse.

Three totally different restaurants, right? Well, not really: You're still giving money to the same company, Darden Restaurants. Grab a sandwich at Pret a Manger, and you're still eating McDonald's, to a certain extent. And even if you've never heard of Yum! Brands, you've eaten plenty of their food: They operate KFC, Pizza Hut, Taco Bell, Long John Silver's, WingStreet, and A&W.

Having so many big restaurant chains guided by just a handful of multinationals does make it easy to figure out what you're eating. But it also steals a little of the magic from dining out. After all, can you really reminisce about that romantic meal you shared at Applebee's in Memphis while you're dining at an identical Applebee's in Minneapolis?

So it makes sense to get out and explore the little guys once in a while—the groovy diners that look like giant RVs, the fish taco joints by the side of the bay, the foodie favorite downtown with the crazy chef who concocts all sorts of bizarre mixtures, and the local sports bar where everybody knows your name and everybody roots for the home team. But once you get there, what do you order? Thanks to this book, you know what's in a McNugget, but how do you know what's in the Blue Plate Special?

It's simple. Use this chapter—our secret menu decoder—as your guide, and you'll swagger like John Wayne into every high-class joint or hole-in-the-wall in your 'hood, always ready to order with confidence.

Breakfast Diner

HUEVOS RANCHEROS

Consider it a culinary blessing that the Mexican take on country-style eggs has spread to the United States. The beans that go on top add belly-filling fiber and, along with the salsa, provide a grab bag of antioxidants. Consider it 500 calories well spent.

STEAK AND EGGS

Protein-based meals like this trounce carb-heavy entrées like French toast and pancake stacks any day. Studies show that a heavy load of protein at breakfast will result in fewer calories eaten throughout the day.

EGGS BENEDICT

Do you really want to burn through an entire day's worth of saturated fat at breakfast? That's exactly what this classic is likely packing. The viscous blanket of hollandaise sauce is actually an emulsion of egg yolks and melted better—both of which are best eaten in moderation. Count on 800 calories and 50 grams of fat for an average serving.

BELGIAN WAFFLE

Meals based on refined flour—all pancakes and waffles included—make for a nutritionally dismal start to the day. The fact that most diner "maple" syrup is nearly pure high-fructose corn syrup only adds insult to injury.

BREAKFAST SPECIALS

Our value-oriented breakfast specials come with your choice of coffee or tea and a small juice.

HAPPY MOUNTAIN
HUEVOS RANCHEROS, with two fresh eggs cooked sunnyside up and topped with beans, avocado, cheddar cheese and fresh salsa on a tortilla 7.95
Add fresh fruit 1.50

WYNDMOOR
STEAK AND EGGS, an 8 oz. strip steak with 2 eggs, hash browns, and choice of whole wheat or white toast 7.95

WAYNE JUNCTION
CLASSIC EGGS BENEDICT Grilled Canadian bacon served under poached eggs and rich Hollandaise neatly stacked on a toasted English muffin. Comes with your choice of home fries, grits or white cheddar grits 8.95

GRAVERS
THREE FLUFFY BUTTERMILK PANCAKES with your choice of breakfast meat 7.45
Add bananas, blueberries or strawberries 1.00

CAPTAIN JANE
FISH & GRITS Cornmeal-dusted Catfish lightly fried and served with Grits or
Cheese Grits 6.95
with Two Eggs 8.45

FRENCH TOAST, PANCAKES, WAFFLES

cooked on our griddle and served with butter and syrup.
Top your griddles with bananas, blueberries, chocolate chips or strawberry topping for 1.00

PANCAKES
FULL STACK (3)
SHORT STACK (2)

BUTTERMILK PANCAKES
Full Stack 4.25
Short Stack 3.75

HONEY BUCKWHEAT PANCAKES
Full Stack 5.50
Short Stack 4.75

WHOLE GRAIN PANCAKES
Full Stack 5.50
Short Stack 4.75

FRENCH TOAST
TEXAS STYLE FRENCH TOAST
Full Stack 3.50
Short Stack 2 .... 2.75

BELGIAN WAFFLE
BELGIAN WAFFLE 3.50

EGG COMBOS

All carefully prepared 3-egg omelettes come with your choice of home fries, cheese grits and white or wheat toast

3 EGG OMELETTES

CHEESE OMELETTE 4.75
HAM OR BACON OMELETTE 4.95
SPINACH & FETA OMELETTE 4.75
VEGGIE OMELETTE 4.95
Mushroom, Onion, Pepper & Tomato
WESTERN OMELETTE 4.95
Ham, Onion & Pepper
SUBSTITUTE EGG WHITES 1.00
ADDITIONAL OMELETTE ITEMS .... 50¢
EACH
Ham, Bacon, Sausage, Potato, Peppers,
Broccoli, Onions, Spinach, Mushrooms,
Tomato, Cheese (American, Swiss,
Mozzarella or Cheddar)

FARM FRESH EGGS
served with home fries or grits & to...
ONE EGG, Any Style, with Toast .. 1...
TWO EGGS, Any Style, with Toast 2.25
with Home Fries & Toast 3.75
STEAK & EGGS 6 oz. Center Cut Strip
Steak with Two Eggs prepared Any Style,
served with your choice of Home Fries or
Grits and toast 12.95

CONTINENTAL CHOICES

BREADS & MUFFINS

TOAST 1.00
ENGLISH MUFFIN 1.00
ASSORTED MUFFINS 1.35
choice of blueberry, bran, apple or corn
BAGEL 1.00
choice of plain, sesame seed, poppy or
everything
with Cream Cheese 1.50
DANISH 1.25

SIDE ORDERS

HASH BROWNS 1.50
BACON, SAUSAGE, SCRAPPLE .. 1.85
CORNED BEEF HASH 2.25

CEREALS & FRUITS

CEREAL with Milk .... 1...
with choice of fruit .... 2...
KETTLE OATS .... 2.2...
with choice of fruit 2.45
GRITS 1.50
with Cheese 2.45
FRESH FRUIT SALAD 3.25
with Cottage Cheese 4.25

BEVERAGES

CHILLED JUICES
Orange, Apple, Grapefruit, or Tomato ...
1.50
BOTTOMLESS COFFEE 1.50
HOT TEA 1.00
ICE COLD MILK 1.50

ALL DAY BREAKFAST

Served from 3:00 p.m. to closing Monday-Saturday 3:30 p.m. to clo...
We feature 100% homemade breads.
Choice of breakfast meat includes: Bacon, sausage links and sc...
Home fries can be prepared with fried onions at no additional c...
An 18% gratuity will be added to parties of six or more.

EGG WHITES

While egg whites have a reputation for being nutritional magic bullets, you should think twice before you nix the yolk. Besides carrying a good dose of healthy fat, yolks are one of the best sources of choline, a nutrient important to brain function that has been shown to help reduce inflammation and improve cardiovascular function. Worried about cholesterol? Don't be. The latest research shows that not only do eggs not raise our bad cholesterol, but that regular consumption may actually improve our overall cholesterol levels.

BAGEL WITH CREAM CHEESE

A bagel is shaped like a zero for a reason. The majority of its 500 calories come from refined carbohydrates, with little redeeming nutrition to justify the price tag. You'd be better off eating a doughnut.

HASH BROWNS

Short order cooks make hash browns in huge batches, using copious amounts of oil to keep the spuds from sticking to the griddle. Figure about 300 calories per side dish; skip the spuds and ask for grits or fresh fruit, instead.

CHILLED JUICE

Not the best way to boost the nutritional value of your meal. A 12-ounce cup of juice can harbor as much as 3 tablespoons of sugar, and that's if the diner serves pure juice with no sugars added in. Better off with coffee or milk.

CORNED BEEF HASH

Corned beef carries a load of salt from the brine it was soaked in, and heavy-handed fry cooks are encouraged to add more at the griddle. Even a side will likely carry more than 1,000 milligrams of sodium.

Burger Joint

TURKEY BURGER

Not always the bona fide safe bet most people believe it to be. Ground turkey, like beef, is classified by the amount of fat found in the grind, and many burger joints, fearing a dry burger, opt for the 80 percent lean variety. This essentially makes it just as caloric as a beef burger.

BUN

Most old-fashioned burger joints will butter their buns before toasting them on a griddle or grill. Save an easy 100 calories by asking for your bun sans butter—you won't even miss it.

MUSHROOM SWISS BURGER

There's a maxim that pertains to the naming of burgers, and it goes like this: The longer the name, the more calories the burger contains. So even though this burger sounds like it's no worse than a regular cheeseburger, chances are it's saddled with a couple hundred extra calories.

MAYONNAISE

Burgers have enough fat as it is, and a routine assault with mayonnaise can add upward of 100 calories to a burger. Make it a personal policy to stick with ketchup and mustard, or even barbecue or steak sauce.

SECRET SAUCE

There's no secret here at all. Nine times out of ten, the recipe amounts to a mix that's three parts mayo, one part ketchup, with a handful of spices thrown in. You're looking at 100 calories a slather— the same price as your average application of cheese.

OUR FAMOUS BURGERS

All Platters Served with Steak Fries, Lettuce and Tomato, English Muffin; Toasted Bun Substitute $0.75 Extra; Semolina Roll $0.75 Extra Baked Potato or Onion Ring Substitute $1.25 Extra, Sandwich / Platter

BEEF BURGER
Our classic burger $8.40

TURKEY BURGER
For a change of pace $8.40

MUSHROOM SWISS BURGER
Smothered with sautéed mushrooms $9.90

ENGLISH BURGER
Served on English muffin $8.40

PIZZA BURGER
With homemade marinara sauce $9.90

CHILI BURGER
Smothered with chili con carne $9.90

SOUTHWEST BURGER
...pped with guacamole and raw onion $11.00

SPECIAL HOUSE BURGER
With Secret sauce, bacon & fried onions $10.15

SANDWICHES & SALADS

CLASSIC BLT
Served on home-baked bread $6.95

HOT DOG
The All-American classic $6

CHICKEN CLUB
Stacked high with chicken, bacon and fresh garden goodness! $7

ROAST BEEF
Topped with provolone cheese $8

PHILADELPHIA CHEESE STEAK
This no-frills sandwich will melt in your mouth $9.50

GRILLED PORTOBELLO SALAD
With sautéed mushrooms, tomatoes, sweet onions, cucumber $6

CRISPY CHICKEN SALAD
With honey-jalapeno vinaigrette $7.50

CENTER CUT ICEBERG
Our version of the wedge, with chopped egg, tomato, bacon bits $11.50

BEVERAGES

Soda $1		Coffee $1	
Milk Shake $3		Tea $1	

BLT

Whether or not it's on the menu, most burger spots are fully equipped to whip up a classic bacon, lettuce, and tomato sandwich. A BLT—even with a swip of mayo—won't stray far past the 400-calorie mark, which makes it a colossal improvement over most of the bloated burgers on the menu.

HOT DOG

Hot dogs trump burgers in 99 percent of nutritional matchups. The reason is simple: portion size. Thanks to an arms race among burger joints, hamburgers today are two to five times bigger than they were 20 years ago. The humble hot dog, however, has remained relatively unchanged in that same time.

CRISPY CHICKEN SALAD

Nobody orders a crispy chicken salad for the lettuce. Common toppings include shredded Cheddar, fried croutons, bacon bits, and ranch dressing. If you plan to go the crispy chicken route, don't do it under nutritional pretenses; it's likely to be as caloric (or more!) than a big burger.

MILK SHAKE

Here's the sad truth: Few desserts in the world are worse than milk shakes. By liquefying cream and sugar, it's possible to inject more calories into the same amount of space, which is why these things commonly hold between 700 and 1,200 calories.

Café

coffee

- ESPRESSO $1.80
- CAPPUCCINO $3.00
- CAFFÈ LATTE $3.00
- STEAMED MILK $3.00
- CAFFÈ MOCHA $3.35
- CAFFÈ AMERICANO $1.95

frozen coffee drinks

- MOCHA $3.75
- TAHITIAN VANILLA LATTE $3.75
- HAZELNUT, ALMOND AND MACADAMIA NUT $3.75
- CRÈME DE MENTHE SYRUP, WHIPPED CREAM $3.75
- PEANUT BUTTER, BANANA AND WHIPPED CREAM $3.75

ALL DRINKS AVAILABLE DECAFFEINATED, WITH SKIM
OR SOY MILK, AND OVER ICE. EXTRA SHOTS OF ESPRESSO,
FLAVORED SYRUPS OR WHIPPED CREAM AVAILABLE
FOR AN EXTRA CHARGE.

SYRUPS: ALMOND, AMARETTO, CARAMEL, CHOCOLATE
MACADAMIA NUT, CHOCOLATE MINT, HAZELNUT, ENGLISH
TOFFEE, IRISH CREAM, RASPBERRY, FRENCH VANILLA

AMERICANO
Made from a few shots of espresso and hot water, this is the best espresso drink on the menu. It's like coffee, with an extra kick.

ESPRESSO
Always choose cappuccinos over lattes. With nearly half the amount of milk, you'll save about 60 calories per medium cup—which adds up fast. Still, when you start adding syrups and whipped topping, both can be dangerous. A large flavored espresso drink made with 2% milk can cost you about 300 calories and 8 grams of fat.

FROZEN COFFEE DRINKS
The worst of all coffee categories. With the heavy reliance on dairy, syrups, and whipped cream kickers, these may as well be labeled "caffeinated milk shakes." Expect to invest between 400 and 700 calories in one of these frozen follies.

FLAVORED SYRUPS
Flavored syrups are made almost entirely of high-fructose corn syrup. Count on 20 calories and 5 grams of sugar per pump. Luckily, health-minded places also carry a good array of sugar-free, zero-calorie syrups like chocolate, hazelnut, and caramel.

QUICHE
Quiche is good for a reliable dose of protein, but it comes at a price. Thanks to an oily pastry shell and an unfettered load of cheese, a slice may carry 500 calories or more. The best part about quiche? The simple salad that is nearly always served on the side.

Breakfast Sandwiches

- SAUSAGE & MELTED AMERICAN CHEESE $4.75
- SMOKED HAM & MELTED AMERICAN CHEESE $4.75
- SMOKED BACON, TOMATO & CREAM CHEESE $4.75
- KIELBASA & MELTED SWISS $4.75
- BREAKFAST BURRITO $4.75
- CANADIAN BACON AND MELTED CHEDDAR $4.75

Muffins
$1.75
- BRAN
- CORN
- BANANA & NUT
- APPLE & CINNAMON
- BLUEBERRY
- RASPBERRY

Biscottis
$1.75
- PREMIUM ALMOND
- CHOCOLATE ALMOND
- HAZELNUT
- CHOCOLATE
- HAZELNUT
- PISTACHIO

Quiche

SERVED WITH A MIXED FIELD GREEN SALAD TOSSED IN OUR LEMON POPPY VINAIGRETTE

- QUICHE LORRAINE $9
- CRAB QUICHE $10
- SPINACH QUICHE $8

Desserts

- YOGURT PARFAIT $3.75
- FRESH FRUIT $3.75
- CHERRY PIE $3.75
- APPLE PIE
- LE

BREAKFAST SANDWICHES

This is a relatively safe spot on the menu, but there's still a strategy to getting the best sandwich. Cap the caloric load at 400 by opting for the smallest bread and avoiding sausage. The best combo? Egg, ham, and American on an English muffin.

BRAN MUFFIN

Putting a fancy name on a pastry is like putting lipstick on a crocodile. No matter how you dress it up, it still bites. A bran muffin might come with a couple grams of fiber, but that's a small pittance for a breakfast that can easily eclipse 400 calories—especially considering that the bulk of those calories comes from the same sugars and starches that make up everything else in the pastry case.

ALMOND BISCOTTI

At 100 calories apiece, this coffee-shop classic makes a reasonable treat—but not if you're pairing it with a sugar-injected latte or blended drink. Pair it with a plain ol' cup of joe or a cappuccino and you'll keep the damage to a minimum.

YOGURT PARFAIT

The healthiest way to satisfy your sweet tooth. The yogurt is loaded with gut-friendly bacteria, protein, and calcium, and to make it a parfait, it's blended with a mix of berries, each of which brings to the cup a unique kick of antioxidants. Just make sure the base is plain—not sugar-laden flavored—yogurt and that the calorie-dense granola is applied with a modest hand. If so, this is a huge coffeehouse green light.

BBQ Shack

BURNT ENDS

The crispy end pieces of brisket. Because the fat from the meat has been fully rendered, they make a much better option than normal brisket, which sports a thick "fat cap."

RIBS

Delicious though they may be, they're the worst option on the menu, with a perilously high fat-to-meat ratio. Split a half slab for the table and make them baby back, which are leaner than spare ribs.

ROTISSERIE CHICKEN

Sans skin, this is the best entrée on the menu. A 6-ounce serving has about 50 grams of protein, plus a load of tryptophan, an amino acid that helps your body regulate appetite.

BRUNSWICK STEW

Depending on which part of the South you order it in, this hearty tomato-based stew may be loaded with chicken, rabbit, or pork, plus a slew of vegetables like corn, lima beans, and okra. An excellent option either way.

OUR MEATS

NORTH CAROLINA PULLED PORK	6.29
KANSAS CITY BURNT ENDS	6.29
TEXAS SLICED BEEF BRISKET	6.29
BARBECUED PORK CHOP	6.29
RED HOT SMOKED SAUSAGE	6.29
MEMPHIS DRY-RUBBED BARBECUED RIBS	
Lone Bone (1 rib)	2.75
Rib Sandwich (2 ribs)	6.29
½ Slab (3–4 ribs)	11.95
½ Slab (5–6 ribs)	13.95
Full Slab (12 Ribs)	21.95
ROTISSERIE CHICKEN	
¼ Chicken	5.95
½ Chicken	9.95
Whole Chicken	16.95
BRUNSWICK STEW	5.29

Generous portions of rabbit and chicken, onions, corn, tomatoes and okra served with a biscuit.

ALL PLATTERS
served with choice of two sides, hush puppies and a biscuit.

OUR MEALS

OUR $60 VALUE

(1) Slab of Ribs

(1) Pint of Pulled Pork, Burnt Ends, Beef Brisket, Pulled Chicken, or Hot Sausage

(1) Barbecued or Jamaican Jerk Half Chicken

(1) Pint each, Baked Beans & Cole Slaw

(4) Biscuits

(2) Quarts of Lemonade or Iced Sweet Tea

Half-pints of BBQ sauces

OUR $97 VALUE

(2) Slabs of Ribs

(2) Pints of Pulled Pork, Burnt Ends, Beef Brisket, Pulled Chicken, or Hot Sausage

SAUCE SELECTOR

● **KANSAS CITY**
Thick, tomato-based sauce with lots of brown sugar. Use sparingly.

● **MEMPHIS**
A well-balanced sauce made with both tomato and vinegar.

● **NORTH CAROLINA**
Vinegar-based sauce with a kick of spice from cayenne pepper. Go nuts.

● **SOUTH CAROLINA**
Also tangy, but made from mustard; a little sweeter than its northern cousin.

● **TEXAS**
Spicy tomato-based sauce blended with peppers and cumin.

OUR OTHERS

BIG GREEN SALAD WITH CORNBREAD 4.75
Choice of Ranch or Italian
With pulled chicken or spicy chicken salad 6.29

HOT OPEN-FACED BRISKET SANDWICH 8.95
With mashed potatoes, pan gravy, collard greens and cornbread

FRIED CATFISH 10.75
Cornmeal crusted and served with cole slaw, hush puppies and mash potatoes

BLACKENED CATFISH 10.75
Grilled in spices and served with cole slaw, mash potatoes and black-eyed corn

PEEL 'N' EAT SHRIMP 12.95

POTLIKKER WITH BISCUITS 1.95
Ask and we'll tell ya

OUR SWEETS

PIE: APPLE, PECAN, LEMON MERINGUE 2.95

KEY LIME PIE 2.95

FRUIT COBBLER 2.95

DREAM BAR 1.95

OUR SIDES

BAKED BEANS 1.95 c / 3.95 p / 6.95 qua

HUSH PUPPIES $.95 / 1.95 p / 3.95 qua

BLACK-EYED CORN 1.95 cup / 3.95 pint / 6.95 quart

HOMEMADE PICKLES 1.95 half pint

PAN GRAVY 3.95 pint

BISCUITS $.75

COLE SLAW 1.9 / 3.9 / 6.95 q

GREEN BEANS 1.95 cup / 3.95 pint

MASH POTATOES

COLLARD GREENS

RICE & BEANS

BAKED BEANS
The one-two combo of brown sugar and molasses used in these beans is more than balanced by a heavy load of protein, fiber, and antioxidants. Even with bacon blended in, this is still a better option than biscuits or French fries.

HUSH PUPPIES
Deep-fried corn bread, often served with a side of whipped butter for dipping. Do you really need to know anything else?

PIE: APPLE, PECAN, LEMON MERINGUE
Meringue pies will generally edge out the other pie choices when it comes to calories. That's because the egg whites and sugar that go into the meringue are whipped with air, so while it feels like a full piece of pie, you're actually eating less.

COLESLAW
Inquire about the coleslaw before you order. If it's mayonnaise-based, it's probably a nutritional dud with hundreds of calories in each scoop. If it's vinegar-based, give it the green light.

COLLARD GREENS
Collards are of the same plant family as broccoli and brussels sprouts, which puts them among the healthiest sides you can order. This side carries a day's worth of vitamin A, 2 days' worth of vitamin K, and a heavy load of sulforaphane, a cancer-fighting antioxidant.

Cajun

GATOR BITES

Alligator meat has a higher proportion of omega-3 fats and more protein than you'll find in chicken. That's why it's a shame so many Cajun chefs don't sell it without first sending it off for a prolonged swim in hot oil. Find a Cajun shack that sells its gator grilled, then eat all you want.

PO'BOY

This Louisiana sub sandwich has the potential to be one of the better meals on the menu, but that potential's shot as soon as you order it stuffed with deep-fried shrimp, oysters, or catfish. Unfortunately, that's the default for most po'boys. Ask to have yours made with grilled or blacked fish or chicken, instead.

FRIED CRAWFISH

Like popcorn shrimp, this Cajun specialty takes a perfectly lean, unadulterated protein and ruins it with a dip in batter and a bath in hot oil. A serving will run about 700 calories, before the side of fries.

DIRTY RICE

No, it's not really dirty, but it is deep brown in color. That's because this rice is cooked with a couple of underappreciated, color-imparting health foods: chicken livers and chicken gizzards, both of which constitute a nutritional leap above sausage. The liver is loaded with vitamins B and A, and the gizzards are rich in iron, which your body uses to transport oxygen through your bloodstream.

APPETIZERS

Gator Bites marinated and fried 5.99

Jalapeno Cheese Bites 5.99

Boudin link grilled 2.59

Popcorn Crawfish 4.99

Oysters on the Half Shell
(6) 3.59   (12) 5.99

Boudin Balls (6)
fried spicy cajun meatballs 5.99

PO'BOYS

ROAST BEEF 'N GRAVY 8.99

CHICKEN 7.99

POPCORN SHRIMP 8.99

FRIED CRAWFISH 8.99

FRIED OYSTER 9.99

CATFISH 9.99

SOFT SHELL CRAB 8.99

PLATTERS & ENTREES

CRAWFISH ÉTOUFFÉE
Crawfish smothered in a spicy rich sauce served over rice. 9.99

SHRIMP AND GRITS
Fresh gulf shrimp and stone-ground gri̱ flavored with bacon. 12.99

RABBIT STEW w/RICE
Cajun Style Rabbit smothered in a spi̱ dark gravy served over rice. 10.99

LOUISIANA RED SNAPPER
Red Snapper smothered in a tomato sauc̱ onions, celery and bell peppers. $14.9

TURTLE SAUCE PIQUANTE
Turtle meat in a spicy sauce. 10.99

BLACKENED CATFISH
Seasoned Catfish fillets grilled to order 10.99

RED BEANS AND RICE
Spicy Red Beans served over rice with grilled smoked sausage. 8.99

INCLUDES OUR HOUSE SALAD AND CHOICE OF:
baked potato (with fixin's .99 xtra), potato salad, red beans 'n rice,
dirty rice, or vegetable of the day (ask your server).

CRAWFISH ÉTOUFFÉE
Both étouffée and gumbo start out with a roux, which is a flour-thickened mix of butter and oil, and both are generally served over white rice. The thicker the étouffée or gumbo, the more fat it has, so quiz your server about whether hers is thin or thick. If it's thick, give it the pass, but if it's thin, go for it.

SHRIMP AND GRITS
Think of this as the South's answer to shrimp scampi. Overall, the dish delivers a good variety of protein, produce, and grain for about 700 calories a serving.

RED SNAPPER
Catch snapper on menus across the Gulf coast, usually blackened or smothered. The latter isn't the type of menu parlance that bodes well for your waistline, but here, it means a spicy tomato stew laced with the Cajun trinity of vegetables.

BLACKENED CATFISH
Blackening adds a massive punch of assertive flavor without sticking your meal with any hidden caloric fees. The basic seasoning blend is garlic, pepper, chiles, and onion powder, all of which bring to the dish their own unique antioxidant profiles. Consider this your best alternative to frying.

RED BEANS AND RICE
The Cajun staple starts with überhealthy kidney beans, which are among the most antioxidant-rich foods in the world. A USDA study showed them to have 10 times as many antioxidants as spinach. In a perfect world, they'd come sans rice, but even with it, this is a solid meal.

Chinese

POT STICKERS

Probably not nearly as bad as you think. Panfrying imparts far less fat than other frying methods do, and the thin dumpling wrapper that holds the meat and vegetables has far fewer carbs than anything made with real bread. As an appetizer split among friends, these stickers are safe.

EGG ROLL

It's not the insides of an egg roll (cabbage, mushrooms, bean sprouts) that will do you in; it's the crunchy, deep-fried carb blanket that forms the exterior. Each roll adds 150 to 200 calories to your plate.

EGG DROP SOUP

Although reliably low in calories, the amount of sodium in egg drop soup varies from high to horrendous. Keep your serving to a small cup rather than a meal-size bowl. Otherwise, you could sacrifice most of a day's sodium allotment in a few spirited slurps.

PEKING DUCK

Duck sits slightly ahead of ground turkey in terms of its overall balance of protein, fat, and nutrients. It's also one of the most authentic Chinese dishes on the menu, with chefs employing painstaking measures to render most of the fat from the bird, ensuring extra-crunchy skin. It dodges the syrupy plague infecting everything else, so it winds up being one of the healthiest entrées.

Noodle Corner

HOURS OF OPERATION
11:00AM–12:00 MIDNIGHT
FREE OUTGOING DELIVERY

TEL 245-5896

APPETIZERS

A1.	PuPu Platter (for 2).	$7.25
	Egg Rolls, Chicken Fingers, Spareribs, Teriyaki Beef, Chicken Wings, Crab Rangoon	
A10.	Chicken Fingers	$7.25
A2.	Mini Pu Pu Platter	$9.95
	Teriyaki Beef (2), Boneless Spare Ribs, Chicken Wings (2), Crab Rangoon (2), Chicken Teriyaki (2).	
A11.	Pot Stickers (Pork or Vegetable) (6)	$3.95
A3.	Beef Teriyaki (6)	$7.55
A12.	Crab Rangoon (6)	$4.25
A4.	Egg Roll (2)	$3.75
A13.	Dim Sim Siu Mi (6)	$4.75
A5.	Shanghai Spring Rolls (2)	$3.95
A14.	Chicken Teriyaki	$7.55
A15.	Vegetable Egg Rolls (2)	$3.95
A7.	Chicken Wings (7)	$5.95
A8.	Fried Shrimps (6)	$7.55
A17.	Scallion Pancake	$3.95
A9.	Spareribs	$7.55
A18.	Boneless Spareribs	$7.25

SOUP

S1.	Wonton Soup	$2.05
S5.★	Hot and Sour Soup	$2.05
S2.	Egg Drop Soup	$1.65
S6.	Chinese Vegetable Soup	$2.05
S3.	House Special Soup	$7.55

BEEF

B1.	Beef with Green Peppers	$9.55
B10.	Beef with Mushrooms	$10.25
	Beef with Broccoli	$9.55
	Beef in Szechuan Sauce.	
	with Pea Pods.	$9.55
	Beef with Peanuts and Peppers	$9.55
	Beef with Pea Pods	$9.55
	Shredded Beef in Garlic Sauce	$9.55

B5.	Beef with Pea Pods and Bamboo Shoots	$10.25
B14.★	Hunan Spiced Beef	$9.55
B6.	Mongolian Barbecued Beef	$10.25
B15.★	Beef with Black Bean Sauce	$9.55
B7.	Beef with Scallions	$9.55
B16.★	Orange Flavored Beef	$10.55
B8.	Beef with Chinese Vegetables	$9.55
B17.★	House Special Lamb	$11.95
B9.	Sesame Beef	$10.95

PORK

P1.	Pork with Pea Pods	$8.95
P5.★	Spicy Double Cooked Pork	$8.95
P2.	Pork with Broccoli	$8.95
P6.★	Spicy Shredded Pork in Garlic Sauce	$8.95
P3.	Pork with Scallions	$8.95
P7.★	Hunan Pork	$8.95
P4.	Three Delights with Pork, Shrimp, or Chicken	$9.55

POULTRY

C1.	Peking Duck	$12.05
C12.★	Kung Pao Chicken	$9.05
C2.	Chicken with Pea Pods	$9.05
C13.★	Tender Chicken w/Black Bean Sauce	$9.05
C3.	Moo Goo Gai Pan	$9.05
C14.★	Orange Flavor Chicken	$9.75
C4.	Eight Treasure Chicken	$9.05
C15.★	Curried Chicken	$9.05
C5.	Chicken with Broccoli	$9.05
C16.★	Jordan Chicken (General Gau's Chicken)	$9.75
C17.★	Chef's Chicken Delight with Spicy Sesame	$8.95
C6.	Chicken with Pineapple	$9.05
C18.★	Sesame Crispy Chicken	$9.95
C7.★	Spicy Szechuan Chicken with Peanuts	$8.05
C19.★	Fresh String Beans with Chicken and Beef	$8.05

LUNCHEON SPECIALS

Served daily 11:30 a.m. to 2:30 p.m. (except Sunday & Holidays). Served with choice of Pork Fried Rice or Steamed choice of Hot and Sour Soup, Egg Drop Soup or Wonton Soup. (Soup not included with Take-Out orders).

1. Chicken Wings (3), Egg Roll $5.25
12. * Kung Pao Chicken $6.55
2. Teriyaki Beef (2), Chicken Wings (2), Egg Roll .. $5.95
13. Eight Treasure Chicken, Teriyaki Beef....... $6.75
3. Boneless Spareribs (4), Egg Roll $5.95
14. Chicken with Pea Pods, Chicken Fingers (3) .. $6.25
4. Teriyaki Beef (2), Spareribs (2), Shrimp (2) $6.95
15. * General Tso's Chicken, Egg Roll.............. $7.25
5. Chicken Fingers (4), Chicken Wings (2) $5.55
16. Combo Lo Mein, Boneless Spareribs........... $5.75
6. Sweet and Sour Pork, Egg Roll $5.25
17. * Shrimp with Garlic Sauce, Egg Roll $7.25

7. Sweet and Sour Chicken, Egg Roll............. $5
18. Shrimp with Lobster Sauce, Egg Roll $7.25
8. Beef with Green Pepper, Egg Roll............. $6.25
19. * Szechuan String Beans, Egg Roll............. $5.35
9. Beef with Broccoli................................
20. Vegetarian's Delight, Egg Roll................ $6.25
10. * Spicy Double Cooked Pork, Egg Roll $5.95
21. * Meatless Chow Mein, Egg Roll $5.55
    (Or choice of Chicken, Shrimp, Beef or Pork Chow $4.25
    Mein).
11. Cashew Chicken $4.45
22. * Shredded Beef Szechuan Style (Or choice of Chicken, $5.75
    Shrimp, or Pork................................. $4.55

WEIGHT WATCHERS

All Weight-Watchers' orders are steamed. There is no seasoning or corn starch used in cooking.

W1. Mixed Vegetables................................ $5.95
W2. Mixed Vegetables (Choice of Pork, Chicken, Beef or Shrimp)................................. $8.95
W3. Steamed Shrimp with Broccoli................ $8.95

MOO-SHI

Moo-Shi is a very popular mandarin dish which contains mushrooms, cabbage, fungus, dried lily flower, eggs and meat served with 6 pancakes and Hoi Sin sauce

MI. Moo-Shi (Chicken, Beef, Pork, Shrimp, or Vegetables)....................................... $7.95
M2. Moo-Shi Peking Style (Spicy) $8.05

VEGETABLES

V1. Vegetarian's Delight $6.55
V5. Stir Fried Pea Pods $6.55
V6. * Spicy Eggplant in Garlic Sauce.............. $6.25
V3. Snow Pea Pods with Water Chestnuts.. $6.55
V7. * Spicy Broccoli.................................. $6.25
V4. Brocoli in Oyster Sauce $6.55
V8. * String Beans, Szechuan Style (Meatless)..... $6.25

SWEET AND SOUR

SW1. Sweet and Sour Pork...............................
SW3. Sweet and Sour Shrimp...........................
SW2. Sweet and Sour Chicken..........................
SW4. Sweet and Sour Combo............................

NOODLES

L1. Lo Mein (Choice of Pork, Chicken, Beef or Shrimp)....................................
L2. Chow Mein.......................................
L4. Shanghai Noodles........................... $7.2
L6. Shanghai Noodles (Meatless)............... $9.25
L7. Cold Noodles in Sesame Sauce.............. $6.95
     .... $4.95

RICE

R1. Steamed Rice.................................... $0.95
R2. Fried Rice (Choice of Pork, Chicken, Beef)..... $5.95
R3. Combo Fried Rice $7.25
R6. Brown Rice $1.50

*spicy

KUNG PAO CHICKEN

Made with roasted peanuts, dried chilies, and a slew of other vegetables, Kung Pao can be one of the best entrées on the Chinese menu. That's because the chicken isn't fried. All but guaranteed to trounce General Tso's, sesame chicken, and sweet and sour anything.

CASHEW CHICKEN

Authentic Chinese? Hardly. The version most common today is reputed to have roots in Springfield, Missouri. Basically it consists of fried chicken, a handful of cashews, and a thick layer of oyster sauce. Not your best choice.

STEAMED SHRIMP WITH BROCCOLI

The best part about ordering meats and veggies steamed is that you can be assured that they haven't spent their last few minutes of kitchen life soaking in a oil-filled wok. What starts out as a low-fat food remains one—a restaurant-world rarity.

LO MEIN AND CHOW MEIN

Noodle dishes like lo mein and chow mein are cooked in the wok right alongside the meat and vegetables. Why is that bad? Because to keep them from sticking, the chef must pour in more oil and more sauce, a careless move that brings to your plate a deluge of extra fat and sugar. A full order may top 1,000 calories.

STEAMED RICE

Just because it's plain doesn't mean it's not dangerous. Even a modest scoop will add about 200 calories of fast-digesting carbohydrates, so limit yourself to a half portion.

Deli

HUMMUS

Most delis keep this Mediterranean spread on hand for their veggie sandwiches, but it's the perfect condiment for meaty subs, too. Swap out mayo for this fiber-rich, flavor-packed puree and save 80 calories a sandwich.

WRAP

Beware the healthy foods that aren't! The tortilla this comes wrapped in packs up to 300 calories on its own and provides ample surface area for a surplus of cheese, meat, and dressing. All told, the average wrap weighs in around 600 calories.

TUNA MELT

It's not the melted cheese that does this sandwich in, it's the cup of mayonnaise that sits beneath it. Sandwich makers treat the tuna as mere flavoring for a mayo sandwich, making this one of the most dubious options on any deli menu.

ITALIAN SANDWICH

A merger of two or more of the biggest hitters in the fatty meat business— salami, pepperoni, bologna, and capicolla. And if that's not scary enough, there's also a carpet of provolone and some sort of oily spread—either mayonnaise or olive oil. No matter how it comes together, one thing's certain: Fat and salt are the primary ingredients.

SANDWICH BREAD TOTEM POLE

ENGLISH MUFFIN
129 calories, 2 g fiber

WHEAT BREAD
132 calories, 4 g fiber

SLICED SOURDOUGH
184 calories, 2 g fiber

CROISSANT
231 calories, 1.5 g fiber

FRENCH ROLL/ PANINI BREAD
233 calories, 2 g fiber

BAGEL
283 calories, 2 g fiber

Sandwich Delights

BLT with mayonnaise on toasted wheat bread $6.2

CUCUMBER AND HERB CHEESE SPREAD with lettuce, tomato, red onion and a splash of oil and vinegar $5.25

VEGETABLE HUMMUS WRAP with cucumber, gree peppers, red onions, lettuce tomato and olives wit roasted garlic hummus in a wheat wrap $6

GREEK WRAP marinated chicken cubes, lettuce, cucumber, tomato, red onion, olives, hot peppers feta cheese, Greek dressing in a wrap ....

CHICKEN CLUB with smoked bacon, brie chees plum tomatoes & ranch dressing

TURKEY BREAST with lettuce, cranberry sauc stuffing on wheat $6.25

ROAST BEEF & TURKEY BREAST with lettuce pepper, tomato and a splash of oil and vinega

TARRAGON CHICKEN SALAD with fresh her tuce, tomato, red onion, and Maitre Tarragon dressing on wheat.................$6.25

BACON CHICKEN SALAD blended with re red onion, fresh herbs, served with lettuce on wheat.................$6.25

CITY DELI CLUB 3 layers of turkey, baco cheddar cheese, tomato & lettuce ....

CAPRI SMOKED TURKEY & PEPPERON lone cheese, cherry peppers and honey

ITALIAN SANDWICH prosciutto, capic provolone, pepperoncini peppers, lettuc Italian vinaigrette on Italian bread .....

DELIGHT FULL HONEY GLAZED TURK cheese with cole slaw and honey must

CORDON BLUE crispy fried chicken brea cheese, tomato and Thousand Island

..COTIA salmon, lake sturgeo

Hot Sandwiches

HOT CORNED BEEF or PASTRAMI with melted Swiss cheese, red onion, sauerkraut, and honeycup mustard on rye............$6.25

PHILADELPHIA CHEESESTEAK with onion & green pepper, topped with melted Jack cheese and served on a French roll $9.25

HOT ROAST BEEF AND GRAVY with herb cheese spread on a bulky roll................$6.25

TUNA MELT with melted Swiss cheese, mayonnaise and tomato on rye bread or an English muffin.....$6.25

Gourmet Salads Sandwiches

All Platters Served with Tossed Salad and Ch
of Coleslaw, Potato Salad or Macaroni Salad

Sandwich/ Platters

Chicken Salad	..........4.99	Italian Tuna	....
Classic Tuna Salad	.4.95	Italian Seafood	....
Seafood Salad	.... 4.50	Dill Chicken Salad	..4.
Egg Salad	................4.95	Shrimp Salad	..........5.50

Build-Your-Own

SERVED WITH LETTUCE, TOMATO AND ONION.
BREAD: Jewish Rye - Wheat - Bulky Roll - White - Wheat - Wraps (Wheat - White).
CHEESE: American - Swiss - Provolone - Cheddar $ .75
EXTRA: Roasted Garlic Hummus - Bacon $ .75 EXTRA
Cucumbers - Green Peppers - Black Olives $ .50 EXTRA

Boiled Ham	.... 3.99	Smoked Turkey	...... 3.99
Turkey Breast	.... 3.99	Virginia Ham	.... 3.99
Roast Beef	.... 4.50	Cappicola Ham	...... 3.99
Pastrami	.... 3.99	Prosciutto	.... 3.50
Corned Beef	.... 3.99	Liverwurst	.... 3.50
Genoa Salami	.... 3.99	Bologna	.... 3.50
Hard Salami	.... 3.99	Spiced Ham	.... 3.50
f Salami	.... 3.99	Black Forest Ham	.. 3.99

HOT SANDWICHES

Calories in the deli rise in direct proportion to the temperature of the sandwich being made. Among the worst offenders in the hot sandwich department: hot pastrami, meatball, sausage and peppers, and, of course, the disastrous cheesesteak.

SALADS

On most menus, salad means a big bowl of greens. On a deli menu, it most likely means a big bowl of mayo. Whether it includes egg, tuna, or chicken, your salad is likely to harbor up to 3 tablespoons of the fatty stuff, which brings the caloric total of even a small order up to around 500 calories.

BUILD YOUR OWN

Always your best bet at a deli, or anywhere else for that matter. As chef, you're in full control of what goes on your sandwich, and you won't fall victim to the high-calorie tolls associated with most house-made "specialties."

CHEESE DECODER
(PER 1 OZ SLICE)

● **PART-SKIM MOZZARELLA:** 72 calories, 4.5 g fat (3 g saturated), 175 mg sodium

● **PROVOLONE:** 100 calories, 7.5 g fat (5 g saturated), 248 mg sodium

● **AMERICAN:** 106 calories, 9 g fat (5.5 g saturated), 184 mg sodium

● **SWISS:** 108 calories, 8 g fat (5 g saturated), 54 mg sodium

● **CHEDDAR:** 114 calories, 9 g fat (6 g saturated), 176 mg sodium

Greek

SPANAKOPITA

The menu will often describe this dish as a "spinach pie." Sounds healthy, right? Turns out it's not. If it were just spinach, egg, and feta, you'd be free to eat, but it's the oil binding and butter-streaked phyllo crust that push this thing dangerously close to the caloric red zone. If you must indulge, split an order with the table.

HUMMUS

Chickpeas form the base of the hummus, and like other legumes, they're packed with protein, fiber, and dozens of vital nutrients. A pita spread thick with this stuff will run you about 200 calories. A sound investment.

TIROPITA

This Greek staple is only one step above an American mozzarella stick. In other words, not your best option. It combines a little egg with a lot of cheese, and then wraps it all in a buttered pocket of phyllo dough. The only advantage it has is that it's baked instead of fried, but even that doesn't save it from nutritional bankruptcy.

BABA GHANOUSH

A true stealth health food, it's made by blending mineral-rich tahini with roasted eggplant. Eat with a few wedges of warm whole wheat pita for a perfect starter.

TZATZIKI

A creamy dip with the consistency of mayonnaise but less than half the fat. How does it manage its lean profile? It employs a mix of garlic-seasoned yogurt and cucumber. Richer varieties might have a drizzle of olive oil, but even then you're looking at a massive improvement over the other white condiment.

MEZEDES (APPETIZERS)

Spanakopita (1) Pastry with spinach & feta cheese	2.25
Loukaniko Homemade Greek sausage with grilled tomato	4.95
Dolmades (1) Grape leaves stuffed with lemon rice	.95¢
Keftedes Seasoned meetballs	7.50
Taramosalata Tamara roe caviar dip	6.95
Hummus Chickpea & garlic dip with Kalamata olive	6.95
Skordalia Pureed potato garlic dip with extra virgin olive oil	6.95
Roasted Eggplant Dip Roasted eggplant, garlic & olive oil	6.95
Grilled Octopus Served with toasted olive bread	10.95
Saganaki Cheese Fried cheese flamed tableside	10.95
Tiropita (1) Pastry with feta cheese & herbs	2.25
Artichokes Tiganites Lightly fried artichoke hearts with lemon, mint & extra virgin olive oil.	8.95
Baba Ghanoush Roasted eggplant, sesame oil, garlic & lemon	4.99
Baked Feta Feta cheese, baked golden brown in a fresh tomato sauce	9.95
Red Pepper Feta Creamy Feta Dip with roasted Red Pepper	7.95
Homemade Olive Bread With feta cheese & olive oil	3.75
Tzatziki Yogurt, cucumber & garlic dip	6.50

SPECIALTIES

Served with a choice of side dish.
Add a Greek salad 1.95.

Moussaka Traditional Greek casserole with layers of potatoes, eggplant, seasoned ground beef, cheese & béchamel sauce	9.95
Pastitsio Traditional Greek casserole with layers of pasta, seasoned ground beef, cheese & béchamel sauce	9.95
Cretan Style Seafood Shrimp, mussels, tilapia, potatoes and seasonal vegetables simmered in a clay pot with wine, garlic & herbs served with grilled olive bread. with mashed potatoes	15.95
Grilled Rack of Lamb Oreganatto Rack of lamb, served with potatoes	22.95

GREEK SALAD

Unlike American salads, so often littered with fried chicken, cheese, and croutons, Greek salads are produce-driven: tomatoes, cucumbers, olives, and onions. Ask them to go light on the feta and take the dressing on the side.

SALAD & SOUP

Greek Salad In a red wine vinaigrette	
Horiatiki Salad Tomato, cucumber, Kalamata olives & feta cheese in a Greek vinaigrette	9.75
Falafel A blend of garbanzo beans mixed with spices and served with a salad of lettuce, tomatoes, and tahini	8.95
Chicken Orzo Soup Family recipe	6.95

GYRO PLATTERS AND SANDWICHES

Choice of meat with Tzatziki sauce, onions & tomatoes. Add a Greek salad 1.95.

Traditional Gyro Beef & Lamb	7.75
Chicken Gyro	7.75
Rotisserie-Carved Beef	8.75
Rotisserie-Carved Lamb	10.25

ROTISSERIE & SOUVLAKI COMBINATIONS

Rotisserie & souvlaki meat served with lemon roasted potatoes & choice of side dish. Add a Greek salad 1.95.

Traditional Gyro Beef & Lamb	7.75
Chicken Gyro	7.75
Rotisserie-Carved Beef	8.75
Rotisserie-Carved Lamb	10.25

DESERTS

Baklava With walnuts	4.95
Baklava Cheesecake	5.95
Chocolate Cake Soaked in raspberry & ouzo	5.95
Homemade Walnut Cake	4.95
Kataifi With pistachio filling	3.95

FALAFEL

The breading-like exterior is actually just the crispy outside of the dough, which is made from seasoned, pureed chickpeas. So when the rolled-up falafel hits the deep fryer, it absorbs far less oil than it would if it were made with true breading. Each falafel contains about 60 calories and 5 grams of fat.

GYRO PLATTER

Get this: The Center for Science in the Public Interest tested gyros across the United States and found that they averaged about 760 calories apiece and packed in a full day's worth of sodium and saturated fat. Shouldering the blame is the compressed lamb-and-beef-combo meat that goes into the pita—it's the grease-loaded Frankenfood of the Fertile Crescent. Find yourself another entrée.

SOUVLAKI

This lean skewer is one of the best entrées on the Mediterranean menu, so try subbing it in place of your usual gyro. Instead of lamb-beef mystery meat, it's made with lean chunks of lamb, chicken, beef, or pork, and usually it's interspersed with grilled vegetables and served over a bed of rice.

BAKLAVA

Sticky layers of phyllo dough interspersed with layers of nuts, honey, and sugar. It's not health food, but it's not nearly as bad as most of the big desserts offered on American menus. (Think brownie à la mode.)

Indian

KACHORI

A pastry ball stuffed with spicy mung beans (khasta kachori) or potatoes (aloo kachori). Ask your server if the restaurant makes one that's baked, instead of fried; otherwise, you can expect that crispy breading to be saddled with a calorie-spiking load of oil.

APPETIZERS

Indian and American restaurants share one thing in common: a reliance on deep-fried appetizers. Given that the rest of the Indian menu is so full of potential, it's best to skip over the oil-soaked starters.

RASAM

The Indian version of tomato soup, rasam is made with fresh tomatoes, tamarind, and a variety of spices. At 100 calories a bowl, it's your best way to start dinner.

MULLIGATAWNY

This soup starts with a healthy base of lentils and a battery of spices, but ask if it's broth- or cream-based. Depending on which, it could range from 100 to 500 calories.

ALOO GOBI

A bright yellow dish made from potatoes and cauliflower, this meal boasts a hefty profile of antioxidants, thanks to a wholesome blend of Indian spices. One of those spices—the one that imparts the yellow coloring—is turmeric, and research has shown that it can help you fight disease by boosting your liver's ability to detoxify blood.

APPETIZERS

VEGETABLE SAMOSA *Two crisp turnovers, stuffed with spiced potatoes, peas, and herbs.* $2.50

VEGETABLE PAKORA *Assorted vegetable fritters gently seasoned and deep fried.* $2.50

PANEER PAKORA *Pieces of homemade cheese, dipped in chickpea flour and fried.* $3.25

CHICKEN PAKORA $3.25

SHRIMP PAKORA *Shrimp dipped in spiced batter, deep fried.* $5.95

KACHORI *A deep-fried, spicy snack. Filled with potatoes or peas.* $5.95

HOUSE SPECIAL PLATTER *A fine presentation of our choice appetizers, recommended for two.* $6.95

SOUPS AND SALADS

GREEN SALAD *Lettuce, tomatoes, green peppers, and onions.* $2.50

VEGETABLE SOUP *Soup made from fresh vegetable, lentils, spices and delicate herbs.* $2.50

RASAM *Soup made from the freshest and juiciest tomatoes with the right amount of spice.* $2.50

MULLIGATAWNY SOUP *A traditional chicken soup with lentils and spices.* $2.50

RICE SPECIALTIES

CHICKEN BIRYANI *Classic mulgai dish of curried rice with chicken, dried fruits and nuts* $9.95

[HOU]SE SPECIAL BIRYANI *Our special [birya]ni cooked with chicken, lamb, [shri]mp, vegetables, dried fruits and [nu]ts* $13.95

OUR CHEF RECOMMENDS

SEAFOOD FANTASY *Start with tandoori fish and tandoori shrimp, followed by your choice of shrimp masala or shrimp curry, dal, naan, pullao and green salad.* $19.95

THALI HOUSE VEGETARIAN *A traditional Indian meal served on a silver platter with dal, chana masala, mattar paneer, rice, poori or roti, raita and gulab jamun.* $12.95

VEGETABLE SEEKHAM *Fresh carrots, cauliflower, green peas, homemade cheese, pineapple chunks cooked with spices, sauce and nuts.* $9.95

LAMB DANSHIK *Tender lamb, chick peas, and lentils cooked with pineapple and herbs.* $11.95

CHICKEN

CHICKEN MAKHANI *The legendary tandoori chicken, cooked in tomato and garlic sauce* $10.95

CHICKEN VINDALOO *Boneless chicken and potatoes in a highly spiced sauce* $9.95

CHICKEN SHAHI KORMA *Tender chicken cooked in a rich sauce with nuts and cream* $9.95

CHICKEN SAAGWALA *Boneless chicken cooked with creamed spinach* $9.95

CHICKEN TIKKA MUGLAI *Tandoori chicken and mushrooms cooked in tomato and garlic* $10.95

CHICKEN TIKKA MASALA *Tandoori roasted chicken tikka, in a tomato and butter sauce* $10.95

CHICKEN CURRY *The original cooked in onions, garlic, ginger, yoghurt, and spices* $9.95

LAMB

LAMB SHAHI KORMA *Tender lamb, in a rich sauce with nuts and cream* $10.95

LAMB SAAGWALA *Chunks of lamb in creamed spinach* $10.95

LAMB BHUNA *Pan-broiled lamb, cooked in specially prepared herbs and spices with a touch of ginger and garlic* $10.95

LAMB VINDALOO *Lamb and potatoes cooked in a sharply spiced tangy sauce* $10.95

KEMMA MATTAR *Ground lamb cooked with peas and herbs* $10.95

VEGETABLE

NAVRATAN CURRY *Nine assorted garden fresh vegetables sauteed in a traditional onion and tomato sauce* $8.95

DAL *Black lentils and beans, cooked in onions, with tomatoes and cream* $8.95

SAAG PANEER *Chunks of homemade cheese in creamed spinach and fresh spices* $8.95

ALOO GOBHI MASALA *Fresh cauliflower and potatoes, cooked dry in onions, tomatoes and herbs* $8.95

ALOO MATTAR *Garden fresh green peas and potatoes with fresh spices* $8.95

MATTAR MUSHROOMS *Garden fresh peas and mushroms cooked with garlic, ginger, and onions* $8.95

CHANNA MASALA PUNJABI *A North Indian specialty, subtly flavored chick peas, tempered with ginger* $8.95

PALAK PANEER *Fresh homemade cheese, cooked with fresh spinach and spices* $8.95

TANDOORI

TANDOORI CHICKEN *Chicken marinated in yoghurt and freshly ground spices, then broiled in the tandoor (half)* $9.95

TANDOORI FISH *Swordfish marinated in an exotic recipe of exciting spices and herbs, broiled on charcoal* $13.95

TANDOORI SHRIMP *Jumbo shrimp seasoned with spices and herbs, bake the tandoor* $14.95

CHICKEN TIKKA *Boneless, tender en, gently broiled* $9.95

RESHMI KABAB *Mild, tender, chicken breast, marinated in mild sauce, barbecued on a sk the tandoor* $10.95

BOTI KABAB *Juicy cubes from leg lamb, broiled to perfection in the ta door* $10.95

SEEK KABAB *Finger rolls of ground lamb, spiced with fresh ginger* $10.95

DRINK SPECIALTIES

LASSI SWEET $2.25

MANGO LASSI $2.75

MANGO JUICE $2.00

STRAWBERRY LASSI *seasonal* $2.75

SODAS $1.25

KESAR PISTA SHAKE *seasonal* $2.75

ACCOMPANIMENTS

MANGO CHUTNEY *Spicy, sweet & sour relish* $4.00

PICKLES *Mango, lemon, chili* $3.00

PAPADUM *Thin bean wafers* $3.00

RAITA *Tomato and cucumber in a yogurt sauce* $3.00

TANDOORI

The tandoor is a clay oven used in traditional Indian cooking, and it uses high heat to produce small, tender slabs of chicken and fish. These are some of the leanest items on the menu, and they include kebabs and chicken tikka, a tandoori dish made from yogurt- and spice-marinated chicken.

DAL

Think of it as lentil soup with spicy Indian seasoning. Eat a cup of this before your meal and the fiber will keep you from overeating when the entrées arrive. Or pair with Tandoori meat for one of the world's healthiest meals.

LASSI

Not unlike an American smoothie, lassis are made by blending yogurt, ice, fruit, and a touch of sugar. The heavy ratio of yogurt means it will be lower in sugar and higher in calcium and protein. A great 300-calorie dessert.

RAITA

Protein-rich, yogurt-based sauce or dip similar to Greek tzatziki. Perfect for dunking kebab meats or one of the various breads, such as naan or papadum.

PALAK PANEER

A decent choice for vegetarians, this dish features mild chunks of cheese tossed in a spinach curry sauce. Proceed with caution, though, as the degree of waistline impact hinges on the chef's use of oil and whether or not the sauce is cut with cream.

Italian

BRUSCHETTA
The Italian version of chips and salsa has much more going for it than the bottomless baskets of fried tortillas. A full order will run about 600 calories—perfect for a table of four. Only the mussels—low in fat, packed with protein—make for a better start to your meal.

PENNE ALLA VODKA
The alcohol gets cooked off, but before it goes it helps to extract flavors that would otherwise remain hidden in the tomatoes. The caliber of the sauce pivots on what's used in the house recipe. Ask your server if it's closer in color to the red of tomato soup or the washed-out pink of white zinfandel wine. If it's the latter, look elsewhere.

BAKED ZITI
Tossed in marinara and then baked with a layer of cheese on top, this pasta falls somewhere between lasagna and spaghetti with red sauce on the calorie meter. But if sausage is mentioned on the menu, avoid it like the plague.

SAUCE DECODER (LISTED FROM BEST TO WORST)

● **MARINARA:** This is virtually fat-free, plus it delivers at least one serving of fruit in the form of antioxidant-packed tomatoes.

● **PESTO:** It's high in fat, but most of that is healthy mono-unsaturated fat from olive oil. Plus basil and garlic both contain strong cancer-fighting compounds.

● **BUTTER AND PARMESAN:** The food of choice for half of this country's young eaters offers just fat from the sauce and quick-burning carbs from the pasta.

● **ALFREDO:** The same as Butter and Parmesan (above), only with the addition of heavy cream. Avoid at all costs.

Appetizers

Homemade Mozzarella with roasted peppers and fresh tomatoes 7.95
Bruschetta with marinated tomatoes, fresh basil and garlic crostini 7.95
Fried Fresh Calamari 8.95
Fried Mozzarella Sticks 8.95
Sautéed Mussels in marinara or fra diavolo sauce 8.95
Combination Platter with fried calamari, mozzarella sticks and eggplant parmigiana 14.95

Soups and Salads

Pasta E Fagioli 7.95
Minestra d'Aglio 6.95
House Salad mixed greens with fresh tomatoes 6.95
Insalata Caprese with mozzarella di bufala campana, plum tomatoes, fresh basil and extra virgin olive oil 7.95
Arugula Salad with goat cheese, roasted pepper, red onions and tomatoes in a citrus vinaigrette 8.95

Pastas

Baked Ziti sausage, mushrooms, peppers, ricotta 9.95
Capellini al Pesto, angel hair pasta in tomato and basil pesto 12.95
Penne alla vodka prosciutto, cream and tomatoes 12.95
Lasagna marinara, lasagna sheets and ricotta cheese topped with mozzarella and baked to perfection 11.95

PARMIGIANA

In Italian, it means "parmesan"; in American, it means a battery of breading, oil, cheese, and sauce. This treatment can turn a harmless vegetable into a 1,000-calorie bomb. Cut that total in half by applying the sauce and cheese to grilled eggplant or chicken, instead.

CHICKEN MARSALA

Healthy in theory only. In practice, chefs get carried away with the prosciutto and oil and this simple staple skyrockets to 900 calories or more.

CANNOLI

This authentic Sicilian dessert consists of pastry dough stuffed with sweetened ricotta, a cheese that shares much in common nutritionally with cottage cheese. As long as the portion size is reasonable, cannoli beats a 700-calorie slice of tiramisu any day. To keep it around 200 calories, look for a piece about as long as two D batteries. If served two to a plate, share.

GELATO

The Italian ice cream is made with milk instead of heavy cream. That doesn't make it a zero-impact food, but it's a massive step above Häagen-Dazs.

ITALIAN SODA

Basically it's carbonated water, coloring, and lots of sugar, which makes it no different than the sodas in your office vending machine.

Entrées

Eggplant Parmigiana grilled with tomatoes, basil, imported mozzarella and Parmigiano-Reggiano cheese 11.95

Grilled Pork Chops served on a bed of grilled polenta 19.95

Grilled Double Breast of Chicken with fresh rosemary and herbs over arugula 11.95

Chicken Marsala sautéed in marsala wine with shallots and mushrooms 13.95

Chicken Balsamic sautéed with onions, mushrooms and fresh tomatoes in a sweet balsamic sauce 13.95

Shrimp and Scallops in fra diavolo or marinara sauce 19.95

Grilled Prawns in Lemon 19.95

Baked Branzino 23.95

Bistecca Fiorentina 24.95

Homemade Sausage with Sweet Peppers 16.95

Neapolitan Beef Ragu 14.95

Neapolitan Meatballs 15.95

Pizzaiola sautéed in marinara with mushrooms and peppers 13.95

Dolce

Cannoli topped with Nutella 4.95

Panna Cotta topped with wild berries 5.95

Tiramisu delicately layered with a hint of coffee 5.95

Gelato in various flavors 4.95

Specialty Drinks

Pellegrino 5.95

Espresso 2.95   Cappuccino 3.95

Italian Soda (Blood Orange, Raspberry, Bianch 3.95

Italian Cremosa 4.50

Japanese

MISO SOUP

Miso is made from fermented soybeans, which means that every bowl brings you a wholesome serving of isoflavones. These powerful compounds have anticarcinogenic properties, and at least one study shows that they prevent your body from overproducing fat cells.

EDAMAME

Consisting of nothing but fresh soybeans, edamame makes a great start to your meal. Working them free from their pods keeps you from eating too quickly, and each bean provides a nourishing mix of protein, fiber, and omega-3 fats. Just ask for your bowl unsalted and add a small pinch at the table.

NOODLE SOUPS

Soba noodles are thin buckwheat noodles, while udon are thick and wheat-based. Think of udon like normal spaghetti, while soba can save you calories and boost your fiber intake.

VEGETABLE TEMPURA

Vegetable or not, this is still the Japanese version of deep-fried food, which makes it essentially the same as Southern staples like fried okra and onion rings. The batter might be slightly lighter than the American version we're used to, but with so many truly healthy items on the menu, why waste your calories on fat?

SUSHI ROLL DECODER (6- TO 8-PIECE ROLL)

● **CUCUMBER ROLL**
110 calories, 0 g fat

● **SPICY TUNA ROLL**
290 calories, 11 g fat

● **TUNA ROLL**
140 calories, 2 g fat

● **DRAGON ROLL**
490 calories, 12 g fat

● **CALIFORNIA ROLL**
255 calories, 7 g fat

● **SHRIMP TEMPURA ROLL**
510 calories, 21 g fat

---

appetizers

Miso Soup

House Salad or Seaweed Salad

Edamame

Gyoza or Yasai Gyoza (6) (shrimp or vegetarian)

Yakitori (choice of chicken, or roasted with special sauce)

Soft Shell Crab with Ponzu sauce

Aged Tofu (deep fried topped with bonito flakes in ginger sauce)

Noodle Soups

Vegetable Udon	Vegetable Soba
Chicken Udon	Chicken Soba
Beef Udon	Beef Soba
Tempura Udon	Shrimp Soba

tempura

Vegetable Tempura 15 pcs. vegetable

Chicken Tempura 7 pcs. chicken & vegetable

Shrimp Tempura 7 pcs. shrimp & vegetable

Salmon Tempura 7 pcs. salmon & vegetable

Tempura Combo 3 pcs. shrimp, 3 pcs. chicken & vegetable

specialty rolls

Black & White (white fish tempura, scallions, black sesame seeds)

Tuna Cubed (blue fin tuna and escolar topped with fatty tuna & wasabi tobiko)

Grand Canyon (unagi, avocado & cucumber topped with broiled escolar, masago & silver sauce)

Green Dragon (Alaska king crab, unagi topped with avocado & tempura crunch)

Hawaiian (spicy salmon, tempura crunch & cucumber topped with avocado & tuna)

Jumbo (crab stick, cucumber, hamachi, unagi & masago)

Fire Island (California roll topped with spicy tuna, scallions & tempura crunch)

Fuji Volcano (shrimp tempura and avocado topped with unagi & spicy masago sauce)

Matsu (unagi, avocado, crab stick, tamago & masago)

sushi nigiri or sashimi

Alaska King Crab

Amaebi (sweet shrimp)

Blue Fin Tuna

Ebi (boiled shrimp)

Escolar (seared fatty white tuna)

Hamachi (yellowtail)

Hirame (fluke)

Hotategai (scallop)

Ika (squid)

Ikura (salmon roe)

Kanikama (crab stick)

Kanpachi (wild yellowtail)

Saba (spanish mackeral)

Shake (fresh salmon)

Shake (smoked salmon)

Spicy Tuna (original or jalapeno)

Suzuki (bass)

Tai (red snapper)

Tako (boiled octopus)

Tobiko (flying fish roe)

Unagi (fresh water eel)

Uni (sea urchin)

sushi or sashimi combinations

Served with Miso Soup & Salad

Sushi Dinner
2 pcs. nigiri sushi consisting of: tuna, salmon, white fish, and 1 pc. yellowtail, spanish mackerel and a California roll or tuna roll

Sushi Deluxe
9 pcs. of Chef's selection and a yellowtail roll

Sashimi Dinner
3 pcs. tuna, 2 pcs. each mackeral, salmon, yellowtail, 4 pcs. white fish

Sashimi Deluxe
Assortment of daily fresh fish

Omakase Dinner
Chef's selection of sushi and sashimi

maki sushi

Alaska Roll (smoked salmon, cream cheese & masago)

California Roll (crab stick & cucumber)

Kappa Maki (cucumber)

Tekka Maki (tuna)

Spicy Tekka Maki (spicy tuna original or jalapeno)

Negi Hamachi Maki (yellowtail & scallions)

Shrimp Tempura Maki 4 pcs. (shrimp tempura, cucumber & crab roe)

Spider Maki 4 pcs (soft shell crab roll & masago)

Tuna Tataki (lightly seared bluefin tuna)

drinks

Green Tea (imported and brewed fresh)

Beer (Sapporo, Kirin, Asahi)

House Sake (versatile with a mellow flavor)

Plum Wine (subtly sweet, a hint of tartness and is truly delightful)

UNAGI

The consumer-awareness organization Seafood Watch has warned consumers to avoid eel for fear of adding more pressure to the already-declining population. Worry not, though; using salmon as a benchmark, eel has less protein and 80 percent more fat, plus it's often prepared with a crust of cooked sugars. Skip it and go straight for the salmon.

OMAKASE

The Japanese equivalent of a multi-course tasting menu. Go ahead, let the chef feed you; he knows what's truly fresh, and unlike American cooks, sushi masters aren't likely to stuff you until you're stuck to the chair.

NIGIRI

This is slabs of raw fish fastened to ice cube–size blocks of rice with pieces of seaweed. Most people find raw fish easier to handle when it's mixed with rice, but beware: That rice acts like a sponge as soon as you dip it in soy sauce. Every tablespoon you eat gobbles up as much as 40 percent of your day's sodium limit.

SASHIMI

Seafood in its purest form, this dish consists of nothing but thin slices of raw salmon, tuna, squid, or whatever else is fresh. No matter which fish you choose, you're guaranteed to get a massive load of protein with relatively little fat.

SAKE

The rice wine might go well with sushi, but you're better off drinking beer or regular wine. A 6-ounce serving of sake has about 230 calories. The same amount of wine—or a 12-ounce beer—has about 150. Choose accordingly.

281

Mexican Cantina

NACHOS

This is the Mexican equivalent of eating a giant plate of chili cheese fries for dinner. And as with the fries, at least half of the 1,000 or more calories come from fat—fat from the oil in the tortilla chips, sour cream, cheese, ground beef, and whatever they plop on top.

SEVICHE

Served all over Latin America, seviche consists of little more than fresh fish or shrimp marinated with diced vegetables and plenty of lime juice, which serves to "cook" the fish. It's a low-calorie, protein-rich start to any meal. Just make sure the fish is spanking fresh.

POZOLE

A delicious broth-based soup built around hominy—the fiber-loaded member of the maize family. Most pozoles are also loaded with chile peppers, which impart antioxidant capsaicins, and pork, which adds high-quality protein. This is one of the lighter meals you can order at a Mexican restaurant.

MOLE SAUCE

A complex sauce that employs half a dozen peppers along with handfuls of different nuts, seeds, spices, and Mexican chocolate.

CHIMICHANGA

Behind every tasty chimi is an ultra-absorbent flour tortilla and a long bath in hot oil. That means it will be saddled with literally hundreds of calories of pure frying oil. Plus there's nothing remotely Mexican about it—it was created in Arizona! We should have known that a 1,200-calorie deep-fried burrito would be an American invention.

Appetizers

SEVICHE *Fish marinated in Felipe's Homade Cocktail Sauce & Limes. Garnished with Cilantro, Tomatoes, Onions, and Avocados. Want it Spicy? Just ask.* 7.50

CHIPS AND SALSA *Made fresh daily in our kitchen*

TAQUITOS *(2) Corn Tortilla or (2) Flour Tortilla Your choice of any meats. garnished with Guacamole* 4.25

FLAUTAS *(2) Corn Tortilla or (2) Flour Tortilla Your choice of any meats. garnished with Guacamole* 4.25

NACHOS *Felipe's Beans, served over a bed of Chips, topped with Melted Cheese and Guacamole   Plain* 5.00   *Meat* 6.00

QUESO FUNDIDO *(Cheese Fondue) Melted Cheese with your choice of meat, garnished with Avocado & Green Onion. Served with Tortillas.   Plain* 5.75   *Meat* 6.75

CHIPOTLE CHICKEN WINGS *(Felipe's Favorite) Wings simmered and sautéed in Alma's Chipotle Sauce. Has a Kick to It!* 7.95

ANTOJITOS PLATTER *A combination of Taquitos, Flautas, Mini Tacos, Quesadillas, Chicken Wings, Tostaditas and Nachos.* 10.50

Entrees

Want it spicier? Just ask! All Mexican Dishes available with your choice of two of any of the following: rice, beans, refried beans, salad or pico de gallo

CHICKEN ENCHILADAS WITH MOLE SAUCE *We use a generous portion of homemade mole topped over our famous chicken enchilada. Delicious*

ASADA *Steak marinated with Felipe's special seasoning and grilled to order*

POLLO *Skinless and boneless chicken marinated with Felipe's Achiote seasonings*

CHILE VERDE *Diced pork cooked in tomatilo sauce*

CHILE RELLENO *A Chile Poblano stuffed with cheese and topped with special sauce*

EN CHIPOTLE *Grilled shrimp sauteed in Felipe's chipotle sauce. Very spicy*

MACHACA *Sautéed strips of pork, eggs, bell peppers, tomatoes, onions*

CARNE DESHEBRADA *Shredded beef simmered with a touch of wine and Felipe's favorite*

POZOLE *Made with pork and topped with a generous portion of sliced avocado*

FAJITAS ASADA *Combination of strips of steak, bell peppers, tomatoes and onions*

FAJITAS POLLO *Combination of chicken, bell peppers, tomatoes and onions*

PICADILLO *Ground beef simmered with diced tomatoes and onions*

VEGETARIANO *A combination of grilled vegetables lightly seasoned*

CHORIZO CON PAPAS *Mexican sausage grilled to order with potatoes and onions*

CHIMICHANGA *Carne adobada, beans, rice and cheese wrapped in a flour tortilla and deep fried. Served with salsa, guacamole and sour cream*

A La Carte

TACOS
All tacos are served on a soft flour tortilla with cheese and lettuce. Hard shell or corn tortilla by request.

Taco filled with...
- Asada, Fajitas Asada 3.50
- Carne Desbebrada, Carne Desbebrada, Carnitas, Pollo, Picadillo, Fajitas Pollo, Chorizo con Papas, Nopales, Machacha, Chile Verde 3.25
- Ensenada or Pescado 3.50

TACO SALAD
Lettuce, rice, beans, jack and cheddar cheese, fresh salsa, guacamole, sour cream served with or without crisp shell

BURRITOS
A meal in itself that starts with a large flour or corn tortilla and your choice of any meat. Then we add rice, beans and cheese all wrapped inside.

Burrito filled with...
- Fajitas Asada, Chile Relleno 8.00
- Carne Desbebrada, Carnitas, Pollo, Picadillo, Fajitas Pollo, Vegetariano, Chorizo con Papas,
- Nopales, Machaca, Chile Verde 7.25
- Ensenada or Pescado 8.50

TOSTADAS
A crisp corn tortilla spread with beans, your choice of entree, topped with fresh lettuce, guacamole and cheese.

Tostadas with...
- Asada, Fajitas Asada 8
- Carne Desbebrada, Ca Picadillo,
- Fajitas Pollo, Vege

QUESADILLAS
Your choice of meat an between two flour torti guacamole.

Quesadillas with...
- Asada 8.00
- Carne Desbebrada, Carnitas, Pollo Picadillo 7.45

ENCHILADAS
A soft corn tortilla, stuffed with cheese or meat, and smothered with enchilada sauce or tomatillo sauce then topped with melted cheese and lettuce.

Enchiladas with...
- Carne Desbebrada, Carnitas,
- Cheese 4.25

Desserts

AVOCADO ICE CREAM Made daily with fresh avocados
FLAN Choice of three flavors: traditional vanilla, pistacio or lemon
SOPAIPILLAS Puffy fried pastries served hot and plain or with a honey glaze
TRES LECHES CAKE Cake made with three milks, evaporated, sweetened condensed, and whole milk.

TOSTADAS
A tostada takes a crispy corn taco shell, irons it flat, and buries it beneath a heap of beans, meat, cheese, and salsa. Ordinarily that sort of pileup approach would lead to trouble, but with the tostada, the perimeter of the corn shell halts the expansion before it gets out of hand. That makes for an awesome lunch for about 300 calories.

GUACAMOLE
With its load of brain-boosting, cancer-fighting healthy fats, guac is a first-class condiment, but it still packs about 100 calories per scoop. Pair it with salsa to replace, not supplement, cheese and sour cream.

FLOUR OR CORN TORTILLA
Finally, a food decision with absolutely no nutritional trade-off. Compared to their flour counterparts, corn tortillas have about half as many calories and twice as much fiber, making them the better option in every instance, especially with tacos and fajitas.

ENCHILADAS
The sleeper hit of the menu. Choose chicken over cheese or ground beef, skip the rice, and trade refried for black beans and you have a top-notch 600-calorie meal.

FLAN
Just like the French dessert crème brûlée, flan is made from a blend of milk, eggs, and sugar. Stick it in the same nutritional category as ice cream—in other words, eat it infrequently and in small portions.

Pizzeria

GARLIC KNOTS

The cheapest item on the menu for good reason: Each knot consists of little more than a pile of flour and a thick smear of butter or oil. That means lots of quick-burning carbs and lots of calorie-dense fats. You'd be better off eating chicken wings.

CHOICE OF CRUST

Your goal here is to minimize the number of empty carbohydrates that go into your pie. Pan crust is by far the worst, and it can easily add 1,000 empty calories to your pie. Thin crust is not only best for you, but it's also the most loyal interpretation of true Italian pizza.

THE TOPPING TOTEM POLE

(nutritional info is for one medium slice)

MUSHROOMS/ONIONS/ OLIVES/TOMATOES/ PEPPERS
~5 cal/0 g fat

HAM
10 calories,
1 g fat (0 g saturated)

CHICKEN
20 calories,
1 g fat (0 g saturated)

GROUND BEEF
30 calories,
2 g fat (1 g saturated)

EXTRA CHEESE
40 calories,
3 g fat (1.5 g saturated)

SAUSAGE
50 calories,
3.5 g fat (2 g saturated)

PEPPERONI
50 calories,
4 g fat (2 g saturated)

PERSONAL PAN

Never fly solo at the pizza parlor, since appropriate portion size is not the sort of consideration that plays into the shaping of most personal pizzas. They're typically sized like serving platters and loaded with 800 calories or more.

CANADIAN BACON

What makes bacon Canadian? It's not the country of origin. But the fact that it comes from the leaner back of the pig means it delivers twice as much protein with 60 percent less fat than normal bacon.

APPETIZERS & SIDES

Garlic Knots *Knotted pizza dough covered with fresh garlic and served with garlic dipping sauce.* 2.99

Pomodoro Bruschetta *Toasted bread topped with roma tomatoes, fresh garlic, basil, and romano cheese* 5.95

Minestrone *Fresh garden vegetables and cannellini beans in a tomato broth* 5.95

Calamari Fritti *Fried golden brown and served with marinara sauce* 7.95

Mozzarella Fritti *Lightly battered fresh mozzarella fried golden brown and served with marinara sauce* 7.95

Buffalo Chicken Wings *Tangy and hot served with bleu cheese dressing* 6.95

House Salad *Fresh chopped Romaine lettuce, red onions, black olives & tomatoes. with blue cheese, ranch or red wine vinaigrette* 5.50

Caesar Salad *Fresh chopped Romaine lettuce, croutons, black olives, and shredded parmesan cheese with Caesar dressing served on the side* 6.50

BUILD-YOUR OWN PIZZAS

Choice of Crust: Pan, Thin, or Original

Personal Pan 8"	Medium 12"	Large 16"
Cheese Only 5.95	Cheese Only 11.95	Cheese Only 13.95
Additional Toppings 1.00	Additional Toppings 1.50	Additional Toppings 1.95

Roasted Peppers	Red Onions	Sliced Hot Sausage
Fresh Garlic	Eggplant	Anchovies
Roma Tomatoes	Mushrooms	Ground Beef
Fresh Jalapeños	Pepperoncini	Chicken
Artichoke Hearts	Sun Dried Tomatoes	Italian Sausage
Bell Peppers	Pineapple	Romano Cheese
Black Olives	Pepperoni	Gorgonzola Cheese
Fresh Basil	Prosciutto	Feta Cheese
Fresh Spinach	Canadian Bacon	Ricotta Cheese
White Onions	Meatballs	Extra Mozzarella Cheese

OUR SPECIALTY PIZZA PIES

3 Cheese Pizza *Mozzarella, Romano, and Gruyere with our marinara sauce 15.99*

Pizza Marinara *No Cheese, Vegan option! 8.59*

Veggie Lover's Pizza *A mountain of fresh vegetables piled high onto our red pie 15.59*

Meat Lover's Pizza *5 toppings - Bacon, Beef, Ham, Pepperoni, and Sausage 15.99*

White Pizza *A delicious blend of fresh garlic, oregano, Romano, Mozzarella, and our special white herb sauce! 9.59*

Cheese Steak Pizza *with Fresh Grilled Rib Eye Steak, Cheese, Mushrooms and Onions 15.59*

Mediterranean Pizza *with olives, artichokes, peppers, and sun-dried tomatoes 15.99*

Hawaiian Style Pizza *A red pie topped with tender diced ham and juicy pineapple chunks 12.99*

Calzone *Traditional style with pepperoni, sausage, meatballs, peppers, onions, garlic, Romano and Mozzarella all wrapped up in our homemade pizza dough! 11.59*

PASTAS

All of our pastas are made fresh to order and served with homemade bread. Multigrain penne and spaghetti pastas are available upon request.

Spaghetti *Spaghetti topped with fresh marinara or meat sauce 7.95*

Penne Bolognese *Ground beef, sausage, tomatoes and carrots, sautéed then simmered in Chianti wine. 10.95*

Fettuccini Alfredo *Fettuccini pasta tossed in a creamy alfredo sauce 10.95*

Lasagna *Fresh pasta layered with meat and cheese 10.95*

Baked Ziti *Penne pasta tossed with fresh marinara sauce and ric[...] topped and baked with fresh mozzarella 9.95*

Cannelloni *Pasta stuffed with fresh spinach and chicken t[...] marinara sauce 10.95*

MEAT LOVER'S PIZZA

The official "Meat Lover's" moniker is owned by Pizza Hut, but you'll find pizzerias all over the country producing their own iterations of the all-meat pie. The reliance on a slew of greasy meats packs each slice with around 400 calories and 10 grams of saturated fat—double what you'll find in a slice of Hawaiian pie.

WHITE PIZZA

The absence of fatty meats puts this pie on the lower end of the caloric spectrum, but it's still just bread and cheese. The hallmark of the white pie is that it's served without sauce, and as it turns out, the sauce is the healthiest part of pizza. Besides being loaded with vitamin C, studies show that cooking tomatoes actually concentrates the disease-fighting lycopene found in raw tomatoes.

MEDITERRANEAN PIZZA

This is generally among the most uniquely flavorful pies on any pizza menu. Instead of sausage or pepperoni, it earns its big flavor through a combination of artichokes, olives, sweet peppers, and sun-dried tomatoes—ingredients characterized by their antioxidants and healthy fats. Sub this in for your normal pie and you'll trade calories for flavor and nutrition.

CALZONE

You can stuff the fat inside, but you can't make it disappear. The pocket-bread approach to pizza construction allows the chef to fold in more grease than you'd ever accept on top of your pie.

PASTAS

Rarely is pasta better for you than pizza. Surprised? The heaping helping of noodles served by most pizza joints provides hundreds of calories' worth of refined carbohydrates, and the sauce that goes on top is generally peppered with the worst of the pizza toppings (i.e., pepperoni and sausage).

Seafood

OYSTERS

Their reputation as an aphrodisiac may be overhyped, but their reputation as a health food certainly is not. Oysters are low in fat, high in protein, and loaded with essential nutrients such as zinc, potassium, and vitamin A. But remember: Order them fried and all bets are off.

SHRIMP COCKTAIL

One of the healthiest starters on any menu. Shrimp have just over 100 calories per 4 ounces, and nearly all of that comes from protein. Just take it easy on the high-sodium cocktail sauce.

COCONUT SHRIMP

Not nearly the clean, healthy appetizer that the name implies. When attached to the word "shrimp," the word "coconut" denotes little more than a few shards of the white fruit blended into a heavy, greasy blanket of breading. You might as well order French fries.

STEAMED SNOW CRAB LEGS

Crab and lobster are both incredibly lean and packed with vitamin B_{12}. This is especially good news for anyone trying to cut back on animal fats. B_{12} is an essential vitamin that can be obtained only from animal proteins, and it helps your body maintain healthy nerve cells and produce new DNA. What's more, crab and lobster are virtually fat-free.

GREAT STARTERS

OYSTERS ON THE HALF SHELL — Six market oysters served with a shallot and vinegar mignonette or cocktail sauce **$7.99**

SHRIMP COCKTAIL — 8 of our butterfly shrimp served with our homemade cocktail sauce **$5.99**

MOZZARELLA STICKS — Mozzarella cheese lightly breaded and golden fried. Served with marinara **$5.99**

SAUTÉED MUSHROOMS — Broiled in lemon, white wine and butter **$5.99**

CIAPPINO — Variety of fresh seafood in a rich spicy tomato broth **$5.99**

COCONUT SHRIMP — Crispy shrimp rolled in a coconut beer batter before frying and served with dipping sauce **$5.99**

APPETIZER SAMPLER — A sharable platter of house favorites. Shrimp cocktail, sautéed mushrooms and popcorn shrimp **$7.99**

SOUP

New England clam chowder **Cup $2.99 Bowl $3.99**

Seafood gumbo **Cup $2.99 Bowl $3.99**

SEAFOOD BUFFET

Features steamed snow crab legs, shrimp, mussels, clams, crawfish, fresh fish, hot and cold pasta dishes, seafood gumbo, fresh fruit, salad bar, and much more **$24.99**

FROM TERRA FIRMA

The following served with one trip to the salad bar and choice of baked potato or fries. Add .50 for sweet potato.

SURF AND TURF — 9 oz. USDA choice ribeye grilled on open flame and one whole steamed lobster served with lemon and melted butter **$MP**

RIBEYE STEAK — Top quality black angus ribeye steak grilled on open flame to your specifications **$21.99**

GRILLED PORK CHOPS — Topped with a garlic-lime sauce **$23.99**

SPECIALTY DISHES

CRAB CAKES · All lump blue crab meat broiled to perfection. Served with remoulade or tartar sauce **$10.99**

SWORDFISH · A thick steak covered in herb butter and broiled. Served over rice pilaf **$12.99**

GARLIC SEA SCALLOPS · Fresh sea scallops perfectly seasoned and broiled. Served over rice pilaf **$15.99**

BUTTERFLY SHRIMP · 12 pieces of shrimp basted in our unique mixture of seasonings, then broiled. Served over rice pilaf **$14.99**

SHRIMP ALFREDO · A generous portion of wild-caught Giant Tiger shrimp simmered in our special alfredo sauce. Served on fettucine pasta

MAKO SHARK STEAK · Baked in an herbed butter. Served with sesame haricot and rice pilaf **$22.99**

STUFFED LOBSTER · Whole lobster oven broiled and stuffed with crab meat dressing **$36.95**

FRIED PLATTERS

Served with slaw, hushpuppies and tartar sauce

Popcorn Shrimp $7.99
Fish & Popcorn Shrimp $10.49
Clam Strips $7.99
Sea Scallops $13.99
Oysters $13.99
Butterfly Shrimp $12.99
Fish & Chips $7.99
Skinless, Boneless Flounder $7.99
Farm Raised Catfish Filets $7.99

CRAB CAKES
In their best iteration, the cakes are light on mayo and breading, cooked in a pan or oven, and served with a bit of cocktail sauce. If they're heavy on filler, cooked in the fryer, and served with tartar, the calorie count doubles from 400 to 800.

GARLIC SEA SCALLOPS
Scallops are an excellent source of lean protein, but considering the way most restaurants prepare them, you might as well order fried chicken. The common approach is to sear and baste them in a butter bath. Order yours steamed, baked, or grilled to save a few hundred calories' worth of fat.

SHRIMP ALFREDO
The key word here is "Alfredo," and no matter how healthy its counterpart—shrimp, chicken, or lobster—it's still going to be the menu's most insulting entrée. The basic Alfredo recipe is some combination of cream, cheese, and butter—something even the leanest protein can't remedy.

SHARK
Toxins become more concentrated as they work their way up the food chain, so the bigger the fish, the more contaminants it contains. Limit consumption of shark, swordfish, king mackerel, and tilefish.

FISH AND CHIPS
There's no faster, more dramatic way to cancel out the benefits of fish than to drop it into the deep fryer. You're looking at 1,000 calories, 50 grams of fat, and up to 10 grams of trans fat in this one plate.

Steak House

APPETIZERS

Depending on how upscale the steak house is, the appetizer list can either be your saving grace or your downfall. Lowbrow steak sellers are most likely pushing wings, potato skins, and cheese fries almost exclusively. But if your restaurant requires a reservation, expect to find first-class starters like raw oysters and shrimp and crab cocktails.

APPETIZERS

SMOKED PACIFIC SALMON

MAINE LOBSTER COCKTAIL

JUMBO LUMP CRABMEAT COCKTAIL

BROILED SEA SCALLOPS WRAPPED IN BACON

COLOSSAL SHRIMP COCKTAIL

OYSTERS ON THE HALF SHELL

JUMBO LUMP CRAB CAKE

COLOSSAL SHRIMP ALEXANDER

LOBSTER BISQUE

BUFFALO WINGS

GRASS-FED

What a novel concept: Feed cows what they were born to eat! Unfortunately, most American steers are raised on corn, which makes for a more mild-tasting, fat-swaddled cut of beef. Grass-fed beef, on the other hand, is lean and loaded with omega-3 fatty acids.

SIDE DISHES

GRILLED JUMBO ASPARAGUS

STEAMED FRESH BROCCOLI

CREAMED SPINACH

SAUTEED FRESH SPINACH & MUSHROOMS

JUMBO BAKED IDAHO POTATO

MASHED POTATOES

POTATOES

A plate of steak house fries or hash browns will likely add 500 calories to your beef entrée, and a large baked potato has nearly 300 calories before factoring in toppings. That means mashed is the way to go, since even a huge scoop rarely tops the 250-calorie mark.

SALAD

CENTER CU

CAESA

MORTO

SLICED BEEFSTEAK

VINAIGRETTE

CHOPPE

PRIME

A term given out by the USDA that means a piece of beef is deeply marbled—which is code for incredibly fat-strewn. Only 3 percent of beef processed in the United States receives this rating, and most of that goes to restaurants. You'll pay for it on the plate, and then again on the scale.

ENTRÉES

*All steaks come with your choice of sauce: bérnaise, peppercorn, or homemade steak sauce

DOUBLE CUT FILET MIGNON

DRY AGED PRIME SIRLOIN STEAK

CHICAGO STYLE BONE-IN RIBEYE STEAK

GRASS-FED BEEF FILET MEDALLIONS

RIBEYE STEAK

PORTERHOUSE STEAK

PRIME NEW YORK STEAK

CHICKEN FRIED STEAK

DOMESTIC DOUBLE RIB LAMB CHOPS

SESAME ENCRUSTED YELLOWFIN TUNA

JUMBO LUMP CRAB CAKES

COLOSSAL SHRIMP ALEXAND

LOBSTER TAIL, WESTERN AUSTR

JUMBO LOBSTER TAIL, WESTERN AU

STEAK BURGER

CHOICE OF SAUCE

A sauce can make or break your hunk of beef. Béarnaise, made almost entirely from egg yolks and melted butter, is the worst of the options. Peppercorn, based on wine or brandy, beef stock, and green peppercorns, is the best.

RIB EYE

A rib eye has one-and-a-half times the fat of a sirloin. If you want a better middle ground, try a strip steak.

SIRLOIN

This is probably the leanest cut you'll find on the menu, and aside from filet mignon, it's the only one you can eat without blasting past 500 calories. Just be sure to cap your serving at 9 ounces.

PORTERHOUSE

This big boy consists of two distinct cuts of beef: The tenderloin and the strip loin. After you cut a 20-ounce porterhouse from the bone, you have about 14 ounces of meat, 1,100 calories, and 32 grams of saturated fat.

CHICKEN FRIED STEAK

Steak faces plenty of challenges without being breaded and fried like a piece of crispy chicken. It's a fat-on-fat crime, with a gravy misdemeanor to top it all off. Just be sure you have your cardiologist on speed dial.

STEAK BURGER

Steak house burgers are juicy for one reason: They're made from leftover steak trimmings, which can carry fat levels in excess of 30 percent. You're much better off with a regular steak.

Thai

SUMMER ROLLS

Lean pork or shrimp mixed with vegetables and rice noodles and wrapped in a thin sheet of rice paper—summer rolls might be accurately thought of as healthy and unfried egg rolls. They have roots in Vietnam, but they're common in other parts of Asia and available on most Thai menus. Just make sure you order a *summer* and not a *spring* roll, or you'll be right back in the fryer.

SATAY

These meat skewers are grilled and then coated in a spicy peanut sauce, which brings to your table lots of flavor and protein with relatively little fat. Consider this one of the good guys: An entrée portion has fewer than 300 calories.

PLA MUOK TAD

It may sound exotic, but this plate is essentially the fried calamari from an Italian joint with a different dipping sauce. That means 800 or more calories per appetizer portion.

TOM YUM

A high-protein, low-calorie soup featuring lean meat and mushrooms simmered in broth with lemongrass, cilantro, and other seasonings. You'll do fine with any bowl of tom yum, but the best options are the ones that feature shrimp or mixed seafood.

COCONUT SOUP

In terms of fat and calories, this soup is on par with a chowder or cream-based soup. Unless it's all you plan on eating, pick something else.

APPETIZERS

SPRING ROLLS Vegetables $5.95

SUMMER ROLLS Shrimp or tofu $6.95

FRIED TOFU
Deep-Fried Fresh Tofu. Served with sweet sauce topped with crushed peanuts $4.50

PEAK GAI YANG
Special Thai B.B.Q. Wings marinated with Thai sauce $5.95

CHICKEN SATAY
Skewered chicken breast with peanut sauce dressing $7.95

PLA MUOK TAD
Deep fried squid served with sweet Chili sauce $6.95

MEE GROB
The most famous Thai crispy noodle with tomato-Tamarind sauce, tofu, bean sprouts $4.50

TOD MAN
Kingfish patties mixed with thai curry and string beans, served with cucumber salad $6.50

SALADS

CUCUMBER SALAD
With sweet and sour sauce $4.00

THAI SALAD
Green salad, bean curd, cucumber, carrot with peanut sauce dressing $4.50

THAI CHICKEN SALAD
With chicken breast and peanut sauce dressing $8.95

THAI GRILLED BEEF SALAD
Grilled flank steak tossed with a delicious Thai dressing $7.95

GREEN PAPAYA SALAD
Lime juice, string beans, tomato, crushed peanuts $4.50

SPICY BBQ BEEF SALAD
Tossed with spicy lime dressing $9.95

SOUPS

TOM YUM
Hot & sour shrimp or chicken with lemon grass, chili and lime juice $5.95

TOM KHA KAI
Chicken soup in coconut milk with mushrooms, chili and lime juice $5.95

THAI COCONUT SOUP
Spicy but not overpowering kick, lemony, earthy flavor, and creamy, silky texture $5.95

PO TAK
Seafood combination soup with lemon grass, mushrooms, chili and lime juice 12.95

SPECIALTIES

ASIAN BARBEQUED STEAK
Steak marinated in Thai seasonings and grilled as desired $10.95

HONEY DUCK
Topped with house honey and hoisin sauce $12.95

GARLIC SCALLOPS $12.95

FISH WITH BLACK BEAN SAUCE $12.95

THAI CHILI FISH
Lightly fried and topped with Thai chili sauce $12.95

PLA LARD PRIK
Crispy snapper with chili, garlic and tamarind $12.95

PAD THAI
Stir-fried Thai noodles with shrimp, chicken, or vegetable, crushed peanuts, beansprouts & scallions $7.95

PAD SEE YU
A traditional Thai broad noodles stir fried with broccoli, egg sweet soy sauce (chicken or beef) $7.95

CURRIES

Please indicate your spice preference: mild, medium or hot

GREEN CURRY
With chicken, basil, peppers, bamboo shoots, string beans in coconut milk 9.50

GAENG PAH
Country-style red curry with chicken or pork, eggplant, long beans, and sweet potato 9.50

PANANG CHICKEN
A rich thick red curry cooked with coconut milk & bell peppers 9.50

PINEAPPLE CURRY SHRIMP
Red curry cooked with coconut milk, basil, pineapple, string beans, bamboo shoots, eggplant, zucchini 11.95

MASSAMAN CURRY
Chicken or beef with potatoes, onion in coconut milk, tamarind juice and roasted peanuts 9.50

MIX VEGETABLE
Mixed veg, tofu with coconut curry sauce 9.50

RICE

THAI FRIED RICE
With onion, carrot, pineapple, choice of chicken or

SPICY BASIL FRIED RICE
With chili, onion, and fresh basil. (chicken or bee

SWEET COCONUT RICE $2.50

RICE $1.00

MILD, MEDIUM, OR HOT

If you can stand the heat, tell the chef to turn it up. That burn on your tongue comes from a class of pepper-based phytochemicals called capsaicins, which have been shown to clear congestion, lower cholesterol, and boost metabolism to reduce body fat. Taiwanese researchers even found that exposing developing fat cells to capsaicins caused them to die before they matured. And hey, who says you can't break a little sweat at the dinner table?

GRILLED

Grilled meats are popular in Thai cuisine, and as far as lean cooking methods go, this is as good as it gets. Instead of letting oils soak into the tissue, the grill's dry heat pulls fats out. Every time you eat Thai, try to squeeze one grilled item onto your family's table.

GAENG PAH

Whereas most curries are made with a base of coconut milk, country-style curries are made with water. For that reason, choosing country-style can cut a couple hundred calories off your meal. Be warned, though: Without the presence of fat from coconut, water-based curries tend to be far spicier than their coconut-based cousins.

MASSAMAN CURRY

A curry that's closer in consistency to the thicker versions of India and generally cooked with crushed peanuts and potatoes. However, like most Thai curries, massaman generally carries a load of high-cal coconut cream.

SWEET COCONUT RICE

It may have fewer calories than the pies and cakes found in American restaurants, but this is no dieter's dessert. The rice contributes nothing but refined starches, the coconut milk packs plenty of fat, and the sugar surge pushes the calorie count over the edge.

THE CAPTIVE EATER'S SURVIVAL GUIDE

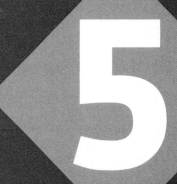

5

EAT THIS NOT THAT!

Restaurant Survival Guide

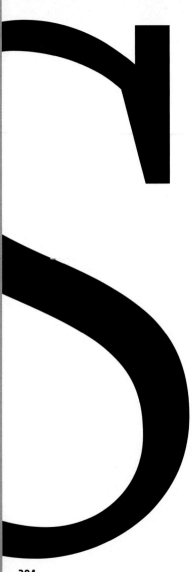

o, been held hostage recently?

No? Are you sure? Because, for a land built on mobility, individuality, and freedom of choice, America sure does a good job of holding its citizens captive— at least when it comes to our nutritional choices. Because while all roads in American culture lead to something cool and interesting, they don't necessarily lead anywhere healthy, foodwise. Too often, when we make the choice to follow our muse, we lose the healthy choices we should be feeding our bellies. Consider what makes us such a great country, and then consider the dietary consequences.

America offers the...

...BEST ENTERTAINMENT IN THE WORLD. But whether you're a girl weeping over a Rachel McAdams tearjerker or a guy pretending to weep over a Rachel McAdams tearjerker so that you can get close to said girl, a trip to the movies can often provide as much fat as it does fun. A towering tonnage of Twizzlers, a prodigious pyramid of popcorn, and a cavernous canyon of Coke will do more than make the theater floor sticky. Sure, it's fun to nosh mindlessly while watching Quentin Tarantino come up with new ways to kill people, but the cost in calories can be considerable.

...BEST SHOPPING IN THE WORLD. Still, 7 out of 10 nutritionists claim they have recurring nightmares of being trapped in a shopping mall. (Okay, that's not actually true, but stay with us here.) When you're burning through a few hundred dollars on the old credit card, it's easy to pack in a few hundred—or even a few thousand—calories at the food court. A limited number of choices—and the ever-present aroma of Cinnabon—make shopping malls some of the most dangerous dietary destinations.

...MOST EXCITING TRAVEL IN THE WORLD. What other country can give you the Grand Canyon and the Big Apple? There are about 5,000 major commercial airports in the United States, and more than 76 million people climb aboard a plane each year at O'Hare International Airport alone. But when it comes to food, airports are like shopping malls with alcohol, and when bad weather hits, you can be trapped in one for hours or even days.

...BEST EDUCATION AND JOB OPPORTUNITIES IN THE WORLD. Okay, so maybe our public school system is lagging a little behind, but the best universities and jobs in the world are still located here. Schools and offices have one thing in common with bus terminals, government buildings, and prison visiting rooms: vending machines. And knowing which lever to pull can make the difference between escaping with a lean waist or an expanding one.

This chapter is your guide to eating in captivity—we'll tell you your best bets for choosing wisely when you're really given no choice at all.

At the Airport
Eat This

Not That!

The bacon alone isn't what gives this sub nearly 600 more calories than its Subway equivalent. A good chunk of the blame lies with the bulkier bread, the oil slick of mayo, and the slices of high-calorie Cheddar.

Quiznos Classic Club with bacon
(regular)

920 calories
54 g fat (15 g saturated)
2,340 mg sodium

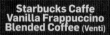

Starbucks Caffe Vanilla Frappuccino Blended Coffee (Venti)

560 calories
16 g fat (10 g saturated)
84 g sugars

The biggest difference between a vanilla Frap and a vanilla latte is in the flavoring—lattes use vanilla-flavored syrup, while Fraps use a more dubious "rich and creamy vanilla" syrup that rings up the calories.

Dunkin' Donuts Blueberry Muffin

510 calories
16 g fat (1.5 g saturated)
51 g sugars

It would be one thing if this muffin brought a ton of nutrition to the table in return for the hefty caloric toll, but with just 3 grams of fiber and more sugar than four Reese's Peanut Butter Cups, the doughnut is clearly the better choice.

A&W Root Beer Freeze
(medium)

530 calories
11 g fat (7 g saturated)
47 g sugars

When it comes to topping your ice cream with something, you're better off choosing a drizzle of melted chocolate and a showering of crushed nuts than you are a huge pour of syrupy sweet root beer.

Auntie Anne's Salted Pretzel

340 calories
5 g fat (3 g saturated)
990 mg sodium

Not only does this pretzel contain 80 more calories than the snack wrap, it's also loaded with refined carbohydrates, which will fuel you in the short term but set you up for a crash later. Not what you need during a long day of travel.

At the Vending Machine
Eat This

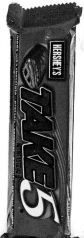

When it comes to America's most popular packaged chocolate treats, Reese's ranks right near the top, with less saturated fat and sugar than almost any bar or cup we've ever come across.

Reese's Peanut Butter Cups
(1 package)

210 calories
13 g fat (4.5 g saturated)
21 g sugars

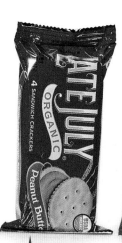
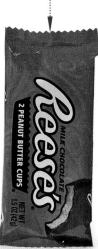
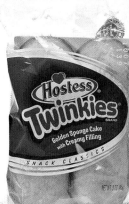
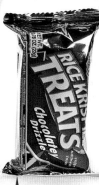

Late July Peanut Butter Sandwich (1 package)

160 calories
8 g fat (2 g saturated)
2 g sugars

Late July is one of our favorite cookie producers, for both its superior nutritional and flavor profiles. These peanut butter sandwich cookies make a perfect snack—just a hint of sugar and less than 200 calories.

Hershey's Take 5
(1 package)

200 calories
11 g fat (5 g saturated)
18 g sugars

The crunch in this bar comes from pretzels, not some mystery nougat concoction, which helps save 70 calories and 10 grams of sugar over the Butterfinger.

Hostess Twinkies
(1 cake)

150 calories
4.5 g fat
(2.5 g saturated, 0 g trans)
17.5 g sugars

Like nearly everything in the vending machine, Twinkies are more science experiment than real food, but when it comes to Hostess treats, this one takes the cake.

Kellogg's Rice Krispies Treats Chocolatey Drizzle
(1 bar)

100 calories
3 g fat (1 g saturated)
8 g sugars

The featherweight Rice Krispies base and the light hand with the sugar is what makes this chocolaty treat so low in calories.

Not That!

Twix Peanut Butter
(2 cookies)

311 calories
19 g fat (9 g saturated)
21 g sugars

This duo of peanut butter bars are the most caloric commercial candy we've stumbled across. They also contain half a day's worth of saturated fat. Stick to the cups and pocket the 100 calories for another occasion.

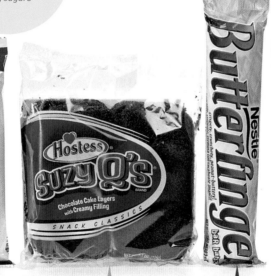

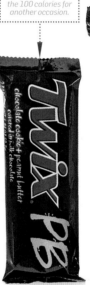

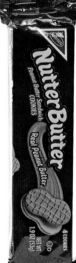

Kellogg's Nutri-Grain Raspberry (1 bar)

130 calories
3 g fat (0.5 g saturated)
12 g sugars

You'd think that a fruity granola bar would beat out a chocolate-drizzled goody, but the Nutri-Grain Raspberry's first ingredient is high-fructose corn syrup. It's second? Regular corn syrup, making it a clear candy bar in disguise.

Hostess Suzy Q's
(1 of 2 cakes)

230 calories
9.5 g fat
(4.5 g saturated, 0.5 g trans)
24.5 g sugars

There's as much sugar in this highly processed dessert as you'll find in nearly 3 scoops of Edy's Slow Churned Rich & Creamy Coffee ice cream.

Nestle Butterfinger
(1 bar)

270 calories
11 g fat (6 g saturated)
28 g sugars

Three of the first 6 ingredients in this candy bar are different forms of sugar, which helps explain why this bar packs as much sweet stuff as 3½ bags of mini Chips Ahoy! cookies.

Nutter Butter Peanut Butter Sandwich
(1 package)

250 calories
10 g fat (2.5 g saturated)
15 g sugars

Make this mistake 3 times a week and you'll gain 4 pounds in a year.

299

At the Amusement Park
Eat This

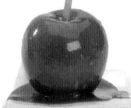

Not only does the hot dog have less than half the caloric load of French fries, it also packs a heavy dose of metabolism-spiking protein.

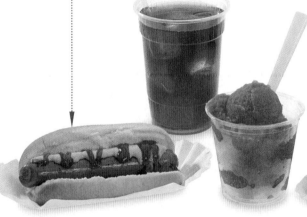

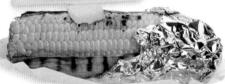

Sweet Tea (8 oz)

58 calories
0 g fat
14 g sugars

This southern specialty can be made even better if you choose to go the unsweetened route. But even when laced with sugar, iced tea has one advantage over almost every other beverage: a potent portfolio of antioxidants.

Italian Ice

120 calories
0 g fat
24 g sugars

Italian ice is nothing more than flavored syrup poured over crushed ice—essentially a Popsicle in a cup. And like Popsicles, the absence of dairy helps keep the calorie counts low, making it a stronger option than any ice cream–like treat.

Caramel Apple

215 calories
0 g fat
38 g sugars

The caramel coating entombing this apple slops on more sugar than we're happy with, but there's still a serving of fruit under all that sweetness. In terms of nutrition, coated apples edge out cotton candy, any day.

Grilled Corn on the Cob with butter

155 calories
3 g fat (2 g saturated)
32 g carbohydrates

Corn isn't an A-list vegetable (like potatoes, it's mostly starch), but in a land of perilous eats, it makes for a safe way to squash your hunger. Don't fear a bit of butter, either; the fat actually helps blunt the impact on your blood sugar levels.

Not That!

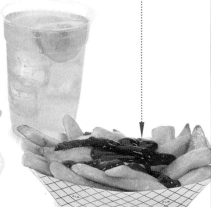
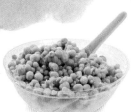
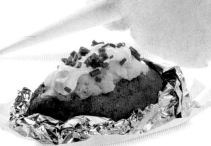

French Fries with ketchup

545 calories
29 g fat
(7 g saturated, 7 g trans)
395 mg sodium

We're not sure which is scarier—the fact that this basket of fries has more calories than any reasonable sandwich should offer, or the fact that it comes with 3½ days' worth of heart-harming trans fat.

Baked Potato
with sour cream and chives

393 calories
22 g fat (10 g saturated)
50 g carbohydrates

A baked potato is a good option in theory, but spuds served outside of your house are too often giant footballs of carbohydrates, dressed with a flurry of fatty toppings. Even with this relatively restrained treatment, it's still trouble.

Cotton Candy

220 calories
0 g fat
56 g sugars

Pure 100% sugar—nothing but a fluffy ball of spun sucrose. Because it's virtually weightless, it still beats out a number of the heftier sweet options, but just know it will do nothing to squash hunger; in fact, the empty sugar surge will only exacerbate your appetite.

Dippin' Dots

190 calories
9 g fat (6 g saturated)
22 g sugars

Dippin' Dots are better than any other type of ice cream (or frozen yogurt, for that matter), but nothing bests Italian ice in the frozen treats category.

Lemonade
(8 oz)

131 calories
0 g fat
33 g sugars

Ever drunk straight lemon juice? It's super bitter. That's why 1 serving of drinkable lemonade is so stuffed with sugar—to mask the actual taste of lemon. At best, this contains just 10% real juice and 90% sugar water.

At the Hotel Breakfast
Eat This

Skim Milk (1 cup)
86 calories
0 g fat
8 g protein
12 g sugars

A study in the *American Journal of Clinical Nutrition* found that people who drank milk at breakfast, instead of juice, consumed 8.5 percent fewer calories at lunch.

Grapes (20)
68 calories
16 g sugars

Grapes pack the same heart-healthy polyphenols found in red wine. Plus, you can pop a whole bunch in your mouth without much of a caloric impact. Double bonus!

Pancakes
(4" in diameter)
2, with 2 Tbsp maple syrup

276 calories
8 g fat (2 g saturated)
48 g carbohydrates

One way to cut back on the calories is to switch to agave syrup instead of maple. Its low glycemic index means your blood sugar will have a gentler ride in the wake of your carb-heavy breakfast.

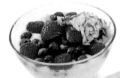
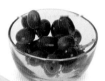
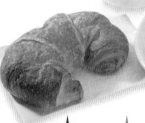
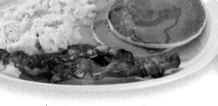
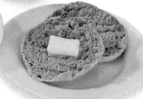

Butter Croissant
(1 medium)
231 calories
12 g fat
(7 g saturated)
26 g carbohydrates

Surprised? A buttered croissant is nutritionally superior to the cranberry muffin in nearly every way.

Plain Yogurt
with almonds and berries
290 calories
13 g fat
(5 g saturated)
13 g protein
20 g sugars

Keep the yogurt plain and control the flavor profile yourself with nuts and fruit.

Scrambled Eggs
(2 large)
204 calories
14 g fat
(4 g saturated)
14 g protein
2 g carbohydrates

Research shows that people who eat eggs in the morning tend to eat less throughout the day.

Bacon
(3 strips)
123 calories
9 g fat (3 g saturated)
9 g protein
564 mg sodium

Both as a side dish and as a garnish for a breakfast sandwich, bacon always beats sausage.

Toasted English Muffin (wheat)
with a pat of butter
162 calories
5 g fat
(3 g saturated)
25 g carbohydrates

English muffins win the battle of the breakfast breads every time.

Not That!

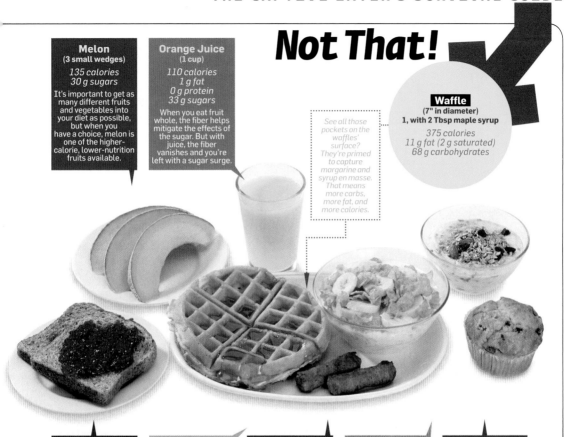

Melon
(3 small wedges)

135 calories
30 g sugars

It's important to get as many different fruits and vegetables into your diet as possible, but when you have a choice, melon is one of the higher-calorie, lower-nutrition fruits available.

Orange Juice
(1 cup)

110 calories
1 g fat
0 g protein
33 g sugars

When you eat fruit whole, the fiber helps mitigate the effects of the sugar. But with juice, the fiber vanishes and you're left with a sugar surge.

See all those pockets on the waffles' surface? They're primed to capture margarine and syrup en masse. That means more carbs, more fat, and more calories.

Waffle
(7" in diameter)
1, with 2 Tbsp maple syrup

375 calories
11 g fat (2 g saturated)
68 g carbohydrates

Toasted Wheat Bread
(2 slices) with jam

262 calories
2 g fat
(1 g saturated)
50 g carbohydrates

Wheat bread is a good start, but most jams are half fruit, half sugar. You'd be better off with peanut butter.

Breakfast Sausage
(2 links)

250 calories
14 g fat
(6 g saturated)
24 g protein
958 mg sodium

Protein-rich though they may be, they're also weighed down by sodium and fat.

Corn Flakes
(1 single-serving box), with skim milk and a sliced banana

267 calories
0 g fat
10 g protein
57 g carbohydrates

Not a bad start to the day, but in our book, nothing beats a few eggs for breakfast.

Fruit-Flavored Yogurt
with granola

388 calories
10 g fat
(3 g saturated)
15 g protein
53 g sugars

Fruit-flavored yogurt is laced with corn syrup, making it sweeter than 3 scoops of ice cream.

Cranberry Muffin
(1 medium)

444 calories
22 g fat
(4 g saturated)
56 g carbohydrates

This cupcake in disguise has as much sugar as a Snickers bar.

303

Eat This

This bar is made from just 6 ingredients: dates, almonds, walnuts, cocoa powder, cocoa mass, and cashews. All Lärabar products are delicious—and nutritious—indulgences.

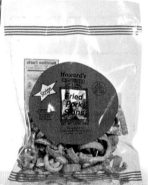

Lärabar Jocalat Chocolate

190 calories
10 g fat (2 g saturated)
5 g protein
5 g fiber
18 g sugars

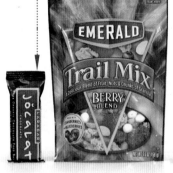
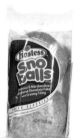
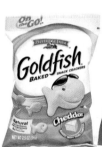
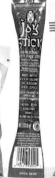

Emerald Trail Mix Berry Blend
(3 Tbsp)

120 calories
6 g fat
(1.5 g saturated)
11 g sugars
45 mg sodium

The berries add antioxidants and displace some of the high-cal chocolate.

Hostess Snoballs
(1 package)

180 calories
5.5 g fat
(3.5 g saturated,
0 g trans)
23 g sugars

These cakes come packed in pairs, so find a friend. But even if you slip up and eat both, you're still better off.

Pepperidge Farm Goldfish Cheddar **(55 pieces)**

140 calories
5 g fat
(1 g saturated)
250 mg sodium

You can eat twice as many individual goldfish crackers for the same caloric bang of half as many Cheez-Its.

Applegate Farms Joy Stick Pepperoni **(1 oz)**

100 calories
7 g fat
(3 g saturated)
700 mg sodium
9 g protein

This is one of the only foods in the mart that will effectively squash hunger.

Howard's Fried Pork Skins **(1 oz)**

160 calories
9 g fat (3 g saturated)
18 g protein
520 mg sodium

The thought of eating pork skins might make you feel like a pig, but unlike normal chips, these babies offer the eater something more: a ton of protein.

Not That!

Kashi GoLean Chewy Malted Chocolate Crisp

*290 calories
6 g fat (4 g saturated)
13 g protein
6 g fiber
35 g sugars*

A candy bar in a protein bar's clothing. This chocolaty mess has twice as much sugar as the Lärabar and 100 extra calories to boot.

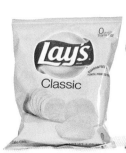

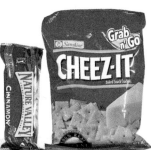

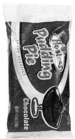

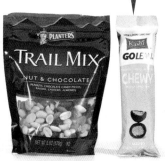

Lay's Potato Chips (1 oz)

*150 calories
10 g fat
(1 g saturated)
2 g protein
180 mg sodium*

Why waste calories on nutritionally void chips when you can get 16 extra grams of protein for 10 calories more?

Nature Valley Crunchy Granola Bar Cinnamon (1 bar)

*180 calories
6 g fat
(0.5 g saturated)
160 mg sodium
4 g protein*

What do you think keeps all that granola held together? Sugar.

Sunshine Cheez-It (27 crackers)

*150 calories
8 g fat
(2 g saturated)
250 mg sodium*

More oil = more fat = more calories. Any questions?

Hostess Pudding Pie Chocolate (1 package)

*520 calories
24 g fat
(12 g saturated,
1.5 g trans)
45 g sugars*

Packed with 75% of your day's saturated and trans fat allowance.

Planters Trail Mix Nut & Chocolate (3 Tbsp)

*160 calories
10 g fat
(2.5 g saturated)
13 g sugars
20 mg sodium*

A high chocolate-to-nut ratio makes this mix a lackluster choice.

At the Movie Theater
Eat This

As long as you're not dipping it into molten cheese, a large soft pretzel makes a reasonable movie theater or street corner snack. Be really good and ask them to skip the salt—mustard packs plenty of sodium as it is.

Soft pretzel with mustard

290 calories
0 g fat
850 mg sodium

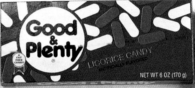
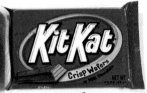
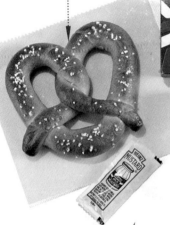
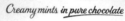
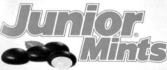
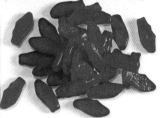

Good & Plenty — LICORICE CANDY · ARTIFICIALLY FLAVORED · NET WT 6 OZ (170 g)

Kit Kat — Crisp Wafers in Milk Chocolate · NET WT

Creamy mints *in pure chocolate* — Junior Mints · Net Wt 4 oz (113 g)

Good & Plenty
(33 pieces)

130 calories
0 g fat
21 g sugars

Many cultures have viewed licorice as a healing herb for centuries, with anti-inflammatory properties. But we're just thankful they have less sugar and fewer calories than traditional chewy fruit candies.

Junior Mints
(½ box)

170 calories
3 g fat (2.5 g saturated)
32 g sugars

Minty candies like Junior Mints and Peppermint Patties tend to be the best of the chocolate choices. Mint, beyond providing antioxidants, has also been shown in studies to improve alertness.

Kit Kat Bar

200 calories
11 g fat (7 g saturated)
20 g sugars

Break this bar up and dole out the pieces. Just because there are four in a package doesn't mean you need to eat them all yourself. (But if you do, take solace in the fact that this is at the top of the candy totem pole.)

Swedish Fish
(2 oz)

200 calories
0 g fat
28 g sugars

In the vast world of pure sugar candies, few are better than the fish from Sweden.

Not That!

Buttered popcorn
(medium; 10–12 cups)

600 calories
39 g fat (12 g saturated)
1,120 mg sodium

Popcorn can be a great, fiber-rich snack, as long as you stay away from the dreaded butter pump. Besides tripling the calories of a bag of popcorn, many movie theater "butters" are teeming with trans fat. Instead, seek flavor from the spice mixes many theaters carry now.

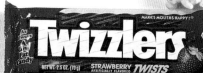

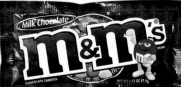

Dots (22 pieces)	**Hershey's** **Milk Chocolate Bar**	**M&M's** (1 bag)	**Twizzlers** (½ 6-oz package)
260 calories *0 g fat* *42 g sugars*	*210 calories* *13 g fat* *(8 g saturated)* *24 g sugars*	*240 calories* *10 g fat* *(6 g saturated)* *31 g sugars*	*240 calories* *1 g fat* *32 g sugars*
They stick to your teeth just like they stick to your waistline. You're better off going for nearly any other gummy product besides these.	If you're going to eat pure chocolate, you're better off picking up a bar with at least 65% cacao. That way, you lower your sugar intake while maximizing antioxidants.	They may seem harmless and fun in their tiny candy-coated vessels, but a few generous handfuls of M&M's can wipe out a meal's worth of calories before you know it.	Ignore the "low fat" claims on the side of the package—these are nothing more than ropes of high-fructose corn syrup.

Index

Boldface page references indicate photographs.
<u>Underscored</u> references indicate boxed text.